Progress
in
Drug Metabolism

Volume 1

Progress in Drug Metabolism

Volume 1

Edited by

J. W. Bridges

Department of Biochemistry,
University of Surrey

L. F. Chasseaud

Department of Metabolism and Pharmacokinetics,
Huntingdon Research Centre

A Wiley–Interscience Publication

JOHN WILEY & SONS

LONDON · NEW YORK · SYDNEY · TORONTO

Library of Congress Cataloging in Publication Data:
Main entry under title:

Progress in drug metabolism.

'A Wiley–Interscience publication.'
Includes bibliographies.
1. Biopharmaceutics. 2. Drug metabolism.
3. Drug interactions. I. Bridges, J. W.
II. Chasseaud, L. F. [DNLM: 1. Drugs—Metabolism.
QV38 P964]
RM301.P73 615'.7 75-19446
ISBN 0 471 10370 5

Printed by A. Wheaton & Company Exeter.

Contributors to Volume 1

J. W. Bridges — *Department of Biochemistry, University of Surrey, Guildford*

L. F. Chasseaud — *Department of Metabolism and Pharmacokinetics, Huntingdon Research Centre, Huntingdon PE18 6ES*

T. A. Connors — *Chester Beatty Research Institute, Institute of Cancer Research, Fulham Road, London SW3*

R. C. Garner — *Cancer Research Unit, University of York, Heslington, York, Y01 5DD*

J. Hunter — *Addenbrooke's Hospital, Hills Road, Cambridge*

B. J. Millard — *The School of Pharmacy, Brunswick Square, London W1*

A. G. E. Wilson — *NIH, National Institute of Environmental Health Sciences, Research Triangle Park, North Carolina, 27709*

Foreword

D. V. Parke
Professor of Biochemistry
University of Surrey, Guildford.

The study of the metabolism of drugs and xenobiotics has developed rapidly during the past few decades, since the importance of these studies to the development of new medicines, and to food toxicology, industrial hygiene, and environmental science, was fully realised. During this period the empirical introduction of selectively toxic chemicals as medicines, food additives and pesticides has progressively given way to a policy of safety evaluation of these chemicals with consequent assessment of benefits to risks, and a more selective and effective usage. Metabolism studies are now an integral part of all programmes of new drug development and are essential to the assessment of safety and efficacy of medicines, and to the determination of appropriate dosage regimens. The study of the pharmacokinetics and the metabolic fate of drugs has contributed, probably more than any other of the medical sciences, to the efficient use of selectively-toxic chemicals as medicines.

The use of food additives which has given us cheaper, more attractive and palatable food has also been questioned in respect of safety, and in the safety evaluation of food additives and assessment of the potential hazards of contaminants, such as nitrosamines and mycotoxins, the study of the metabolism of these chemicals has been of paramount importance. Pesticides and herbicides, which play so valuable a role, in increasing food production and in the eradication and control of vector borne diseases, are now carefully evaluated for safety and persistence, studies which are highly dependent on a knowledge of the metabolic fate of these compounds in man and other animals, and in plants and soil microflora. Furthermore, the current widespread concern with environmental pollution has led to an escalation of ecotoxicity studies of these chemicals and of their metabolism and distribution kinetics in the ecosystem. The environmental burden of toxic chemicals is greatly added to by the multitude of industrial chemicals and intermediates that are marketed, disposed of as waste products, or discharged in industrial effluents. Legislation to protect the industrial worker and to preserve a healthy environment has been enacted recently in many countries, and will require safety evaluation of industrial chemicals and the consequent study of their metabolic fate and chemobiokinetics.

Increasingly, it is now becoming appreciated that the metabolism of xenobiotic chemicals is fundamental to many toxic processes such as carcinogenesis, teratogenesis and tissue necrosis, and that the enzymes involved in drug metabolism may also carry out the metabolism of a number of endogenous substrates, such as steroids, fatty acids and haeme. The inhibition and induction of these enzymes by xenobiotics may consequently have profound effects on the normal processes of intermediary metabolism, such as tissue growth and development, haemopoiesis, calcification and lipid metabolism.

The widespread development in safety evaluation of drugs and other chemicals and its consequent stimulation of metabolism studies, has resulted in a proliferation of publications in this field which makes it extremely difficult for the non-specialist to keep abreast of recent advances. The need for selective, critical reviews of this plethora of new information is therefore very great, and in this new work, *Progress in Drug Metabolism* monographs on topics of drug metabolism, selected for their current importance, meets this need most appropriately.

This first volume of *Progress in Drug Metabolism* contains contributions on some of the most topical aspects of this field of study. The recently renewed interest in the metabolism of xenobiotics into toxic and carcinogenic intermediates, is covered by a chapter on the Role of Epoxides in Bioactivation and Carcinogenesis by Dr. Garner. For a chemical to be sufficiently reactive to alkylate DNA and to initiate carcinogenesis it is now widely believed that it must first be transformed into a metastable carcinogenic intermediate within the cell. Similarly, it would seem that for many cytotoxic, anticancer drugs to be sufficiently reactive to poison and kill the malignant cell, they too have to be activated within the host's tissues, by a similar process of metabolism. This concept of drug activation by metabolism was at first not fully appreciated, but subsequent realisation of the need for activation and of its consequences on the therapeutic regimen have contributed to the recent more successful treatment of malignancy. This fascinating aspect of therapeutics is reviewed in the chapter on Bioactivation and Cytotoxicity by Dr. Connors.

Many drugs and other xenobiotic chemicals are known to be highly bound to proteins, especially those of the blood plasma such as serum albumin. This protein binding effectively removes a major portion of these drugs from the sphere of pharmacological activity, and factors which disturb this binding can profoundly modify the kinetics of drug distribution and the consequent therapeutic response. A knowledge of these interactions is of considerable consequence to the safety of drug therapy, as is illustrated in the chapter on Drug-Serum Protein Interactions and their Biological Significance by Drs. Bridges and Wilson. A further aspect of drug metabolism that is known to affect the safety of drug therapy is the induction of the enzymes involved in metabolism. This induction, which involves the increased *de novo* synthesis of the enzyme proteins, is a physiological response to the administration of certain drugs and other chemicals, such as the pesticide DDT and the food additive, butylated hydroxytoluene (BHT), to provide more enzyme and to increase the rate of metabolism, and hence excretion, of these chemicals. The consequences of this phenomenon affect not only the therapeutic response to drugs, but may also disturb certain processes of intermediary metabolism and may even be implicated in the mechanism of carcinogenesis. This most important aspect is effectively described in the chapter, Clinical Aspects of Microsomal Enzyme Induction, by Drs. Hunter and Chasseaud.

The great impetus given to drug metabolism studies by the needs of safety evaluation procedures has been matched by comparable developments in experimental techniques. Among these new developments mass spectrometry has contributed greatly to the identification of metabolites, which was previously achieved by laborious procedures involving synthesis of authentic materials for comparative identification, or by less-specific, equivocal, chromatography techniques. This elegant identification procedure of mass spectrometry and the more recent advances in this technique, are reviewed in the opening chapter by Dr. Millard.

The philosophy of this volume has been to review advances in the general fundamentals of drug metabolism, namely, the reactions involved, the phenomena observed, and the techniques employed, rather than to deal with the metabolic fate of individual chemicals, which is more the purpose of *Foreign Compound Metabolism in Mammals*, published by the Chemical Society. In this respect it fulfils a real need, and makes for a most readable book.

The editors of this present work are already planning a second volume, and indeed a succession of volumes, under the series title of *Progress in Drug Metabolism*. They are to be congratulated on their enthusiasm and industry, though they may find it no easy matter to match the topicality and excellence of the contributions to this their first creation. The non-expert in drug metabolism, the pharmacist and clinical pharmacologist, the toxicologist and environmental scientist, should have cause to thank the authors and editors of this fine volume for bringing to them in a succinct and readily assimilable form this distillate of such a rich harvest and diverse vintage.

August, 1975.

Preface

Drug metabolism may be defined in its widest sense as the biological fate of a drug or xenobiotic in terms of absorption, distribution, biotransformation and excretion. Many techniques and scientific approaches are required to investigate these processes.

Rational drug development and regulatory requirements have made the study of drug metabolism and its allied techniques one of the more rapidly expanding areas in the life sciences. Despite the advent of specialized journals dealing with drug metabolism studies, the multiplicity of disciplines involved has caused much of the data to become published in widely diverse journals with subject matter ranging, for example, from clinical, to endocrinological, to pharmacological, to biochemical and to chemical: indeed a herculean reading list.

Progress in Drug Metabolism is a review series intended to provide comprehensive, authoritative, readable, up-to-date and critical accounts by experts in the respective subject areas. The reviews will be concerned with newer developments, the progress in established areas, or, alternatively, they may retrieve and review the widely disseminated literature on a particular subject. Thus it is hoped that *Progress in Drug Metabolism* will enable the reader to keep more easily informed of the many and varied developments in drug metabolism.

No discipline can progress without constant communication and the editors welcome suggestions as to future reviews that ought to be included in the series.

J. W. BRIDGES
L. F. CHASSEAUD

Contents

CHAPTER 1

Newer developments in the mass spectrometry of drugs and metabolites

B. J. Millard

INTRODUCTION

The virtues of high sensitivity, compound specificity and, especially when combined with gas chromatography, the ability to deal with complex mixtures, renders mass spectrometry particularly advantageous to workers in the field of drug metabolism. Indeed, mass spectrometry has now become almost a routine technique for the identification and quantification of a wide range of compounds of biological interest. Several reviews (Stenhagen, 1966; Foster, 1969; van Lear and McLafferty, 1969; Hammar *et al*, 1969; Hammar, 1971; Millard, 1971; Gordon and Frigerio, 1972; Knapp and Gaffney, 1972; Jenden and Cho, 1973; Burlingame and Johanson, 1972) and textbooks (Milne, 1971; Frigerio, 1972; Waller, 1972; Castagnoli and Frigerio, 1974) on such applications have appeared.

The requirement of workers in the biochemical field that ever decreasing amounts of compound in mixtures of ever increasing complexity should still yield structural and quantitative information has provided the impetus for several newer developments in mass spectrometry. The purpose of this review is to discuss the more important or potentially important of these and in particular newer methods of ion formation, such as chemical ionization, field ionization and field desorption, multiple-ion monitoring, the use of stable isotopes and the use of high-resolution mass spectrometry for the study of biological mixtures without prior purification. However, before proceeding to these more detailed aspects, it is necessary to outline the main features of conventional mass spectrometry in order to understand why such developments have come about.

A mass spectrometer is a device that can produce ions from an organic compound and then separate these ions according to their mass-to-charge ratio (m/e value). The majority of present-day instruments use an electron-impact source to produce these ions. A typical magnetic sector instrument of the single-focussing type is shown in figure 1.

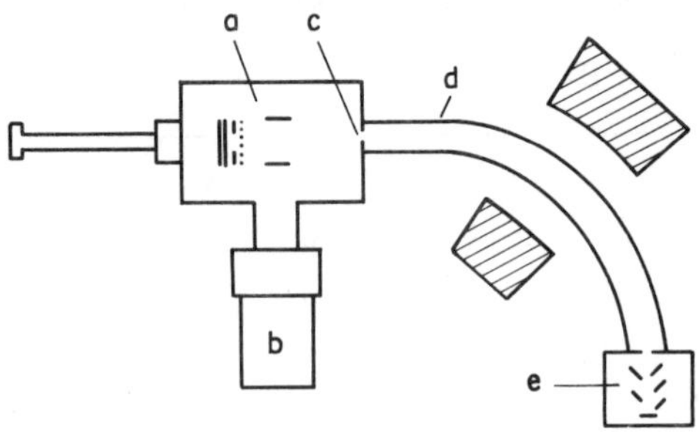

Figure 1 A typical single-focussing magnetic sector mass spectrometer

Solid compounds are evaporated from a direct inlet probe via a vacuum lock into the source a which is kept at low pressure (10^{-7} mm) by the pump b; liquid or gaseous samples are allowed to leak from a reservoir at a higher pressure. The effluent from a gas chromatograph can be introduced directly in the case of capillary columns (McFadden *et al*, 1963; Dorsey *et al*, 1963; Heins *et al*, 1966) or have the carrier gas preferentially removed by means of separators (Watson and Biemann, 1964; Ryhage, 1964; Lipsky *et al*, 1966; Llewellyn and Littlejohn, 1968) in the case of packed columns. The problems of integrating gas chromatography and mass spectrometry have been reviewed by Stallberg-Stenhagen and Stenhagen (1970) as have applications of integrated gas chromatography–mass spectrometry (g.c. m.s.) in pharmacology and toxicology (Jenden and Cho, 1973).

Whatever the inlet system, the compound, now in the vapour phase, is bombarded with electrons, usually at an energy of 70 eV. This process produces a small number of negative ions but a much larger number of positive ions. Most of the positive ions produced are singly charged, although some doubly and even triply charged ions may be formed. In the case of an organic compound M, these processes may be summarized as:

$$M + e \rightarrow M^{+\cdot} + 2e$$
$$M + e \rightarrow M^{++} + 3e$$

The species $M^{+\cdot}$, sometimes written M^{+}, is known as the molecular ion, the

+· symbol signifying an ion with a single positive charge and an odd number of electrons. Such molecular ions will possess a few electron volts of energy in excess of their ionization potential. As a result, some or all of the molecular ions will break down further by loss of neutral molecules or radicals to form fragment ions such as A^+ and $B^{+\cdot}$:

$$\begin{array}{l} M^{+\cdot} \rightarrow A^+ \rightarrow C^+ \\ \qquad\qquad\qquad\quad \searrow \\ M^{+\cdot} \rightarrow B^{+\cdot} \longrightarrow D^+ \end{array}$$

These may themselves fragment further to C^+, D^+, etc. Some of these ions (e.g. D^+) may have several precursors. Some ions will be odd-electron species ($B^{+\cdot}$) while others may be even-electron species (A^+, C^+), depending on the nature of the uncharged part of the precursor ion which is eliminated in the fragmentation.

The result of these processes is that the source contains a mixture of mainly singly charged ions of different masses. These ions are accelerated out of the source because the ion chamber in which they are formed is at a high positive potential with respect to the source exit slit c. The ions then pass down the flight tube d. In this magnetic sector instrument, ions are deflected in a circular path by the magnetic field and hence the flight tube describes an arc of a circle. Ions of different m/e values are deflected to different extents, the equation which describes this being:

$$m/e = \frac{H^2R^2}{2V}$$

where m = mass of the ion
e = charge on the ion
H = strength of the magnetic field
V = accelerating voltage
R = radius of the ion path

Since the ion path is a flight tube of fixed radius, for given values of V and H an ion of only one particular m/e value will pass down the centre of the tube and reach the collector *e*. The signal produced by the arrival of this ion is amplified by an electron multiplier and passed to a recorder. By scanning the magnetic field a mass spectrum can be obtained, this being an analogue or digital display of the mass-to-charge ratio and relative abundance of all the ions produced from the compound in question. Since the charge on most ions is unity, m/e values are usually referred to as 'masses'. With modern instruments a mass spectrum from say m/e 500 down to m/e 28 can be scanned in 10 s or less using about a microgram of compound.

It can be seen from the above equation that a mass spectrum could be scanned by keeping the magnetic field (H) constant and varying the accelerating voltage (V). This method is not used for obtaining a complete spectrum, but is used for accurate mass measurements at high resolution in that the voltage (V) is switched between the two values necessary to focus an unknown ion and a reference ion, the ratio of these voltages being the ratio of the two masses. It is also the basis of the technique known as multiple-ion monitoring, where the voltage is rapidly switched between the values necessary to observe several masses (typically three or four) simultaneously.

With magnetic sector spectrometers the normal ions appear as sharp peaks at nearly integral mass values. Sometimes, however, broad peaks, usually of low intensity, occur at integral or non-integral masses. These are called metastable peaks and are due to ions which fragment as they enter the first part of the flight tube prior to entering the magnetic field. These ions have been accelerated as one mass m_1 but enter the magnetic field as a smaller mass m_2 so that they appear at neither m_1 nor m_2 on the mass scale but at a mass m^* given by the equation:

$$m^* = \frac{m_2^2}{m_1}$$

The observation of such a metastable ion amounts to proof that an ion m_2^{+} is derived directly from an ion m_1^{+}, but the absence of such a metastable ion does not imply that m_2^{+} does not come from m_1^{+}. The fragmentation has to occur in the early region of the flight tube, so extremely rapid or extremely slow fragmentations do not give observable metastable ions. The great usefulness of metastable ions is that they help in building up the overall fragmentation scheme for a particular molecule, and such schemes are necessary if structural information is to be deduced from a mass spectrum.

In the case of quadrupole mass spectrometers, the ions emerging from the source are passed into a mass filter. This consists of four parallel rods arranged at the corners of a square. Diagonally opposite rods are connected to radiofrequency (r.f.) and d.c. voltage generators, with one pair of rods being out of phase with the other. For a given value of r.f. and d.c. voltage, only ions of a certain m/e value will pass down the centre of the filter arrangement without colliding with the rods. Detection is similar to that for magnetic instruments with an electron multiplier and recording system. A mass spectrum is scanned by sweeping the d.c. voltages from zero to a maximum. The advantage of quadrupoles is twofold: they are fairly inexpensive compared with magnetic sector instruments and they are capable of very fast scanning, which makes them particularly useful for coupling to gas chromatographs. The main disadvantages are in (*i*) the restricted mass range, usually up to about m/e 900, (*ii*) low resolving power, (*iii*) mass discrimination so that high masses are less intense than they should be (although this can be overcome), and (*iv*) lastly that no metastable ions are observed.

The resolving power R of a mass spectrometer can be expressed by the equation:

$$R = \frac{M}{\Delta M}$$

where M is the mean of two adjacent masses and ΔM is the mass separation between them. In this expression two adjacent masses are said to be resolved when the height of the valley between them is 10% of the peak height. An instrument quoted as having a resolving power of 1000 (10% valley definition) would be able to separate two ions of m/e 100·0 and 100·1 to this extent.

Single-focussing magnetic sector instruments of the type discussed and quadrupole instruments have resolving powers of between 500 and 3000. The m/e values of ions in the mass spectra produced from such spectrometers can only be determined to the nearest integer. This is not a serious limitation as far as drug-metabolism studies are concerned, since the structure of the original drug is known and metabolic transformations are limited in number and often predictable. Thus if a drug has a molecular weight of 300 and gives a molecular ion (at m/e 300) while the metabolite has a molecular ion at m/e 286, this loss of 14 mass units would reasonably suggest that demethylation has occurred. It should be stressed here that some molecular ions, for example in the barbiturate series, fragment so rapidly that they are not observed in the mass spectrum, thus making interpretation difficult. However, the m/e value of this invisible ion can sometimes be inferred from calculations on metastable ions or from study of high-mass fragment ions. Alternative methods of ionization discussed later often give molecular or quasi-molecular ions for such sensitive compounds.

If the mass of an ion can be determined with sufficient accuracy, an unequivocal elemental composition can be assigned to it. Thus the masses of the molecular ions from carbon monoxide, nitrogen and ethylene, are 27·99491, 28·00615 and 28·03130 respectively. In a low-resolution mass spectrometer, a mixture of these compounds would appear to give one ion at m/e 28. However, a high-resolution instrument would show the presence of three ions. Moreover, the mass of each of these ions could be determined with sufficient accuracy (1–10 ppm) to enable the correct assignment to be made. Although single-focussing spectrometers are in a few instances capable of a 10 ppm mass measurement accuracy, for very high resolving powers (100,000) and high accuracy of mass measurement, double-focussing mass spectrometers are necessary. These are called double-focussing because they have an electrostatic sector between the source and the magnetic sector. The electrostatic sector ensures that all ions of the same m/e value leaving it do so with the same energy, thus increasing the resolution. Such mass spectrometers are of two types, so-called Nier–Johnson geometry and Mattauch–Herzog geometry. In the latter type, photoplate as well as electrical recording of the mass spectrum can be used.

By a manual technique of comparing the accelerating voltages necessary to observe both a reference ion of known mass and the unknown ion, while the magnetic field is kept constant, it is possible to obtain the mass of the unknown to about 1 or 2 ppm. However, this is an extremely time-consuming operation, taking several minutes per peak. The use of small dedicated computers has now made it possible to obtain accurate mass measurements on all the peaks in a mass spectrum (frequently 200 peaks) which have been obtained in a 10 s scan at say 10,000 resolving power (McMurray *et al*, 1966; Bower *et al*, 1968; Burlingame *et al*, 1968; Milne, 1971; Waller, 1972). Only about a microgram of compound is required for such a determination.

Perhaps the biggest impact of computers in mass spectrometry has been in the field of g.c.–m.s. The vast amount of information obtained with such systems (usually at low resolution) cannot be realistically handled without computers. The advantages are that masses and intensities for each gas-chromatograph peak are rapidly available, spectra can be subtracted from each other, thereby eliminating column bleed as a problem, and spectra can be printed out as bar diagrams if necessary (Hites and Biemann, 1967; Waller, 1972). If a visual-display unit is available, the mass spectrum of a g.c. peak can be displayed on the top half of the screen while spectra can be displayed from a library on the lower half until these have been matched. Several procedures have been described for matching unknown low-resolution spectra with files of reference spectra (Talroze *et al*, 1964; Crawford and Morrison, 1968; Abrahamsson, 1967; Petersson and Ryhage, 1967; Knock *et al*, 1970). The Mass Spectrometry Data Centre at Aldermaston makes available 10,000 spectra on magnetic tape. The Self-Training Interpretative and Retrieval System (STIRS) has 24,000 spectra on file (Venkataraghavan *et al*, 1969), the National Institutes of Health at Bethesda holds a large file (Heller, 1972; Heller *et al*, 1973), the Environmental Protection Agency has 11,000 spectra while other organizations such as the American Petroleum Institute, the Manufacturing Chemists' Association and ASTM Committee E-14 also hold large files of spectra.

Many excellent textbooks are available which discuss the fragmentation of various classes of compounds, and how structural information may be obtained from a knowledge of such fragmentations (Beynon, 1960; Biemann, 1962; Budzikiewicz *et al*, 1964a–c, 1967; Hill, 1966; Reed, 1966, 1968; Spiteller, 1966; McLafferty, 1967; Williams and Howe, 1972; Johnstone, 1972), so this aspect of mass spectrometry will not be discussed in this review. Where simple fragmentations are discussed, even-electron ions will be denoted by the symbol + and odd-electron ions by $]^{+\cdot}$. Fission of bonds can occur by one-electron shifts (⌒) or two-electron shifts (⌒).

SINGLE AND MULTIPLE ION MONITORING (MASS FRAGMENTOGRAPHY)

With a few exceptions it is true to say that no two compounds give identical mass spectra. Hence a mass spectrometer is the ultimate specific detector which can be coupled to a gas chromatograph. When used in a scanning mode, a good quality mass spectrum can be obtained in a 10 s scan on between 100 ng and 1 μg of compound. However, if the mass spectrometer is allowed to monitor only one ion continuously, the detection sensitivity is increased dramatically to some tens of picograms. In g.c.–m.s. systems a flame-ionization detector is not normally used, but the total ion current (t.i.c.) produced by the ions leaving the source of the mass spectrometer is monitored. Since this current increases as more sample enters the source, it can be used to obtain the usual g.c. trace and is of a similar sensitivity. Substances present in such low concentration that they are not observed in this t.i.c. trace can be detected by the single-ion monitoring (s.i.m.) technique if the ion to be monitored is chosen with care.

The s.i.m. technique was first used by Henneberg (1959, 1961) and Schomburg and Henneberg (1968) in a study of hydrocarbons, alcohols and esters. Although the greatest sensitivity in s.i.m. is obtained by monitoring the most intense peak in the spectrum (the base peak), greater selectivity may be obtained by monitoring an ion which is not formed by other compounds present in a complex mixture, or is formed by a minimum of such interfering substances. If the mass spectrum of a compound, such as a metabolite, is not available, because the compound has not yet been synthesized, it is necessary to choose the molecular ion, hoping that the compound has one, or alternatively to predict how fragmentation will occur so that a diagnostic fragment ion may be monitored. In the case of the hallucinogen 2,5-dimethoxy-4-methylamphetamine (STP) (**1**), the mass spectrum was available (Frigerio *et al*, 1972a). The base peak in the mass spectrum was at m/e 44 ($CH_3CH{=}\overset{+}{N}H_2$) but greater selectivity was obtained by monitoring an intense ion at m/e 166 (figure 2) formed as follows:

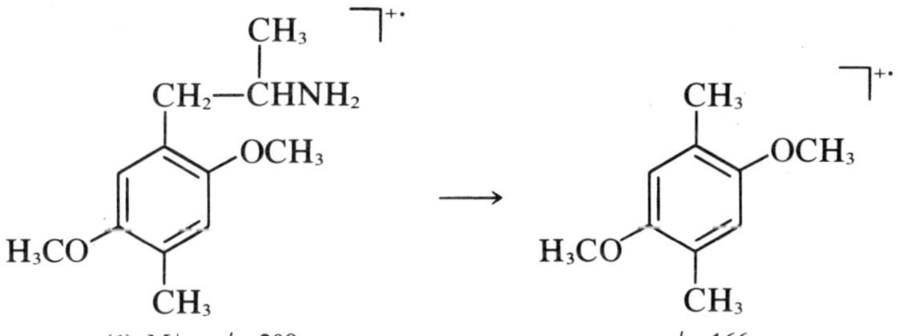

(**1**) M^{+}, m/e 209 → m/e 166

Although no g.c. peak was evident on the t.i.c. trace, there was a response for m/e 166 in the mass spectrometer at the correct retention time for STP. Less than 100 pg of STP (**1**) could be detected in this way.

Naturally, s.i.m. produces a response for all those compounds that give that ion, hence the technique can be used to monitor a series of compounds which give that ion. Thus an extract from the pseudoenzymic oxidation of the antihistamine mepyramine (**2**) was injected into a g.c.–m.s. system and the ion at m/e 58 monitored (Lee and Millard, 1973). This ion was produced from all those mepyramine derivatives in which the side-chain was unaffected. In this case the compounds were produced on a scale large enough

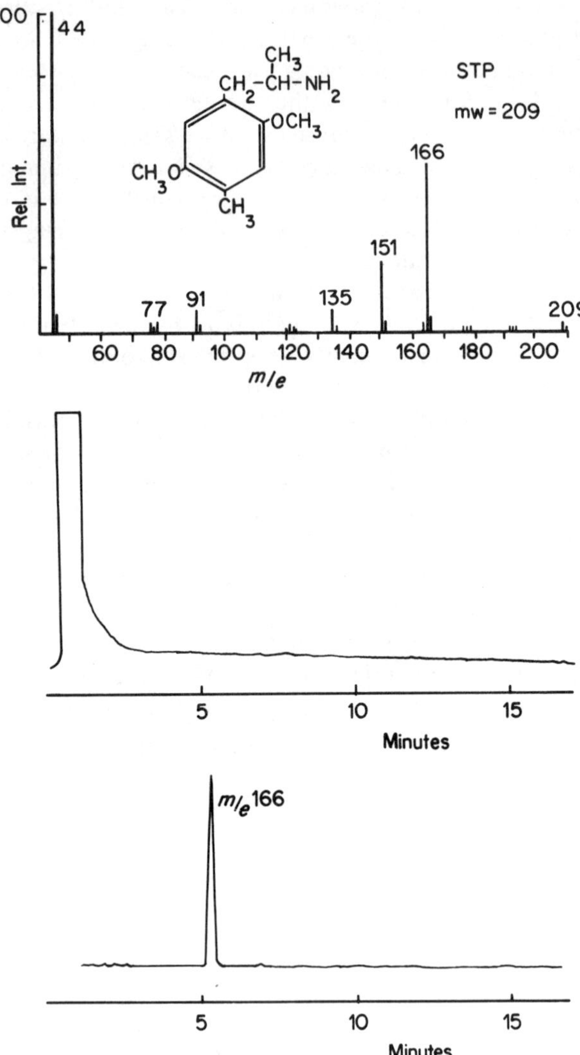

Figure 2 Top panel: Mass spectrum of STP (2,5-dimethoxy-4-methylamphetamine). Middle panel: g.l.c. of 1 ng of STP. Column; *OV 17* (3%) on *Gas-Chrom Q*; isothermal conditions at 140°; detector, total-ion monitor of mass spectrometer [reproduced with permission, Frigerio *et al* (1972a)]. Lower panel: Single-ion monitoring at *m/e* 166 for 1 ng on-column injection of STP

for unequivocal location of ring substituents by n.m.r., but the possibilities for monitoring urine extracts from patients taking the drug are obvious.

As well as being able to detect small amounts of drugs and metabolites, it is also extremely important to be able to quantify them. In order to achieve this by s.i.m. it is necessary to add an internal standard which gives an ion of

H_3CO — CH_2—N— (pyridyl) | $CH_2CH_2N(CH_3)_2$ $]^{+\cdot}$ ⟶ $CH_2{=}\overset{+}{N}(CH_3)_2$

(**2**) M^+, *m/e* 285 *m/e* 58

the same *m/e* value as the substance to be determined. The two retention times should be close but not overlapping. Thus Draffan *et al* (1973) were able to determine down to 10 ng/ml of amylobarbitone and 50 ng/ml of its metabolite 3′-hydroxyamylobarbitone in as little as 100 μl of plasma. Butobarbitone was used as an internal standard for amylobarbitone and the ion at *m/e* 169 monitored. However, as the retention times of the hydroxy compound and butobarbitone were too far apart, phenobarbitone had to be used as an internal standard. This entailed monitoring *m/e* 169 for the hydroxy compound and then switching to *m/e* 175 which was derived from phenobarbitone. This procedure obviously introduces additional error since the setting of the magnet has to be changed and hysteresis might cause the position of focus to drift from the top of the peak.

The major disadvantage of the s.i.m. technique is that it is not very specific for compounds of low molecular weight, since many other substances will be present in biological extracts which give ions at virtually every *m/e* value up to about *m/e* 400. Furthermore, the ideal internal standard, which would be an isotopically labelled version of the compound to be measured, cannot be employed for quantitative work because it would

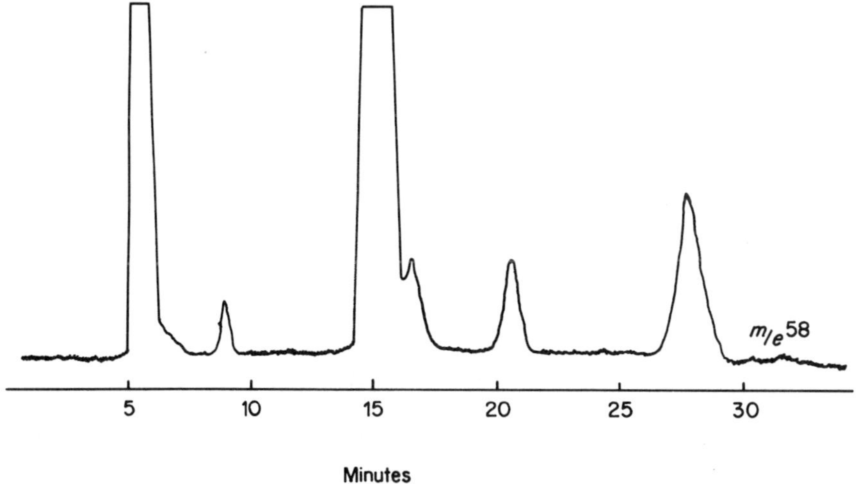

Figure 3 Single-ion monitoring (s.i.m.) of *m/e* 58 from a methylated extract of mepyramine after oxidation in a pseudo-enzyme system (Lee and Millard, 1973)

have the same retention time. However, the ability to monitor say three ions simultaneously would be a great advantage. The technique would be highly selective, since there would be virtually no chance that two compounds with the same retention time would give the same three ions with exactly the same ratio of intensities. It would also be possible to build up the mass spectrum of a compound when insufficient quantity was available for a normal mass-spectral scan or where one component of a mixture could not be completely resolved from another. Different groups of three ions could be monitored until the complete spectrum was obtained.

The possibility of multiple-ion monitoring (m.i.m.)—sometimes called mass fragmentography—was first indicated by Sweeley *et al* (1966) who used a device called an accelerating voltage alternator (a.v.a.) to switch the accelerating voltage of a single-focussing mass spectrometer between two values. By this means two m/e values could be monitored simultaneously, and the procedure was used to resolve mixtures of glucose and glucose-d_7 which eluted simultaneously from a gas chromatograph. From this work was developed an a.v.a. allowing three ions to be monitored simultaneously, although the mass range was limited to a 10% difference between the lowest and highest masses (Hammar *et al*, 1968).

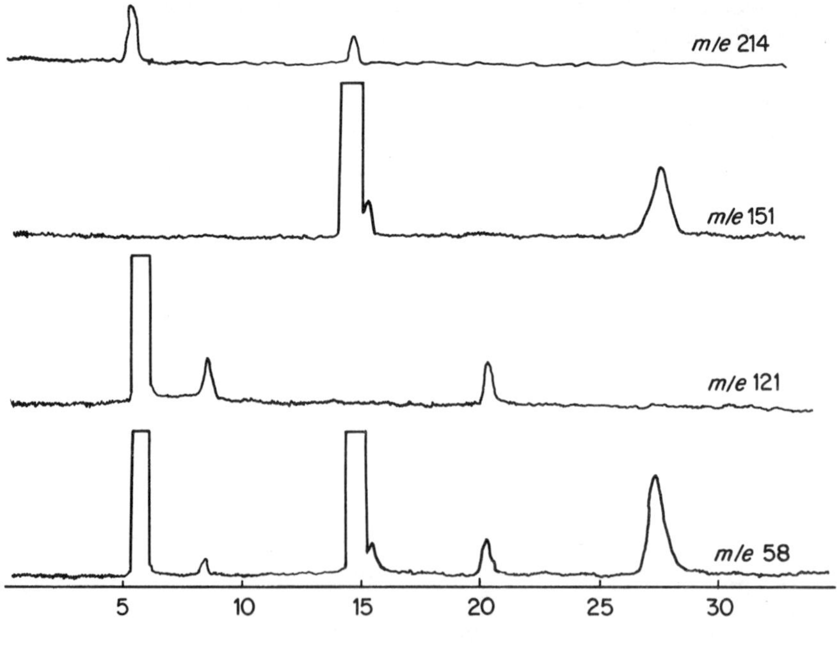

Figure 4 Multiple-ion monitoring (m.i.m.) of m/e 58, 121, 151 and 214, from a methylated extract of mepyramine after oxidation in a pseudo-enzyme system (Lee and Millard, 1973)

A typical application of multiple-ion monitoring is shown in figure 4, where the mepyramine extract mentioned previously (Lee and Millard, 1973), after methylation with diazomethane, has been injected into a g.c.–m.s. system and the ions *m/e* 58, 121, 151 and 214, monitored.

Since mepyramine fragments as follows:

H_3CO — CH_2—N(pyridyl)—$CH_2CH_2N(CH_3)_2$ $]^{+\cdot}$

(**2**) *m/e* 285

→ $CH_2{=}\overset{+}{N}(CH_3)_2$ *m/e* 58

→ H_3CO — CH_2—$\overset{+}{N}$(=CH_2)—(pyridyl) *m/e* 227

→ H_3CO — CH_2—NH—(pyridyl) $]^{+\cdot}$ *m/e* 214

→ H_3CO — (tropylium +) *m/e* 121

m/e 58 can be used to indicate all those compounds present having an intact side chain, *m/e* 121 all those with a methoxybenzyl group, *m/e* 151 all those with a dimethoxybenzyl group and *m/e* 214 should only come from mepyramine itself.

Hammar *et al* (1968) used the technique, which they called mass fragmentography, to study the metabolism of chlorpromazine (**3**). A plasma extract was prepared from a patient taking the drug, and derivatized by formation of the trifluoroacetyl compounds. The ions at *m/e* 232, 234 and 246, were monitored and three peaks emerging from the gas chromatograph were shown to contain these three ions and also have the two ions *m/e* 232 and 234 in the ratio 3 to 1 (due to the ^{35}Cl to ^{37}Cl ratio being 3 to 1). The experiment was repeated and the ions *m/e* 154 and 168 monitored. As these ions would be formed from the trifluoroacetyl compounds **4** and **5**, the three g.c. peaks were thus seen to belong to chlorpromazine and its N-desmethyl and N-didesmethyl metabolites (**6** and **7**). This technique was so sensitive that picogram quantities of chlorpromazine could be detected.

Since this early version of a multiple-ion detector from Hammar and co-workers, steady improvements have been made both to the quality of the response and to the mass range which can be covered. Thus Hammar and Hessling (1971) achieved a mass range of 20% on an LKB instrument while

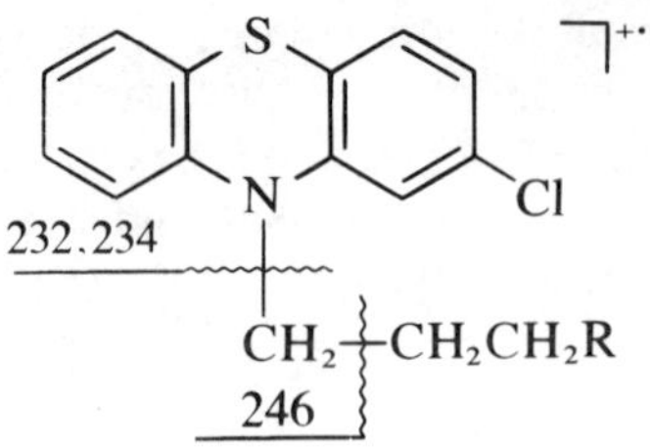

232.234

CH_2–CH_2CH_2R

246

(**3**) $R = N(CH_3)_2$

(**4**) $R = NCH_3COCF_3 \rightarrow \overset{+}{C}H_2CH_2CH_2NCH_3COCF_3$
m/e 168

(**5**) $R = NHCOCF_3 \rightarrow \overset{+}{C}H_2CH_2CH_2NHCOCF_3$
m/e 154

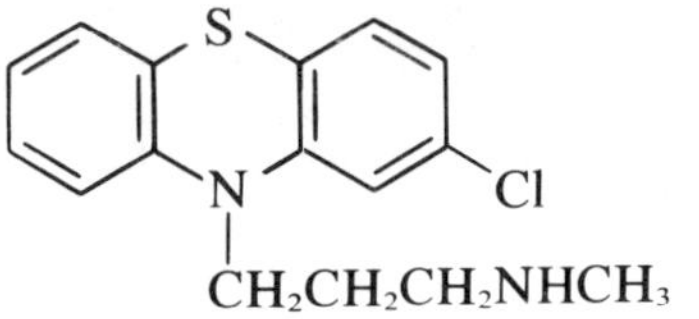

$CH_2CH_2CH_2NHCH_3$
(**6**)

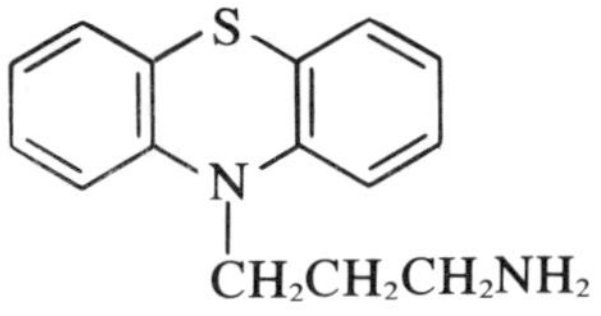

$CH_2CH_2CH_2NH_2$
(**7**)

more recently a range of 30% has been attained (Klein *et al*, 1972). Multiple-ion monitors on the double-focussing double-beam GEC–AEI *MS* 30 instrument are claimed to operate over a 2–300% range by varying the electrostatic analyser voltage.

In the case of accelerating voltage alternators, there are some problems of stability to be overcome. In the high-mass range, using high magnet currents, temperature increases occur which can defocus the ions being monitored. It is thus necessary to refocus during a g.c. run. One approach to this problem has been to use a computer to continually add or subtract a small offset voltage to the coarse accelerating voltages chosen by the a.v.a. This results in optimal focussing of the ions (Holland *et al*, 1973), with improvements in the precision in stable isotope abundance measurements to better than 1% on 100 ng samples of prostaglandin methyl esters.

Quadrupole mass spectrometers are not subject to any limitation in the mass range covered in m.i.m. mode, it being perfectly possible to monitor *m/e* 28 and *m/e* 280 at the same time. With some quadrupole mass spectrometers it is possible to monitor eight ions simultaneously (Knight, 1971). This wider mass range of quadrupoles was utilized by Strong and Atkinson (1972) to measure simultaneously the plasma concentrations of lidocaine (**8**) and its bioactive de-ethylated metabolite (**9**). By fragmentation at the bonds shown, **8** produces ions of *m/e* 86 and 120, while the analogous fragmentation in **9** gives ions of *m/e* 58 and 120. Using trimecaine (**10**) as an internal standard, the ions *m/e* 58, 86 and 120, were monitored. By this means a precision of 3·1% for **8** in the range 0·5–10 μg/ml of plasma and 7·4% for **9** in the range 0·3–5 μg/ml of plasma was obtained.

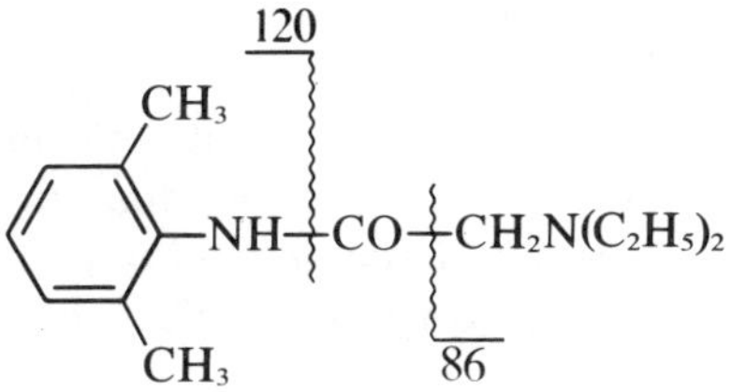

120
CH_3
—NH—CO—$CH_2N(C_2H_5)_2$
CH_3
86

(8)

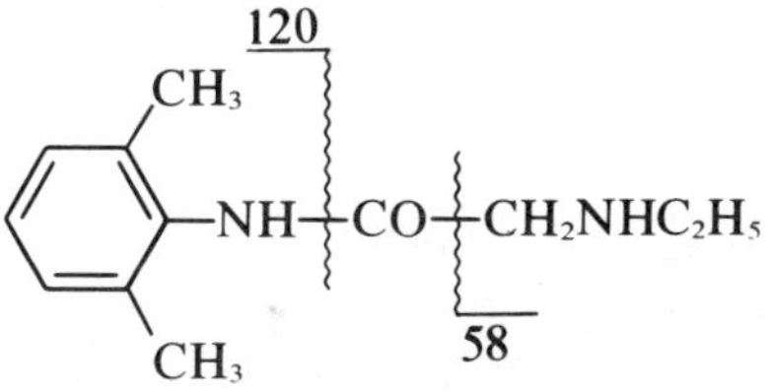

120
CH_3
—NH—CO—$CH_2NHC_2H_5$
CH_3
58

(9)

CH_3
H_3C—⟨ ⟩—NH—CO—$CH_2N(C_2H_5)_2$
CH_3
86

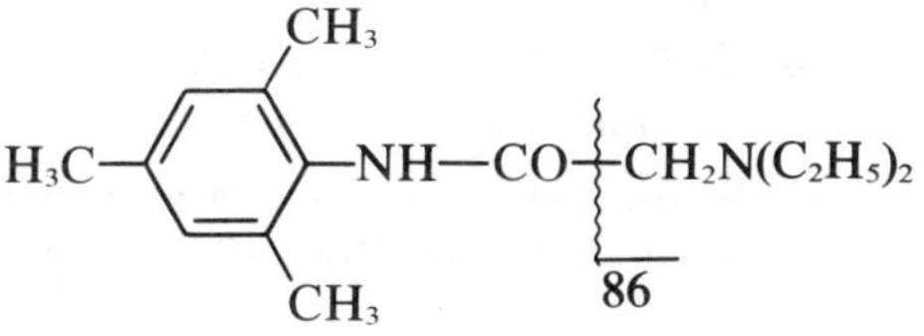

(10)

It has already been stated that the ability to monitor say three ions would mean the capability of building up the mass spectra of inaccessible compounds. This technique has been successful in the hands of Hammar *et al* (1968; 1969) to obtain the mass spectra of the demethylated and deaminated metabolites of chlorpromazine (**3**).

The quantitative use of mass fragmentography has tended to overshadow its use in a qualitative sense. If the mass spectra of synthetic metabolites are available, diagnostic ions can be chosen and extracts of body fluids monitored to see if such ions are detectable at the correct retention time and with the correct intensity ratios. Even if such metabolites cannot be synthesized, their major fragment ions can be predicted from a knowledge of how the parent drug fragments, and a search can be made for these ions. These methods have been applied to the identification of 10-hydroxynortriptyline, desmethylnortriptyline and 10-hydroxydesmethylnortriptyline (Hammar *et al*, 1970 1971), to the identification of (-)Δ^9-6*a*,10*a*-*trans*-tetrahydrocannabinol and two of its metabolites after β-glucuronidase treatment of rat urine, faeces and bile (Mikes *et al*, 1971) and to the detection of normorphine in the urine of humans after the ingestion of codeine (Ebbighausen *et al*, 1973).

In a study of the metabolism of allobarbitone (**11**) in humans (Millard *et al*, 1973a), the deallylated metabolite (**12**) was detected. It was shown that a

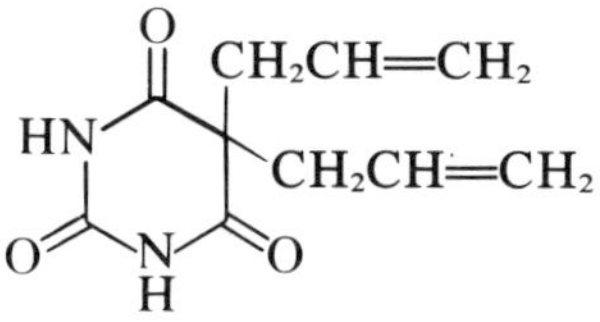

O
HN — $CH_2CH{=}CH_2$ / $CH_2CH{=}CH_2$
O — N — O
H

(11)

O
HN — H / $CH_2CH{=}CH_2$
O — N — O
H

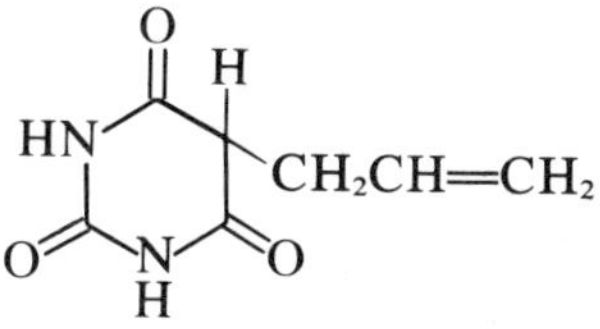

(12)

synthetic sample of (**12**) on methylation of hydroxyl and amino groups with diazomethane gave two trimethyl derivatives of molecular weight 210. On monitoring *m/e* 210 and 195 ($M{-}CH_3\cdot$) a response was obtained at the same two retention times for a methylated extract from a patient taking the drug, the intensity ratios being the same as for the synthetic compounds. It was also shown that **12** was not an impurity present in the original sample of **11**.

The majority of publications on multiple-ion monitoring (or mass fragmentography) at the present time feature its use to measure small quantities of compounds by reference to an internal standard. The ideal internal standard should be chemically similar to the compound to be determined and should be extractable from complex mixtures by the same solvents. The two compounds should either be separable on the gas chromatograph because they have different retention times or they can have the same retention time but be separable by virtue of the fact that they give different ions. Thus Kelly (1971) used 4-methyl-oestra-1,3,5(10)-triene-1,15α,16α,17β-tetrol as a standard for oestetrol. The brain amines dopamine and noradrenaline have been measured by using the corresponding methyl homologues (Knight, 1971) and the pentafluoropropionic anhydride derivatives (Koslow *et al*, 1972). Biologically active amines, such as amphetamines, catecholamines and certain hallucinogens, have also been analyzed by Brandenberger and Schnyder (1972).

In the quantitative determination of imipramine (**13**) in human plasma (Frigerio *et al*, 1972b), promazine (**14**) was used as an internal marker. Figure 5 shows the response obtained from the fragment ions *m/e* 235 formed from **13** and *m/e* 238 formed from **14**. It was possible to detect down to 10 ng of imipramine per ml of plasma. Bertilsson and Palmer (1972) were able to quantify indole-3-acetic acid in cerebrospinal fluid (CSF) by using the

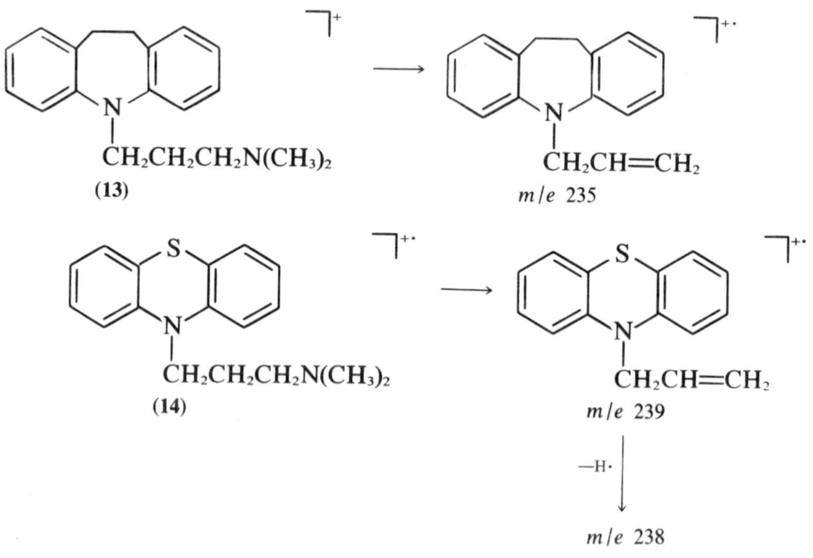

$CH_2CH_2CH_2N(CH_3)_2$ $\longrightarrow$ $CH_2CH{=}CH_2$

(**13**) *m/e* 235

$CH_2CH_2CH_2N(CH_3)_2$ $\longrightarrow$ $CH_2CH{=}CH_2$

(**14**) *m/e* 239

$-H\cdot$

m/e 238

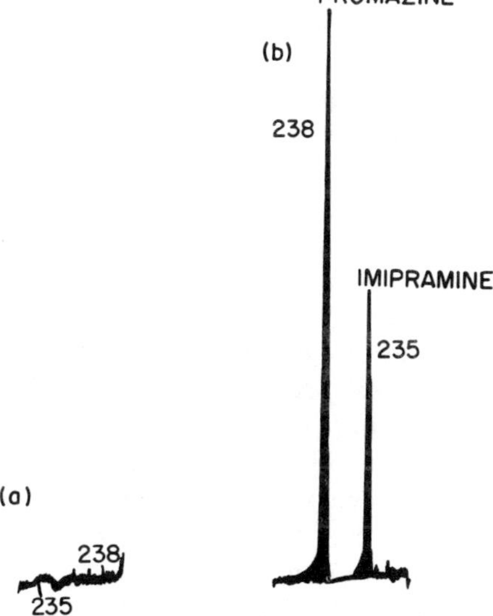

Figure 5 Mass fragmentograms of human-plasma extracts: (a) plasma blank (b) plasma after addition of 100 ng/ml of imipramine and 1 ng/μl of the internal marker promazine [reproduced with permission, Frigerio *et al* (1972b)]

5-methyl analogue as an internal marker. The methyl esters of the heptafluorobutyryl derivatives (**15** and **16**) were used. By monitoring *m/e* 385 and *m/e* 326, 340, which were formed by the fragmentation shown below, quantities of the order of 2 ng/ml of indole-3-acetic acid in CSF could be estimated.

326
CH_2—$COOCH_3$
N
COC_3F_7
(**15**) M^+, *m/e* 385

340
H_3C CH_2—$COOCH_3$
N
COC_3F_7
(**16**) M^+, *m/e* 399

Since small changes occur in the operating conditions of both the gas chromatograph and the mass spectrometer between the time of elution of two peaks, errors may arise where a different chemical compound is used as an internal reference. If, however, it can be arranged that the two compounds are eluted simultaneously, these errors are obviously eliminated. Such a state of affairs can be brought about by the use of compounds labelled with stable isotopes such as ^2H, ^{13}C, ^{15}N and ^{18}O. Usually such compounds have the same retention time as the unlabelled compounds on the gas chromatograph, although it has been reported that d_{45}-penta-O-trimethylsilyl-D-glucose was separable from the unlabelled material (Waller *et al*, 1969). However, due to the increase in mass of the stable isotope over the normal isotope of the particular element, the two compounds will give molecular and fragment ions of different mass. The first use of such a technique was reported by Samuelsson *et al* (1970) who used a deuterated methoxy derivative of prostaglandin E_1. Quantification of nanogram amounts was easily carried out. Picomole amounts of prostaglandins E_2 and $F_{2\alpha}$ were also determined by such a technique (Axen *et al*, 1971). By using a large amount of the labelled material compared to the amount of unlabelled material to be determined, the carrier effect reduced substantially on-column adsorption of these small quantities of unlabelled compounds.

Labelled compounds can either be a labelled version of the compound under study, or derivatives can be made utilizing labelled reagents. The advantage of employing a labelled version of the compound itself is that as well as its use in quantification the label facilitates studies of the metabolism of the compound. This aspect is discussed later. Bertilsson *et al* (1972) used a labelled version of 5-hydroxyindole-3-acetic acid to determine the latter in cerebrospinal fluid. These compounds were studied as the heptafluorobutyryl derivatives of the methyl esters **17** and **18**. Although primarily intended for electron-capture gas chromatography, these derivatives

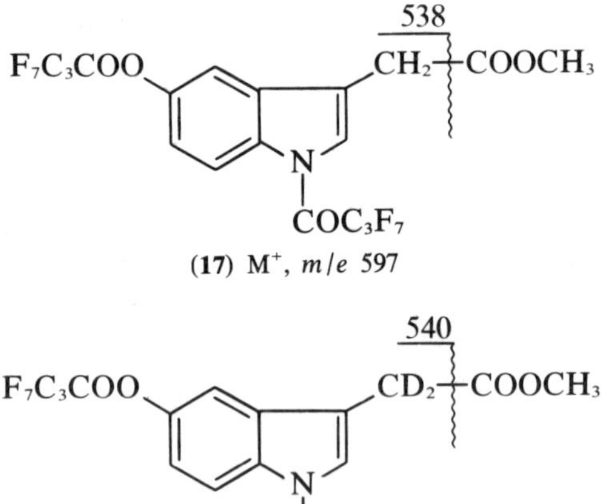

538

F_7C_3COO CH_2—$COOCH_3$

N

COC_3F_7

(**17**) M^+, *m*/*e* 597

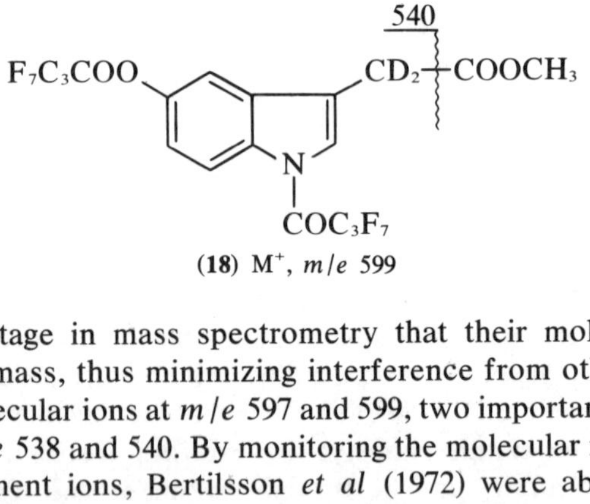

540

F_7C_3COO CD_2—$COOCH_3$

N

COC_3F_7

(**18**) M^+, *m*/*e* 599

have the advantage in mass spectrometry that their molecular ions are shifted to high mass, thus minimizing interference from other compounds. Besides the molecular ions at *m*/*e* 597 and 599, two important ions were also produced at *m*/*e* 538 and 540. By monitoring the molecular ion *m*/*e* 597 and these two fragment ions, Bertilsson *et al* (1972) were able to determine 2–50 ng/ml of the compound using 2 ml of CSF for the analysis. The standard deviation was about 7% in the 8–20 ng range.

In a study of nortriptyline (Gaffney *et al*, 1971) both deuterium and ^{15}N labelling was used. The trifluoroacetyl derivatives of nortriptyline (**19**), the deuterium analogue (**20**), the ^{15}N analogue (**21**) and an unlabelled standard

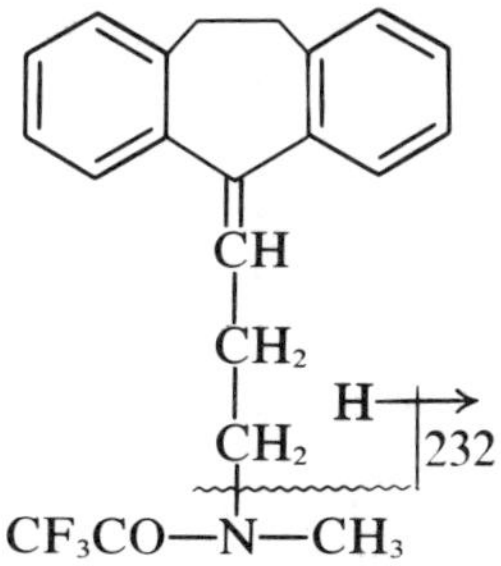

(19) 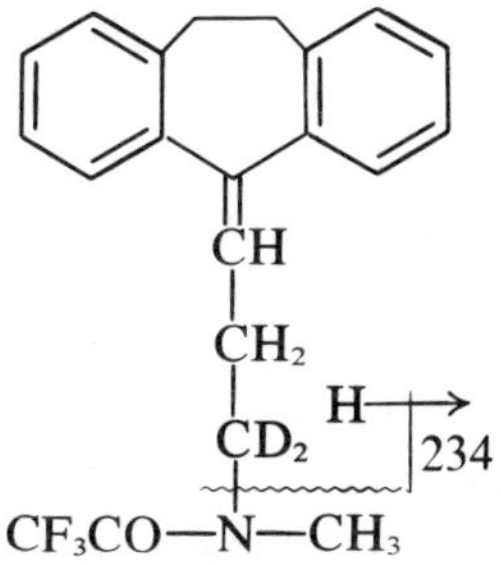 (20)

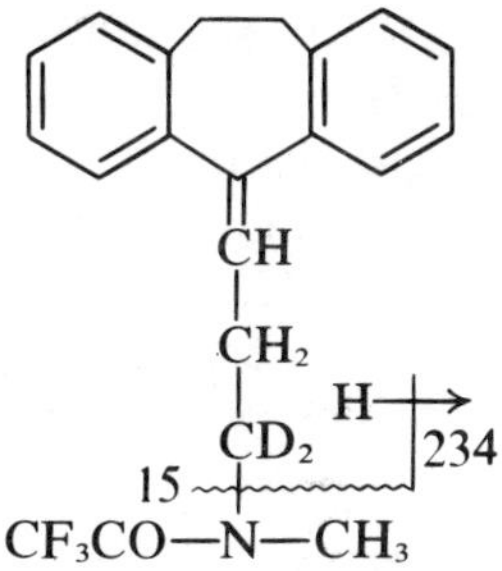

(21) 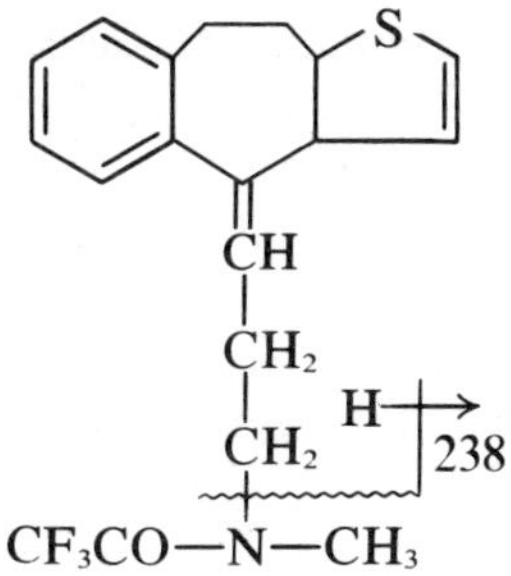 (22)

(**22**) was utilized for the determination. 50 picograms of **19** were easily detectable. It appeared that the alternative standard (**22**) was partially lost by on-column adsorption, since much lower signals were obtained at *m/e* 238 for **22** than those at *m/e* 234 in the case of **20** and **21**. However, since the authors did not state how much of the total ion current in each of the spectra was due to these ions in question, it could be that the lower signal from *m/e* 238 was due to the low intensity of this ion in the mass spectrum.

In a study on the levels of Δ^1-tetrahydrocannabinol in the plasma of cannabis smokers, Agurell *et al* (1973) have been able to quantify down to 5 ng/ml of plasma by using Δ^1-THC-d_2 as an internal standard. The ions *m/e* 299 and 314 from Δ^1-THC and *m/e* 301 and 316 from the dideutero compound were monitored.

Carriers that are labelled versions of the substances to be measured have the advantage that they can be added to the crude biological extract before work-up and derivatization. However, since the major losses in dealing with small amounts of compounds are often on the gas-chromatograph column rather than in the initial work-up, the use of labelled reagents for the formation of derivatives is still an important application yet to be fully exploited. This method has already been utilized for the estimation of prostaglandins (Samuelsson *et al*, 1970). The possibility exists of using silylating agents labelled with deuterium (Narasimhachari and Vouros, 1972), methylating agents such as trideuteromethyl iodide and acylating agents such as perdeuteroacetic anhydride (van Heijenoort *et al*, 1967).

In our laboratories diazomethane in O-deuteromethanol is employed as a methylating agent for barbiturates. Since an exchange reaction is involved, complete deuteration is not achieved, instead a mixture of d_0- up to d_6-dimethyl derivatives are formed. However, the amount of d_0 material is extremely small, and if the extent of labelling in the standard is checked no confusion arises.

Since, as has already been mentioned, quadrupoles have the capability of monitoring many more ions simultaneously than magnetic instruments using a.v.a.s, it is not surprising that computers have been used to change the quadrupole voltages. Thus it is only necessary to type-in on the input terminal the masses it is desired to monitor, and these are immediately focussed. This technique has been extended by Green and Hertel (1973) who have used a quadrupole mass spectrometer under computer control to monitor contracted mass spectra. They argue, correctly, that in scanning a complete mass spectrum, much time is wasted in scanning portions of the mass spectrum in which no information resides. If, for example, it is desired to monitor a mixture for the presence of chlorpromazine, as few as ten correctly chosen ions would give an unequivocal identification. By examining each of these ions in turn while ignoring other portions of the spectrum, such a contracted spectrum can be obtained in 0.1 s, nearly 30 times faster than a conventional scan of a complete mass spectrum. In the case of methadone, 15 m/e values were considered to give an unequivocal identification. In an effort to overcome the lengthy time necessary for analysis with a g.c.–m.s. system, Green and Hertel (1973) used a flash evaporator with a membrane separator. Liquid samples were injected into the evaporator and carried into the separator by a stream of nitrogen. Using this system, useful results on street drug mixtures and urine samples were obtained in seconds as opposed to perhaps 30 min for a typical g.c.–m.s. determination.

Instead of using an a.v.a. to examine selected ions, the use of computers with a large tape or disc-storage system has meant that mass spectrometers can be used in a repetitive scanning mode when used in a g.c.–m.s. combination. With magnetic instruments up to four spectra per minute may be obtained, while quadrupoles are very much faster. Instead of monitoring the total ion current from the mass spectrometer in order to obtain a gas chromatogram, the computer can be programmed to sum the total ion intensities in each scan and so reconstruct its own total ion-current trace. More important, however, is the fact that the intensity of a particular ion can be plotted as a function of time, thus constructing a mass chromatogram, this being a computer equivalent of s.i.m. Since complete spectra are on file, requests can be made for mass chromatograms of any other ions within the mass range scanned by the mass spectrometer. This is the basis of a system reported by Hites and Biemann (1970) which permits total mass fragmentography to be carried out after one column injection. Since the spectrum has been scanned through the entire mass range, it would be expected that the response to a particular m/e value would be less than in conventional s.i.m., where one ion is monitored continuously. For this reason Baczynskyj *et al*, (1973) adopted the procedure of scanning a narrow mass range of 20–30 mass units in an effort to give more flexibility than m.i.m. These workers used the technique for steroids and prostaglandins. However, according to Middleditch and Desiderio (1973), repetitive scanning (r.s.) and s.i.m. are of similar sensitivity when each is used under optimum conditions. They point out that r.s. is superior for screening of body fluids for drugs since any ion can be followed from a single injection.

Additional examples of the applications of mass fragmentography can be found in a recently published list (Costa and Holmstedt, 1973).

USE OF STABLE ISOTOPES

From the previous section, it is obvious that stable isotopes are finding an increasing use in the quantification of low levels of compounds of biological importance. But isotopes have been used for over fifty years as biological tracers; for example the use of ^{212}Pb by Hevesy (1923). The use of deuterium in metabolic studies was pioneered by Schoenheimer and Rittenberg in the 1930's (Waller, 1972) and is now widespread in biochemical studies (Popjak *et al*, 1962; Eidenoff, 1953). ^{13}C has been used in biosynthetic work (Pomerantz and Ward, 1958) and in mechanistic studies on enzymic conversions (Kellermeyer and Ward, 1962), while ^{15}N has been used in investigations of intermediary metabolic processes (Shemin and Henbergh, 1946) and in studies of the metabolism of pentobarbitone (Maynert and van Dyke, 1950a), amylobarbitone (Maynert and van Dyke, 1950b) and barbitone (Maynert and van Dyke, 1950c). More recently ^{18}O has been used for studies of enzymic oxidation (Jerina *et al*, 1968).

In the study of drug metabolism the chief advantage of stable isotopes over radioactive tracers is the lack of radiation hazards for humans which is especially important in the case of pregnant females. With currently available instrumentation, however, stable isotopes are much less conveniently measured than radioactive ones. The use of mass spectrometry usually enables the position of the label in the molecule to be determined. This can be done by reference to fragment ions which either may or may not contain the isotope in question. Furthermore it is possible to employ multiple labelling at different sites of the molecule with either the same isotope or even mixtures of isotopes. However, the widespread use of stable isotopes such as ^{2}H, ^{13}C, ^{15}N and ^{18}O, has awaited the development of more sensitive mass spectrometers, especially g.c.–m.s. systems, and only in the last few years have papers begun to appear which describe this technique. These have recently been reviewed by Knapp and Gaffney (1972).

Because of the typical isotope patterns of bromine- and chlorine-containing compounds, the presence of one or more of these elements in a compound can be inferred at a glance from its mass spectrum. Thus one of the attractions of a mass-spectrometric investigation of the metabolism of a drug, such as chlorpromazine or chlordiazepoxide, is that it is easy to recognize the spectra of those compounds derived from the drug so that other spectra can be ignored. Unfortunately only a few drugs contain chlorine or bromine, so that the use of stable isotopes to create recognizable patterns in the mass spectra has much attraction. The use of perdeuteroacetic anhydride has been mentioned earlier in connection with peptides (van Heijenoort *et al*, 1967). This reagent was used with an equimolar amount of acetic anhydride to create recognizable clusters of ions. All fragment ions containing the acyl group consisted of doublets three mass units apart and so were easily noticed.

Perhaps the first application of this technique to the field of drug metabolism was a study of the metabolism of a mixture of 7β-d-testosterone and testosterone in the canine perianal gland (Morfin *et al*, 1970). The metabolic fate of 1-n-butyl-5,5-diethylbarbituric acid in the rat was studied by using an ^{15}N label (Vore *et al*, 1971). Doublets were produced one mass unit apart for all those ions which still contained the nitrogen atom. Natural isotopic contribution, mainly from ^{13}C, and ion–molecule collisions in sources operating at higher pressures can, however, both affect the M, M + 1 ratio and such M, M + 1 doublets may not therefore be ideal for this application. Nevertheless, Braselton *et al* (1973) used monodeuterium-labelled compounds to produce M, M + 1 ions of equal intensity when studying the metabolism of androstenedione and testosterone by the aromatizing enzymes of human placenta. After applying the products to a g.c.–m.s. system, they examined every peak emerging from the chromatograph to determine whether twin ions were present. They claimed that the sensitivity of the technique was such that it was possible to detect as little as 5% of contaminating compounds which were not resolved on the column. As a result of using this technique, they were able to identify 17β,19-dihydroxyandrost-4-en-3-one, 19-hydroxyandrost-4-ene-3,17-dione, 17β-hydroxy-3-oxoandrost-4-en-19-al, 3,17-dioxoandrost-4-en-19-al, oestradiol-17β and oestrone.

Prox *et al* (1973) also used an M, M + 1 doublet in a study of the metabolic transformations of 4-morpholino-2-piperazinothieno[3,2]pyrimidine labelled in the 2-position of the pyrimidine ring (**23**).

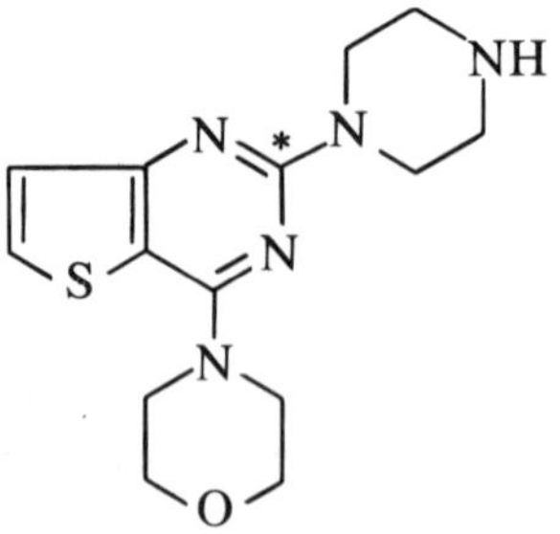

(23)

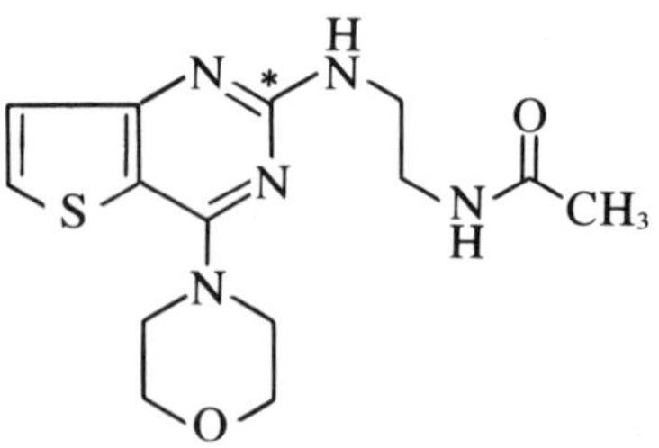

(24)

The synthesis started with 60% enriched ^{13}C-KSCN, so the molecular-ion region of **23** had an M + 1 ion somewhat more intense than the M^+ ion. A methanol extract of rat urine containing the metabolites was subjected to two dimensional thin-layer chromatography. The spots from the thin-layer plate were all subjected to mass spectrometry and metabolites readily detected by the presence of twin ions. For example, figure 6 shows the consecutive mass spectra of one metabolite (**24**) as the inlet probe temperature was increased. By the end of the distillation the mass spectrum of this metabolite could be obtained almost free from impurity. From the molecular ions at *m/e* 321 and *m/e* 322 and a consideration of the fragmentation, the structure (**24**) was deduced for this metabolite. The structures of several other metabolites were determined similarly. In a later paper, Zimmer *et al* (1973) described the use of simultaneous labelling with ^{13}C and ^{14}C at the same position of **23**. The synthesis was started with a mixture of 60% enriched ^{13}C—KCN and ^{14}C—KCN. The authors pointed out that an advantage of simultaneous labelling was that the pharmacokinetics and structure elucidation could be carried out together. This approach should find widespread use, since usually both the ^{13}C- and ^{14}C-labelled drugs can be synthesized simultaneously employing mixed labels in the starting material.

Knapp *et al* (1972a) have preferred to use M and M + 3 doublets created by using trideuterium- and dideuterium-^{15}N-labelled drugs. An equimolar mixture of nortriptyline (**25**) and deuterium labelled nortriptyline (**26**) was given to rats and the extracted urine was derivatized with trifluoroacetic anhydride. The mixture was injected on the column of a g.c.–m.s. system and mass spectra obtained on all the peaks emerging from the chromatograph. One of these spectra contained a doublet three mass units apart at *m/e* 357 and *m/e* 360 (figure 7) so indicating that a compound derived from the

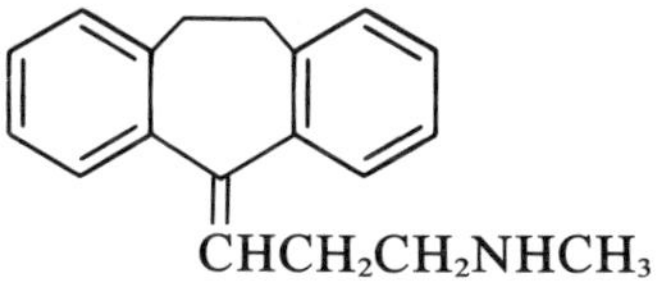

$CHCH_2CH_2NHCH_3$

(25)

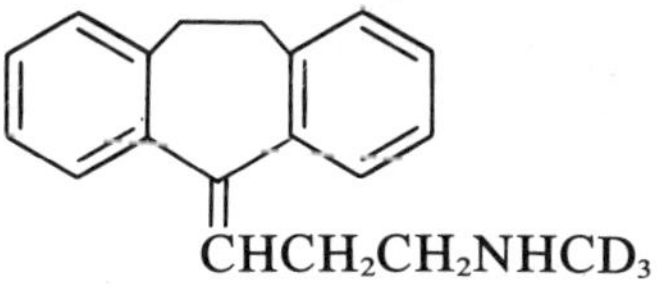

$CHCH_2CH_2NHCD_3$

(26)

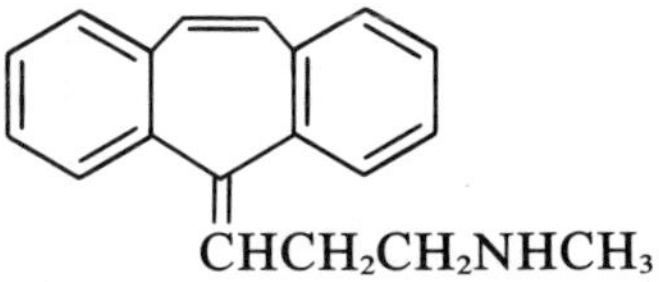

$CHCH_2CH_2NHCH_3$

(27)

labelled (**26**) and unlabelled (**25**) mixture was present. A mass spectrum was taken at the same position in a g.c. trace from an experiment in which unlabelled nortriptyline had been used, since such a spectrum was much easier to interpret than the mixed one. The structure of the metabolite was

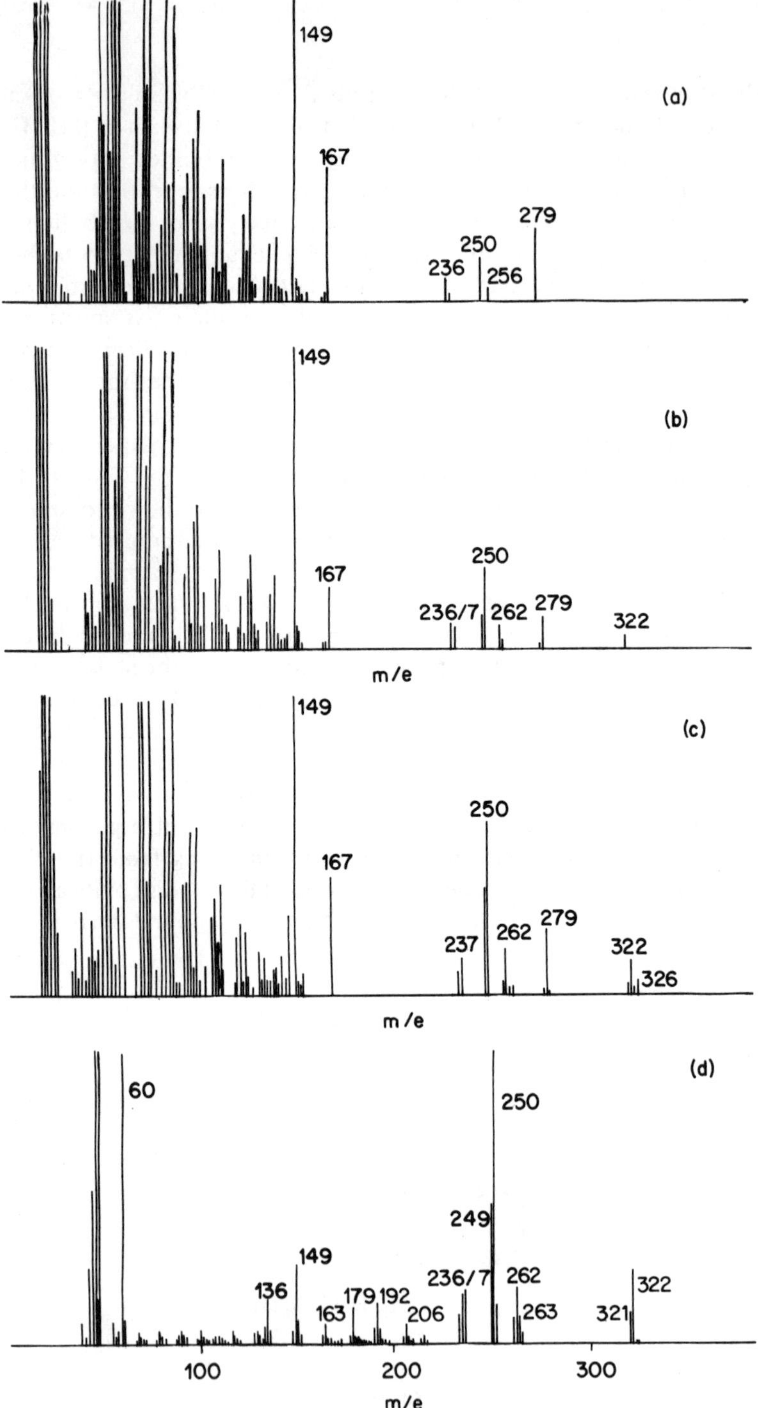

Figure 6 Consecutive mass spectra (70 eV) of the metabolite M_4 as observed with increasing sample probe temperature. Probe temperatures were: (a) 100°, (b) 110°, (c) 130°, (d) 150° [reproduced with permission, Prox *et al* (1973)]

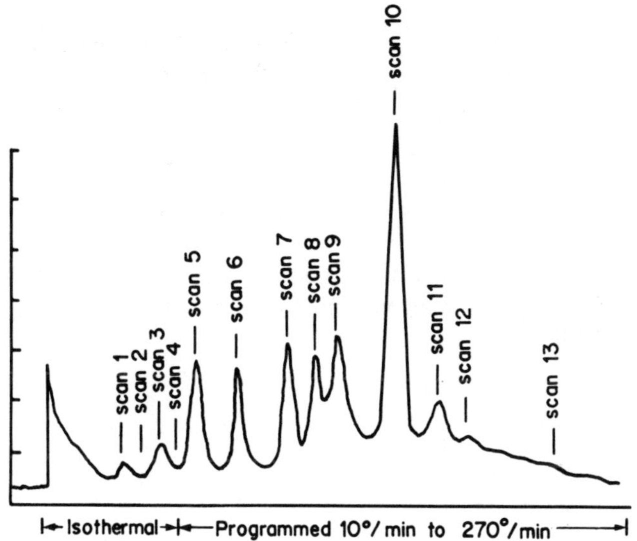

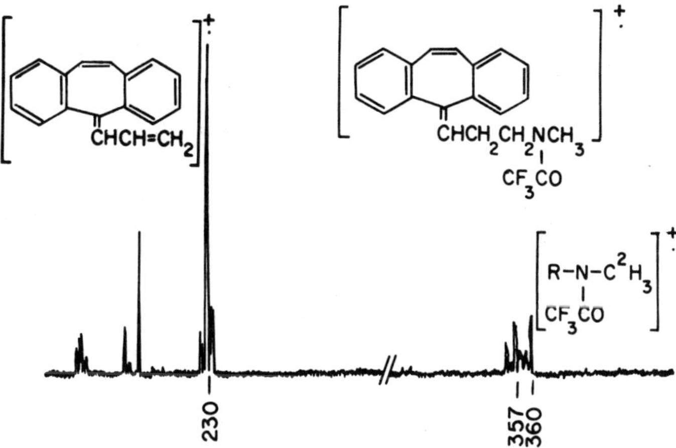

Figure 7 Upper panel: Total-ion current reading from separation of trifluoroacetylated basic urine extract showing mass-spectral scan points. Lower panel: Partial mass spectrum from scan 10 (20 eV) [reproduced with permission, Knapp *et al* (1972a)]

OH

$CHCH_2CH_2NHCH_3$

(28)

$CHCH_2CD_2{}^{15}NHCH_3$

(29)

deduced to be **27**, but it was argued that **27** was most probably derived from the trifluoroacetate of **28** by the loss of trifluoroacetic acid.

The same authors (Knapp *et al*, 1972b) also investigated the urinary and biliary metabolites of **25** in humans. Having recognized that the CD_3 group in **26** was a poor choice for a labelling position since it was in a metabolically labile position, they utilized the ^{15}N and ^{2}H labelled compound **29**. By the technique used in the previous paper, they identified the desmethyl compound (**30**) and its hydroxy derivative (**31**) in addition to the 10-hydroxy derivative of **25**. **30** had previously been reported to be a metabolite of nortriptyline present in human plasma by Hammar *et al* (1971) who also tentatively identified **31**.

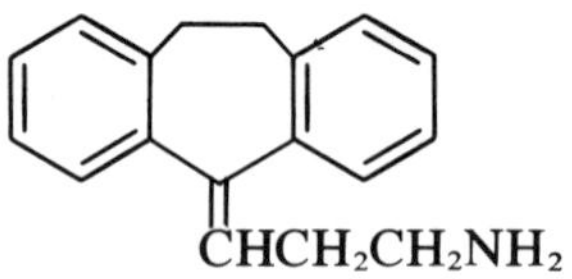

$CHCH_2CH_2NH_2$
(**30**)

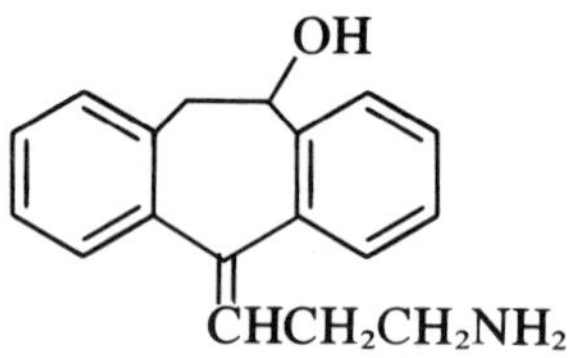

OH
$CHCH_2CH_2NH_2$
(**31**)

Walle *et al* (1972) studied the metabolism of propanolol (**32**) and hexadeuteropropanolol (**33**) in the dog. A urine extract was reacted with 2,4-dinitrofluorobenzene in order to form the dinitrophenyl derivatives. By this means isopropylamine and d_6-isopropylamine were detected as metabo-

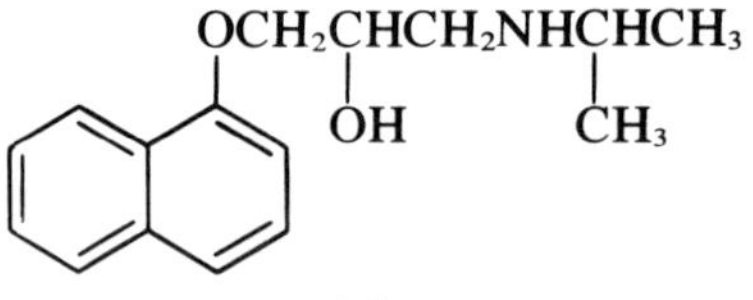

$OCH_2CHCH_2NHCHCH_3$ (OH, CH_3)
(**32**)

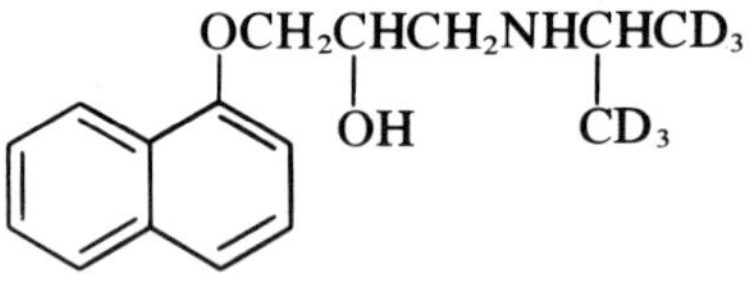

$OCH_2CHCH_2NHCHCD_3$ (OH, CD_3)
(**33**)

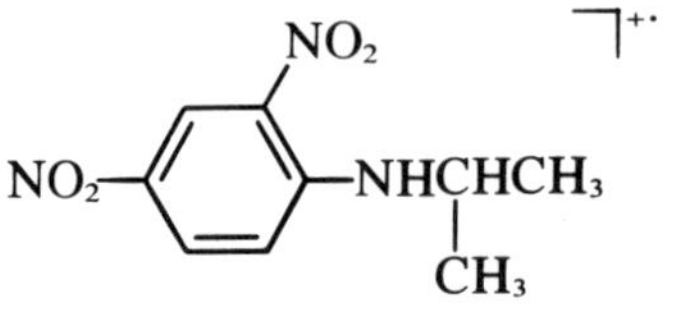

NO_2, NO_2, $-NHCHCH_3$ (CH_3) $]^{+\cdot}$
(**34**) *m/e* 225

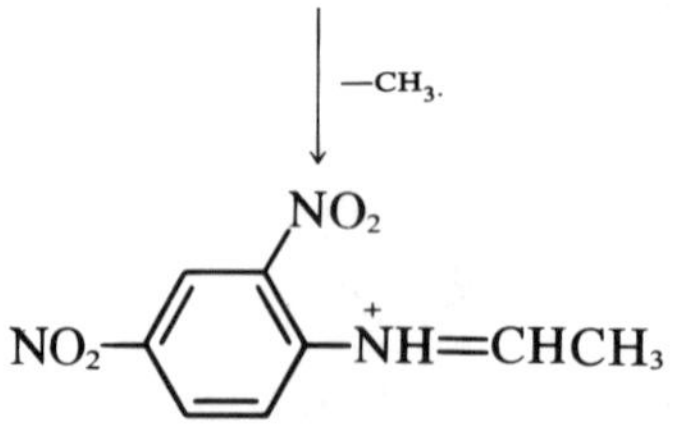

NO_2, NO_2, $-NHCHCD_3$ (CD_3) $]^{+\cdot}$
(**35**) *m/e* 231

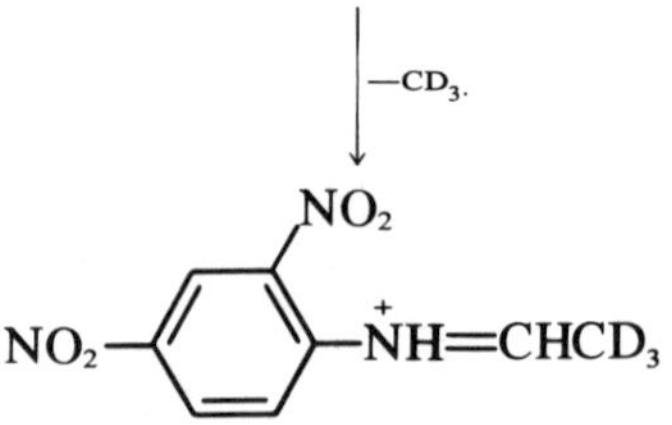

$-CH_3\cdot$

$-CD_3\cdot$

NO_2, NO_2, $-\overset{+}{N}H{=}CHCH_3$
m/e 210

NO_2, NO_2, $-\overset{+}{N}H{=}CHCD_3$
m/e 213

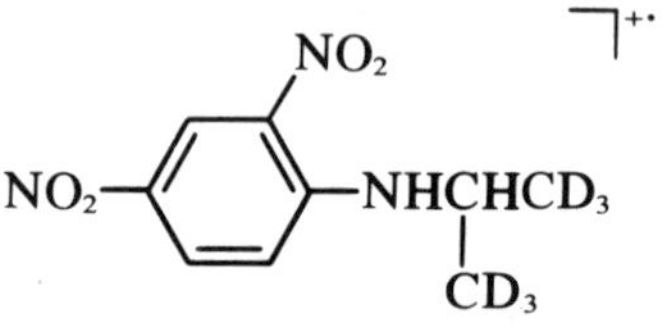

lites. The DNP derivatives (**34** and **35**) fragmented as shown, so that it was possible to monitor m/e 210 and 225 from **34** and m/e 213 and 231 from **35**.

When administering labelled compounds to animals or humans, the operation of isotope effects should not be overlooked. These are sometimes quite large, as discovered by Vree *et al* (1971), who compared the elimination of deuterated amphetamines and N-substituted deuterated amphetamines with the unlabelled compounds.

NEWER METHODS OF IONIZATION

In the applications discussed so far, mass spectra have been obtained using an electron-impact source. This method of ionization results in the formation of large numbers of fragment ions because substantial amounts of energy are transferred to the molecule. It often happens that fragmentation occurs so readily that a molecular ion is not observed, making interpretation of the spectrum difficult. Although fragment ions are useful from an interpretative point of view, the most useful piece of information to be obtained from a mass spectrum is the molecular weight of the compound concerned. It is not surprising therefore that alternative methods of ionization have been sought which would result in much less energy being transferred to the molecular ion with consequent reduction in fragmentation and enhancement of the intensity of the molecular ion. The most important of these are chemical ionization, and field ionization and desorption.

Chemical Ionization

Chemical ionization (Milne, 1972; Waller, 1972) employs a set of reagent ions to ionize the organic compound under study (Munson and Field, 1966; Field, 1968; Munson, 1971). The most common reagent is methane gas which, at a pressure of about 1 mm of Hg, is ionized by electron bombardment. This results in the formation of the following ions:

$$CH_4 + e \rightarrow CH_4^{+\cdot}, CH_3^+, CH_2^{+\cdot}$$
$$CH_4^{+\cdot} + CH_4 \rightarrow CH_5^+ + CH_3\cdot$$
$$CH_3^+ + CH_4 \rightarrow C_2H_5^+ + H_2$$
$$CH_2^{+\cdot} + CH_4 \rightarrow C_2H_3^+ + H_2 + H\cdot$$
$$C_2H_3^+ + CH_4 \rightarrow C_3H_5^+ + H_2$$

At a pressure of 1 mm, over 90% of the total ions consist of CH_5^+ and $C_2H_5^+$. The organic compound is present at a concentration of about 0·1% in the source, and as a result of collisions with the reagent ions, protonated and adduct ions are formed. Since little excess energy is transferred by these processes, fragmentation is very much less pronounced than in electron-impact (e.i.) mass spectrometry. Reagent ions have also been formed from helium, argon–water mixtures (Hunt and Ryan, 1972) and isobutane (Milne *et al*, 1971). The reagent gas can also be used as a carrier in g.c.–m.s. systems, so that molecular separators are not necessary.

As well as the virtue of giving much simpler spectra (because of reduced fragmentation), chemical ionization (c.i.) mass spectrometry has been particularly useful in studying those compounds which give no molecular ions in their e.i. spectra. Several workers have found that barbiturates often give no molecular ions (Costapanagiotis and Budzikiewicz, 1965; Grutzmacher and Arnold, 1966; Coutts and Locock, 1968). Fales *et al* (1970) have shown that, with methane as reagent gas, barbiturates give intense quasi-molecular ions at $(M+1)^+$, i.e. MH^+. This can be seen in figure 8, where the c.i. and e.i. mass spectra of ortal (hexethal) (**36**) are compared. The molecular ion at m/e 240 in the e.i. spectrum is virtually nonexistent, the major fragmentation resulting in the formation of m/e 156 as follows:

(**36**) $\longrightarrow$ m/e 156

This ion would be formed from any barbiturate with an ethyl group at the 5 position. Identification of such barbiturates based on their e.i. spectra is at best difficult and at worst impossible. However, the MH^+ ion in the c.i. spectrum gives the molecular weight as 240 and identification is simple.

Isobutane holds an advantage over methane gas, since the only significant protonating species is the *t*-butyl ion $C_4H_9^+$, which compared with CH_5^+ transfers a proton with much less energy. Therefore isobutane c.i.-spectra are characterized by much less intense fragment ions, often less than 5% of the intensity of MH^+. The isobutane c.i. spectra of some 48 drugs have been determined by Milne *et al* (1971). For the most part these gave only MH^+ ions (except notably aspirin) and hence, for example, the identification of drugs present in the stomach washings of an overdose patient is a simple problem of using a table of molecular weights of common drugs (figure 9).

The c.i. spectra of macrolide antibiotics (Mitscher and Showalter, 1972) showed prominent MH^+ ions. The fragmentation patterns of, for example, erythromycin B were simple, the glycosidic bonds being particularly subject to cleavage.

However, in many cases in c.i. spectra, MH^+ ions may be absent or of low intensity. Thus for the prostaglandins, MH^+ ions were much less intense than those due to the loss of one and two molecules of water from MH^+ (Desiderio and Hägele, 1971). In the case of steroids, the presence or otherwise of MH^+ ions depends on the type of steroid. Thus Michnowicz and Munson (1972) reported that for 17-hydroxysteroids, with methane as reagent gas, little fragmentation is observed except for loss of water from

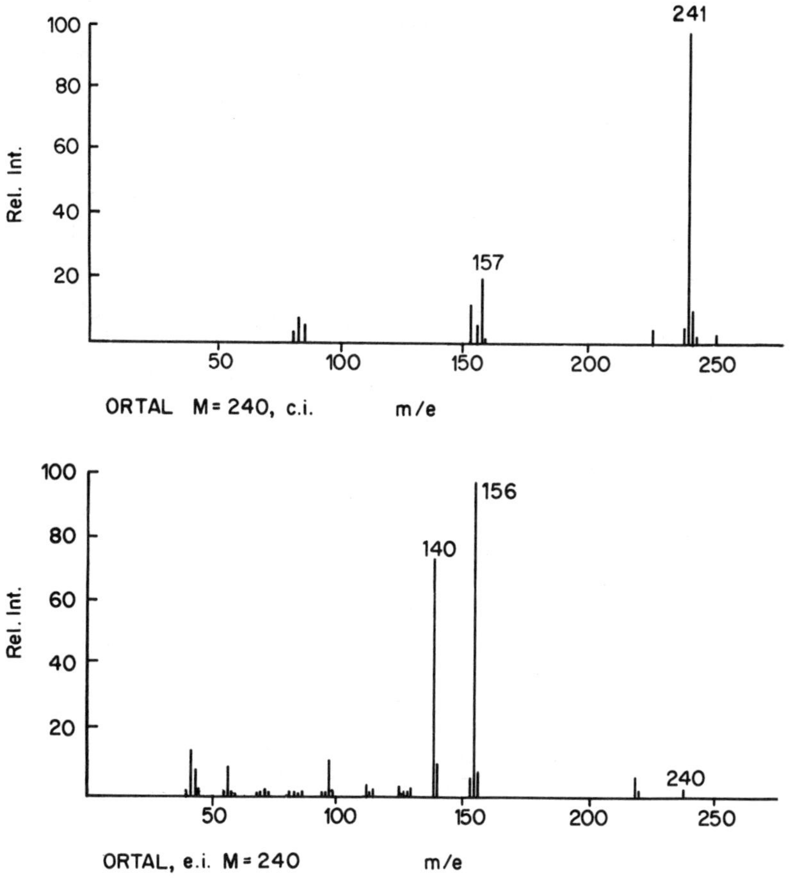

Figure 8 Electron-impact (c.i.) and chemical-ionization (c.i.) mass spectra of *Ortal* [reproduced with permission, Fales *et al* (1970)]

MH^+ ions. Those steroids with 3-keto functions appear to form $(M + C_2H_5)^+$ ions. Horning and Horning (1972) studied the trimethylsilyl derivatives of androsterone methyl oxime, dehydroepiandrosterone methyl oxime and pregnanediol and found significant fragmentation involving loss of trimethylsilanol, and additionally methanol, from the methyl oxime derivatives. These authors also utilized c.i. mass spectrometry for an investigation of phenobarbitone metabolism, using a g.c.–m.s. system with methane as the carrier gas. They looked for MH^+ ions which would be derived from the methylated derivatives of *p*-methoxyphenobarbitone, *m*-methoxyphenobarbitone and 3,4-dimethoxyphenobarbitone. These derivatives would be formed from the corresponding hydroxy compounds by the methylation procedure used. Such ions were indeed detected, providing evidence that these compounds were formed as metabolites of phenobarbitone in the rat.

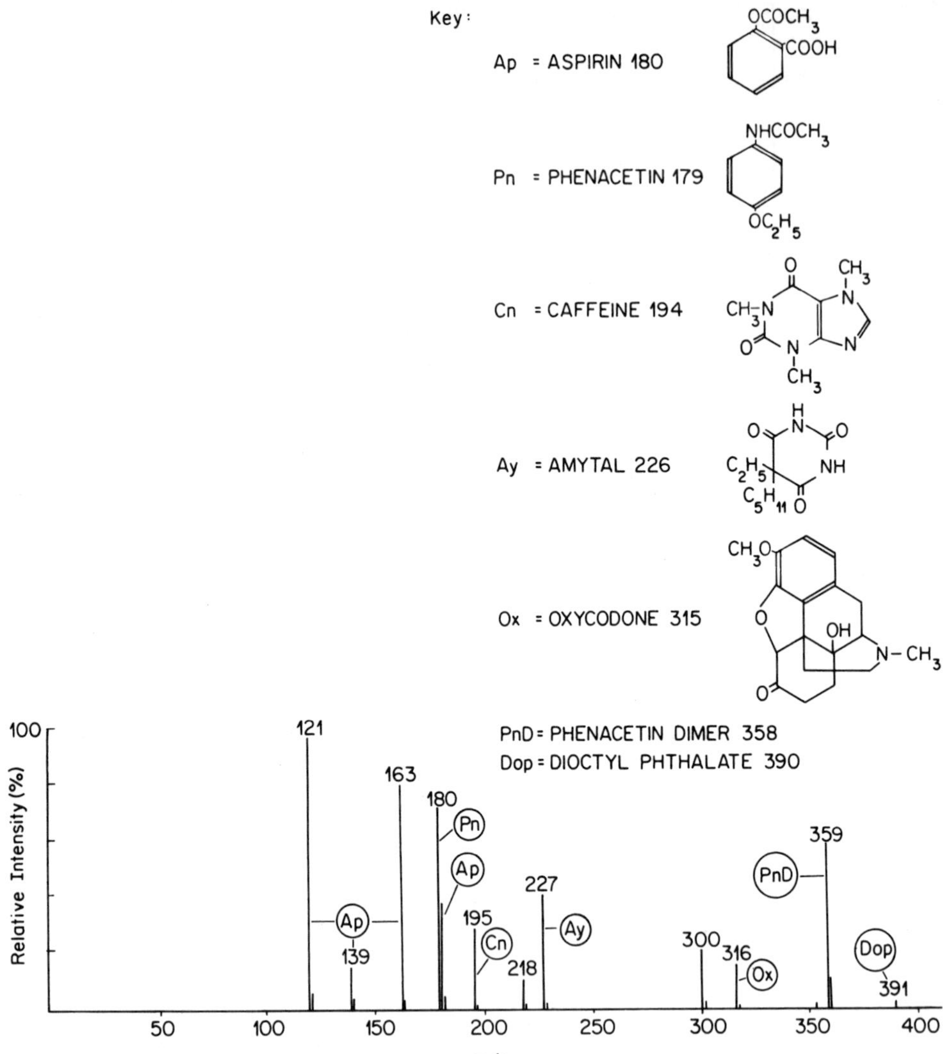

Figure 9 Isobutane chemical ionization mass spectrum of gastric contents in an overdose case [reproduced with permission, Milne *et al* (1971)]

E.i. and c.i. mass spectrometry was used in a study of the metabolism of the antiarrhythmic agent 2-[*o*-(3-dimethylaminopropyl)thio]phenyl-3-methyl urea (**37**) in the dog (Cohen *et al*, 1972). Although an N-desmethyl derivative was readily identified from its e.i. mass spectrum, the identification of **38**, **39** and **40**, was difficult due to the low intensity of their molecular ions. Thus **38** gave apparently the same molecular ion (m/e 267) as **37**, while **39** gave an ion (m/e 266) one mass unit lower, and **40** an ion (m/e 282) 15 mass units higher. This was due to the loss of oxygen from **38**, behaviour in the mass

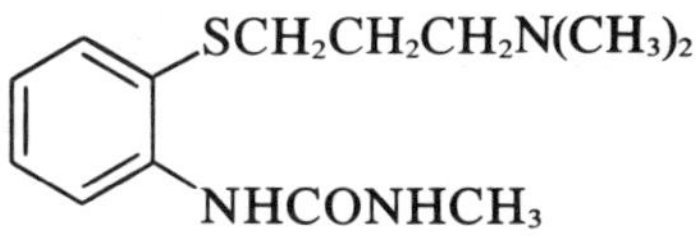

$SCH_2CH_2CH_2N(CH_3)_2$ / $NHCONHCH_3$
(37)

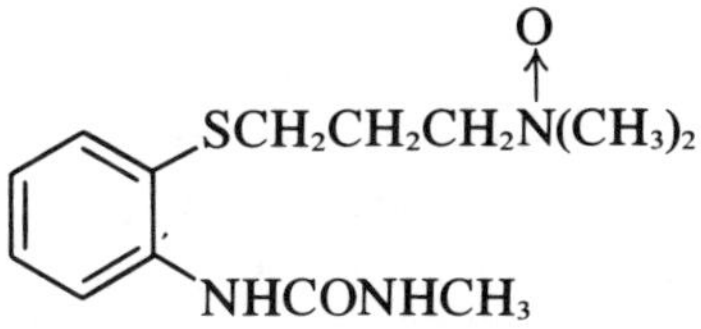

$SCH_2CH_2CH_2\overset{O}{\overset{\uparrow}{N}}(CH_3)_2$ / $NHCONHCH_3$
(38)

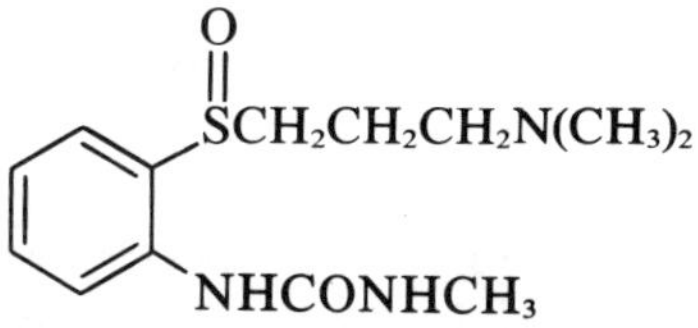

$\overset{O}{\overset{\|}{S}}CH_2CH_2CH_2N(CH_3)_2$ / $NHCONHCH_3$
(39)

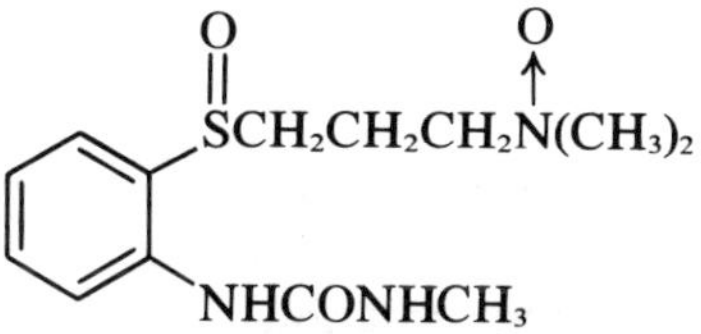

$\overset{O}{\overset{\|}{S}}CH_2CH_2CH_2\overset{O}{\overset{\uparrow}{N}}(CH_3)_2$ / $NHCONHCH_3$
(40)

spectrometer typical of N-oxides, while **39** and **40** lost OH·, behaviour typical of sulphoxides. The c.i. mass spectra of these metabolites (**38–40**) contained greatly enhanced high mass ions enabling better interpretation of the data. These structures were finally confirmed by n.m.r. spectroscopy.

A chemical-ionization mass spectrometer has also recently been used for experiments which involved linking a liquid chromatograph to a mass spectrometer (Baldwin and McLafferty, 1973). It was found possible to introduce 10 μl solutions in capillary tubes into the source via the direct inlet system. Under the source vacuum conditions the liquid sprayed out into the source. Solvents chosen on the basis of being good c.i. reagents included liquid ammonia, n-hexane, methanol and methanol–water mixtures. Using these approaches, a mass spectrum has been readily obtained from an underivatized tetrapeptide such as Ala.Ala.Ala.His.

Field Ionization and Field Desorption

Although the technique of field ionization (f.i.) has been known for a number of years (Block, 1968) and a number of applications to organic structural determination described (Beckey, 1969a), only recently with improvements in sensitivity have field ionization and field desorption been applied to biologically significant molecules.

The field ionization source consists of an anode, which may be a sharp blade, wire or point, and a cathode with a slit or hole, depending on the type of anode. A high voltage between the two electrodes provides an electric field approaching 2 volts/Å. Organic molecules introduced into such a field can lose an electron by the tunnelling processes to form positive ions which are accelerated out of the source through the hole in the cathode.

The crucial difference between the f.i. source and the electron-impact (e.i.) source is that in the former case no energy is transferred to the molecule under these conditions and residence times in the source are very much shorter than the 10^{-6} s common to e.i. sources. Those ions that are seen in f.i. spectra are formed extremely rapidly after field ionization near the tip or edge. The initial criticism of f.i., that it was very much less sensitive than e.i. mass spectrometry, has now been overcome by Beckey *et al* (1969) who treats the anodes with benzonitrile to sensitize them. It is possible to use f.i. in high resolution mass spectrometers with resolving powers up to 20,000 (Chait *et al*, 1969; Brunée *et al*, 1967). This means that the elemental composition of submicrogram quantities of organic compounds can now be obtained (Chait *et al*, 1968) whereas previously this was only possible for those compounds that gave molecular ions in their e.i. spectra.

An alternative to admitting samples in the vapour phase is to deposit the compound on the anode in solution (Beckey, 1969b). The spectra obtained by this method are known as field-desorption (f.d.) spectra. In the case of glucose, the f.d. spectra consisted of M^+ and MH^+ ions, while extensive dehydration was noticed in the corresponding f.i. spectra. Thus f.d. mass spectrometry seems to offer the most potential for simplifying mass spectra. It may be noted here that MH^+ ions are typical of both f.i. and f.d. mass spectra since ionization takes place in a highly concentrated layer of the organic compound.

At the present time there are few reports in the literature that f.i. or f.d. mass spectrometry has been used to study drugs or metabolites, due to the fact that not many laboratories possess mass spectrometers with f.i. sources. Such sources are being made available by a number of manufacturers and no doubt many workers in the field of drug metabolism will upgrade their instruments and incorporate these sources. There are several applications of f.i. to the study of carbohydrates and peptides which serve to show the potential that the technique will have in drug-metabolism studies, particularly for the identification and analysis of drug conjugates.

The behaviour of several groups of simple functionalized organic compounds under f.i. conditions has been described (Beckey *et al*, 1966; Robertson and Viney, 1966; Wanless and Glock, 1967). Damico and Barron (1971) investigated the g.c.–f.i.m.s. of a number of aldehydes, ketones and lactones, showing that some compounds were more sensitive than others to field ionization. Combined g.c.–f.i.m.s. has also been used in a study of natural coumarins (Games *et al*, 1974). In this group of compounds the molecular ions were the base peaks in the spectra.

In an f.i. study of cardenolides (Brown *et al*, 1970), digitoxin gave an intense molecular ion at m/e 764 with sequence ions corresponding to cleavage at each glycoside link with simultaneous hydrogen transfer. However, when cardenolides with sugars containing more free hydroxyl groups were examined, the high mass peaks of structural significance tended to be lost. In a later study of the aglycones (Brown *et al*, 1971), it was shown that digitoxigenin for example gave only three ions of note, M^+, $M^+–H_2O$ and a small $M^+–2H_2O$. This simple spectrum contrasts with the complex electron-impact spectrum as shown in figure 10.

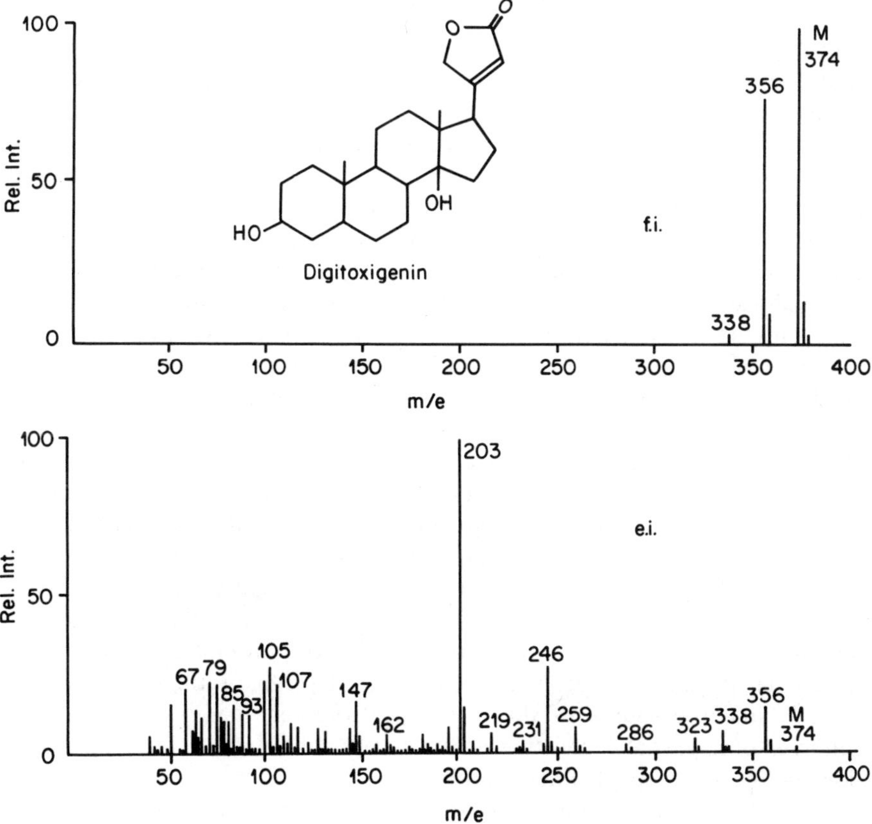

Figure 10 Field-ionization (f.i.) and electron-impact (e.i.) mass spectra of digitoxigenin [reproduced with permission, Brown *et al* (1971)]

More polar compounds such as strophanthidin tended to give more complex spectra with intense MH^+ ions

Other Methods of Ionization

A recent paper by Horning *et al* (1973) described the use of a mass spectrometer fitted with an external ionization source at atmospheric pressure. Compounds such as cocaine and methadone were introduced in a solvent, such as chloroform, to a source containing ^{63}Ni. By a complex series of ion–molecule collisions MH^+ ions were formed from these compounds. In the case of 2,6-dimethyl-γ-pyrone, for example, as little as 5 pg could be detected. Further developments have already improved the sensitivity of the system so that amounts of the order of 100 femtograms (0·1 picogram) can be detected. The availability of such a sensitive and specific detector means that the metabolism of drugs which are administered in the microgram range can readily be studied.

HIGH RESOLUTION MASS SPECTROMETRY

In order to analyse a complex mixture, it is necessary either to separate each component by extraction procedures, thin-layer chromatography or gas chromatography etc, or to measure some property unique to each component of interest, such as its ultra-violet absorption at a particular wavelength. A g.c.–m.s. system can utilize both of these principles, using the gas chromatograph to achieve a substantial separation, then monitoring m/e values which are chosen so as to be as unique as possible for each component. Without such prior gas-chromatographic separation, the integral m/e values obtained from a low-resolution mass spectrometer operating on a mixture are not sufficiently unique except in the simplest of cases. A urine sample, for example, run via a direct inlet on a mass spectrometer leads to a mass spectrum with a peak at virtually every mass unit up to about m/e 500.

However, the molecular and fragment ions derived from drugs have elemental compositions which are often different from those of naturally occurring components present in urine or plasma samples. This is particularly true if the drug either has large numbers of elements such as nitrogen or sulphur, or contains more unusual elements (in a biological sense) such as chlorine or fluorine. Since a high-resolution mass spectrometer can determine the elemental compositions of ions, it offers the possibility of monitoring mixtures directly (without prior extraction or chromatography) for ions which are diagnostic of drugs or metabolites. By evaporating such mixtures directly into the source of the mass spectrometer, it is often possible to achieve some partial separation of the components by differential evaporation off the mass-spectrometer probe.

Once the particular ion diagnostic of the drug or metabolite has been chosen, a quantitative estimation of the compound can proceed by evaporating known amounts from the direct inlet probe while integrating the response at the particular m/e value. This gives a calibration curve which can be used to determine that compound present in the biological mixture. Since the sensitivity and resolution of mass spectrometers can be traded against each other, the instrument should be operated at the lowest resolving power commensurate with separation from interfering ions (at the same nominal m/e value) produced by other substances.

This 'integrated ion current' technique was first utilized by Boulton and Majer (1970a, 1970b, 1971) in a study of *p*-tyramine (**41**) present in rat brain. The base peak in the mass spectrum of **41** occurs at m/e 108:

$$\left[HO-C_6H_4-CH_2CH_2NH_2\right]^{+\cdot} \longrightarrow \left[HO-C_6H_4-CH_3\right]^{+\cdot}$$

(**41**) m/e 137 m/e 108

Examination at high resolution of the *m/e* 108 region of the spectrum obtained from a rat-brain extract showed the presence of a doublet at *m/e* 108·0939 due to $C_8H_{12}^{+\cdot}$ and *m/e* 108·0575 due to $C_7H_8O^{+\cdot}$ from (**41**). The ion current at *m/e* 108·0575 was integrated during evaporation of the extract from the mass-spectrometer probe and the amount of *p*-tyramine inferred from a calibration curve previously obtained. Errors of only $\pm 5\%$ ($P = 0.95$) were obtained in the useful working range of 10^{-12} to 10^{-5} g.

However, such a method is subject to inaccuracies caused by changes in operating conditions in the mass spectrometer source between successive determinations. This can be overcome by the use of internal standards. Thus in a determination of diphenylhydantoin in rat brain at various times after dosage, phenyl *p*-tolylhydantoin was used as an internal standard and the respective molecular ions at *m/e* 252·0899 and 266·1055 integrated during sample evaporation (Millard *et al*, 1973c, 1973d).

In the case of urine samples monitored directly, many more interfering ions are present than in brain extracts, and in general higher resolving powers are necessary to remove the contribution which these make to the ion current at that mass value. Thus in figure 11 where a blank urine sample is compared with a urine sample obtained from a patient taking heptabarbitone (**42**), several ions are present at *m/e* 221 in addition to the ion

(42)

$C_{11}H_{13}N_2O_3^+$ at 221·0926 which is derived from **42** by loss of an ethyl radical. In order to quantify both **42** and its metabolites, 3-keto, 3-hydroxy- and 7-hydroxyheptabarbitone (Gilbert *et al*, 1974), 2-chlorophenothiazine was

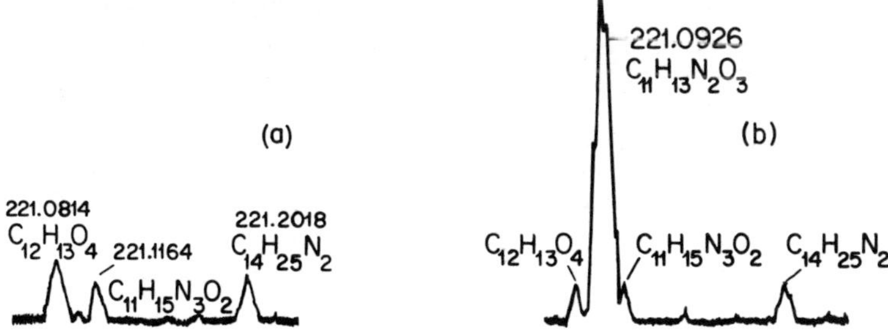

Figure 11 (a) *m/e* 221 region from the mass spectrum of a urine blank (10,000 resolving power). (b) *m/e* 221 region from the mass spectrum of urine from a patient taking heptabarbitone (Millard *et al*, 1973a)

added as internal standard (Millard *et al*, 1973a). The molecular ion from this ($C_{12}H_8NSCl^{+\cdot}$) and the $M{-}C_2H_5$($C_{11}H_{13}N_2O_3^{+}$) ion from **42** and its metabolites were monitored. After calibration it was possible to determine quantities down to 2 ng on the probe with a coefficient of variation of 4.6%.

Although the use of multiple-ion monitoring is to be preferred for drugs, such as barbiturates, which pass easily through gas-chromatographic columns, the high-resolution method holds promise for those drugs and metabolites which are relatively nonvolatile or are subject to thermal degradation. Thus Millard *et al* (1973b) have successfully used the method to monitor conjugated metabolites of piribedil.

The integrated ion-current technique can also be utilized for the quantification of compounds in tissue without prior extraction, as shown by Parker *et al* (1969, 1970) and Snedden and Parker (1971). These workers determined simultaneously hypoxanthine, xanthine, uric acid, allopurinol and oxipurinol in tissue by monitoring at high resolution, diagnostic ions produced from 5 mg quantities of desiccated tissue placed in the direct inlet system. Accuracies of ±20% were common at the 10–100 ppm level.

CONCLUSION

Mass spectrometry has followed closely the almost classical development of spectroscopic techniques in general. Once its potential for structural elucidation was recognized by a few early pioneers such as Beynon, Biemann, Djerassi and McLafferty, there followed a period of consolidation in which the guidelines to the subject were laid down. During this time, the mass spectra of tens of thousands of compounds were determined so that the relationship between structure and fragmentation could be elucidated. We are now well into the phase in which mass spectrometry is being used to solve problems, and the area of drug research is one of the major growth points at the present time.

Since instrument manufacturers have not been slow to recognize this fact, there is at present intense competition to sell mass spectrometers to the major pharmaceutical companies and the clinical pharmacology departments of hospitals. This competition has had the result that the cost of instruments of low resolving power has tended to remain fairly static or even fall slightly in real terms. Thus a typical low-resolution instrument equipped for g.c.–m.s. work would cost considerably less than £40,000. Paradoxically, the cost of high-resolution mass spectrometers has soared over the last few years, so that most of these cost in the region of £1000,000. Since some form of data-acquisition system is essential if the maximum information is to be obtained from such instruments, the total system cost is now approaching £120,000.

In a review such as this in which the state of the art at the present time has been outlined, the concluding paragraphs should attempt to predict as far as possible developments to be expected over the next few years. This is perhaps easiest in the case of instruments themselves. Improvement of instrumentation appears to lie in two directions. Firstly, attention will be paid to the design of sources, whether they are of the electron-impact, chemical-ionization or field-ionization type. At the moment sources are highly inefficient, with only a small proportion of the molecules entering them becoming ionized. Good design should increase the sensitivity of the modern source by at least a factor of ten, perhaps even more. Secondly, mass spectrometers will be made much easier to operate. To obtain high-quality spectra is still an art, highly dependent on the skill of the operator. Improvements here may take place through the use of magnetic or punched cards which will automatically set up such functions as source temperature, scan speed, multiplier gain and electron-beam energy to predetermined values. Since more and more mass spectrometers will be sold complete with data systems, it is to be expected that operating parameters will be entirely controlled from the teletype keyboard.

It is less easy to predict how applications of mass spectrometry to drug research will develop in the future. Although the more important developments at the present time have been discussed fully in this chapter, some of these may peter out and be superseded by others. Thus, although the techniques of field desorption and field ionization have been shown to yield valuable results, it may well be that they will not be suitable for routine use where a large throughput of compounds is desired, due to difficulties in maintaining maximum sensitivity. Chemical ionization may become the front runner in alternative ionization techniques because of the ease of incorporating gas chromatography. Capillary columns may find increasing use, since molecular separators, with their problems of adsorption of polar compounds and variable efficiency, are then not needed. This may be one method of improving the overall sensitivity of g.c.–m.s. systems.

Increasing the sensitivity of mass spectrometers will have the effect of improving the accuracy of quantification of drugs and metabolites at the levels discussed in this review. It will also mean that minor metabolites at present quite inaccessible by any technique will become amenable to mass-spectrometric investigation.

Whatever happens, mass spectrometry has been anything but a static subject over the last ten years, and will not become so over the next decade. The contents of a chapter written five years hence on 'New developments in the mass spectrometry of drugs and metabolites' will be very different from this one.

REFERENCES

Abrahamsson, S. (1967), *Science Tools*, **14**, 29.

Agurell, S., Gustafsson, B., Holmstedt, B., Leander, K., Lingren, J.-E., Nilsson, I., Sandberg, F. and Asberg, M. (1973), *J. Pharm. Pharmacol.*, **25**, 554.

Axen, U., Green, K., Hörlin, D. and Samuelsson, B. (1971), *Biochem. Biophys. Res. Commun.*, **45**, 519.

Baczynskyj, L., Duchamp, D. J., Zieserl, J. F. and Axen, U. (1973), *Anal. Chem.*, **45**, 479.
Baldwin, M. A. and McLafferty, F. W. (1973), *Org. Mass Spectrom.*, **9**, 1111.
Beckey, H. D. (1969a), *Angew. Chem. Int. Edn.*, **8**, 623.
Beckey, H. D. (1969b), *Int. J. Mass Spectrom. Ion Phys.*, **2**, 500.
Beckey, H. D., Knöppel, H., Metzinger, G. and Schultze, P. (1966), *Adv. Mass Spectrom.*, **3**, 35.
Beckey, H. D., Krone, H. and Roelgen, F. W. (1969), *Int. J. Mass Spectrom. Ion Phys.*, **3**, 167.
Bertilsson, L. and Palmer, L. (1972), *Science*, **177**, 74.
Bertilsson, L., Atkinson, jr., A. J., Altheus, J. R., Hartast, A., Lingren, J.-E. and Holmstedt, B. (1972), *Anal. Chem.*, **44**, 1434.
Beynon, J. H. (1960), *Mass spectrometry and its application to organic chemistry*, Elsevier, Amsterdam.
Biemann, K. (1962), *Mass spectrometry, applications to organic chemistry*, McGraw-Hill, New York.
Block, J. (1968), in Kendrick, E., (ed.) *Advances in mass spectrometry*, Institute of Petroleum, London.
Boulton, A. A. and Majer, J. R. (1970a), *J. Chromatogr.*, **48**, 322.
Boulton, A. A. and Majer, J. R. (1970b), *Nature*, **225**, 658.
Boulton, A. A. and Majer, J. R. (1971), *Can. J. Biochem.*, **49**, 993.
Bower, H. C., Clayton, E., Shields, D. J. and Stanier, H. M. (1968), *Adv. Mass Spectrom.*, **4**, 257.
Brandenberger, H. and Schnyder, D. (1972), *Z. Anal. Chem.*, **259**, 210.
Braselton, W. E., Orr, J. C. and Engel L. C. (1973), *Anal. Biochem.*, **53**, 64.
Brown, P., Bruschweiler, F., Pettit, G. R. and Reichstein T. (1970), *J. Amer. Chem. Soc.*, **92**, 4470.
Brown, P., Bruschweiler, F., Pettit, G. R. and Reichstein T. (1971), *Org. Mass Spectrom.*, **5**, 573.
Brunée, C., Kappus, G. and Mauser, K. H. (1967), *Z. Anal. Chem.*, **232**, 17.
Burlingame, A. L., Smith, D. H. and Olsen, R. W. (1968), *Anal. Chem.*, **40**, 13.
Burlingame, A. L. and Johanson, G. A. (1972), *Anal. Chem.*, **44**, 337R.
Budzikiewicz, H., Djerassi, C. and Williams D. H. (1964a), *Interpretation of mass spectra of organic compounds*, Holden–Day, San Francisco.
Budzikiewicz, H., Djerassi, C. and Williams, D. H. (1964b), *Structure elucidation of natural products by mass spectrometry*, part 1, Holden–Day, San Francisco.
Budzikiewicz, H., Djerassi, C. and Williams D. H. (1964c), *Structure elucidation of natural products by mass spectrometry*, part 2, Holden–Day, San Francisco.
Budzikiewicz, H., Djerassi, C. and Williams D. H. (1967), *Mass spectrometry of organic compounds*, Holden–Day, San Francisco.
Castagnoli, N. and Frigerio, A. (1974), *Proceedings of the International Symposium on Mass Spectrometry in Biochemistry and Medicine, Milan*, Raven Press, New York.
Chait, E. M., Shannon, T. W., Amy, J. W. and McLafferty, F. W. (1968), *Anal. Chem.*, **40**, 835.
Chait, E. M., Shannon, T. W., Perry, W. O., van Lear, G. E. and McLafferty, F. W. (1969), *Int. J. Mass Spectrom. Ion Phys.*, **2**, 141.
Cohen, A. I., Dreyfuss, J. and Fales, H. M. (1972), *J. Med. Chem.*, **15**, 542.
Costapanagiotis, A. and Budzikiewicz, H. (1965), *Monatsh. Chem.*, **91**, 1900.
Coutts, R. T. and Locock, R. A. (1968), *J. Pharm. Sci.*, **57**, 2096.
Crawford, L. R. and Morrison, J. D. (1968), *Anal. Chem.*, **40**, 1469.
Damico, J. N. and Barron P. P. (1971), *Anal. Chem.*, **43**, 17.
Desiderio, D. M. and Hägele K. (1971), *Chem. Commun.*, 1074.
Dorsey, J. A., Hunt, R. H. and O'Neal M. J. (1963), *Anal. Chem.*, **35**, 511.

Draffan, G. H., Clare, R. A. and Williams, F. M. (1973), *J. Chromatogr.*, **75**, 45.

Ebbighausen, W. O. R., Mowat, P. and Vestergaard. P. (1973), *J. Pharm. Sci.*, **62**, 146.

Eidenoff, M. C., Peri, G. C., Knoll, J. E., Marano, B. J. and Arnheim, J. (1953), *J. Amer. Chem. Soc.*, **75**, 248.

Fales, H. M., Milne, G. W. A. and Axenrod T. (1970), *Anal. Chem.*, **42**, 1432.

Field, F. H. (1968), *Accounts Chem. Res.* **1**, 42.

Foster, A. B. (1969), *Lab. Practice*, **18**, 743.

Frigerio, A. (1972), *Proceedings of the International Symposium on Gas Chromatography–Mass Spectrometry*, Tamburini Editore, Milan.

Frigerio, A., Fanelli, R. and Danieli, B. (1972a), *Chem. Ind.*, 769.

Frigerio, A., Belvedere, G., De Nadai, F., Fanelli, C., Pantarotto, C., Riva, F. and Morselli, L. (1972b), *J. Chromatogr.*, **54**, 201.

Gaffney, T. E., Hammar, C.-G., Holmstedt, B. and McMahon, R. E. (1971), *Anal. Chem.*, **43**, 307.

Games, D. E., Jackson, A. H., Millington, D. S. and Rossiter M. (1974), *Biomed. Mass Spectrom.*, **1**, 7.

Gilbert, J. N. T., Millard, B. J., Powell, J. W. and Whalley, W. B. (1974), *J. Pharm. Pharmacol*, **26**, 123.

Gordon, A. E. and Frigerio, A. (1972), *J. Chromatogr.*, **73**, 401.

Green, D. E. and Hertel, R. H. (1973), *Symposium on Analytical Advances in Clinical and Medicinal Chemistry*, American Chemical Society, Chicago.

Grützmacher, H.-F. and Arnold, W. (1966), *Tetrahedron Lett.*, 1365.

Hammar, C.-G. (1970), in Bacq, Z. M., (ed.), *Fundamentals of biochemical pharmacology*, Pergamon, Oxford.

Hammar, C.-G. (1971), *Acta Pharm. Suec.*, **8**, 129.

Hammar, C.-G. and Hessling, R. (1971), *Anal. Chem.*, **44**, 490.

Hammar, C.-G., Holmstedt, B. and Ryhage, R. (1968), *Anal. Biochem.*, **25**, 532.

Hammar, C.-G., Holmstedt, B., Lingren, J.-E. and Tham, R. (1969), in Garattini, S., Goldin, A., Hawking, F. and Kopin, I. J. (ed.), *Advances in pharmacology and chemotherapy*, vol. 7, pp. 53–89, Academic Press, New York and London.

Hammar, C.-G., Alexandersson, B., Holmstedt, B. and Sjoqvist, I. (1971), *Clin. Pharmacol. Ther.*, **12**, 496.

Heins, J. T., Maarse, H., de Brauw, M. C. T. N. and Weurmann C. (1966), *J. Gas Chromatogr.*, **4**, 395.

Heller, S. R. (1972), *Anal. Chem.*, **44**, 1951.

Heller, S. R., Fales, H. M. and Milne, G. W. A. (1973), *Org. Mass Spectrom.*, **7**, 107.

Henneberg, D. (1959), *Z. Anal. Chem.*, **170**, 365.

Henneberg, D. (1961), *Z. Anal. Chem.*, **183**, 12.

Hevesy, G. (1923), *Biochem. J.*, **17**, 439.

Hill, H. C. (1966), *Introduction to mass spectrometry*, Heyden and Son, London.

Hites, R. A. and Biemann, K. (1967), *Adv. Mass Spectrom.*, **4**, 37.

Hites, R. A. and Biemann, K. (1970), *Anal. Chem.*, **42**, 855.

Holland, J. F., Sweeley, C. C., Thrush, R. E., Teets, R. E. and Beiber, M. A. (1973), *Anal. Chem.*, **45**, 308.

Horning, E. C. and Horning, M. G. (1972), *International symposium on gas chromatography–mass spectrometry*, Elba.

Horning, E. C., Horning, M. G., Carroll, D. I., Dzidic, I. and Stillwell, R. N. (1973), *Anal. Chem.*, **45**, 936.

Hunt, D. F. and Ryan J. F. (1972), *Anal. Chem.*, **44**, 1306.

Jenden, D. J. and Cho A. K. (1973), *Ann. Rev. Pharmacol.*, **13**, 371.

Jerina, D. M., Daly, J. W., Witkop, B., Zaltzmann-Nirenberg, P. and Udenfriend, S. (1968), *J. Amer. Chem. Soc.*, **90**, 6525.

Johnstone, R. A. W. (1972), *Mass spectrometry for organic chemists*, Cambridge University Press, London.

Kellermeyer, R. W. and Ward, H. G. (1962), *Biochemistry*, **1**, 1124.
Kelly, R. W. (1971), *J. Chromatogr.*, **54**, 345.
Klein, P. D., Haumann, J. R. and Eisler, W. J. (1972), *Anal. Chem.*, **44**, 490.
Knapp, D. R. and Gaffney, T. E. (1972), *Clin. Pharmacol. Ther.*, **13**, 307.
Knapp, D. R., Gaffney, T. E. and McMahon, R. E. (1972a), *Biochem. Pharmacol.*, **21**, 425.
Knapp, D. R., Gaffney, T. E. and McMahon, R. E. (1972b), *J. Pharmacol. Exp. Ther.*, **180**, 784.
Knight, J. B. (1971), *Finnigan Spectra*, **1**, No. 1.
Knock, B. A., Smith, I. C., Wright, D. E., Ridley, R. G. and Kelly, W. (1970), *Anal. Chem.*, **42**, 1516.
Koslow, S. H., Cattabeni, F. and Costa, E. (1972), *Science*, **176**, 177.
Lee, M. G. and Millard, B. J. (1973), unpublished work.
Lipsky, S. R., Horvath, C. G. and Murray, W. J. (1966), *Anal. Chem.*, **38**, 1585.
Llewellyn, P. M. and Littlejohn, D. (1968), *Conference on Analytical and Applied Spectroscopy*, Pittsburgh.
Maynert, E. W. and van Dyke, H. B. (1950a), *J. Pharmacol. Exp. Ther.*, **98**, 174.
Maynert, E. W. and van Dyke, H. B. (1950b), *J. Pharmacol. Exp. Ther.*, **98**, 180.
Maynert, E. W. and van Dyke, H. B. (1950c), *J. Pharmacol. Exp. Ther.*, **98**, 184.
McFadden, W. H., Teranishi, R., Black, D. R. and Day, J. C. (1963), *J. Food Sci.*, **28**, 316.
McLafferty, F. W. (1967), *Interpretation of mass spectra*, Benjamin, New York.
McMurray, W. J., Green, B. N. and Lipsky S. R. (1966), *Anal. Chem.*, **38**, 1194.
Michnowicz, J. and Munson B. (1972), *Org. Mass Spectrom.*, **6**, 765.
Middleditch, B. S. and Desiderio D. M. (1973), *Anal. Chem.*, **45**, 806.
Mikes, F., Hofmann, A. and Waser, P. G. (1971), *Biochem. Pharmacol.*, **20**, 2469.
Millard, B. J. (1971), in Simmonds, A. B. and Harper, N. J. (ed.), *Advances in drug research*, vol. 6, pp. 157–231, Academic Press, London and New York.
Millard, B. J., Lee, M. G. and Haskins, N. J. (1973a), *6th International Symposium on Mass Spectrometry*, Edinburgh.
Millard, B. J., Campbell, D. B., Jenner, P. and Taylor, A. R. (1973b), *International Symposium on Mass Spectrometry in Biochemistry and Medicine*, Milan.
Millard, B. J., Lascelles, P., Goldberg, V. and Tickner, T. (1973c), *Hensberger Centenary Symposium on Epilepsy*, Edinburgh.
Millard, B. J., Lascelles, P., Goldberg, V. and Tickner, T. (1973d), *4th International Meeting of the Society of Neurochemistry*, Tokyo.
Milne, G. W. A. (1971), *Mass spectrometry. Techniques and applications*, Wiley, New York.
Milne, G. W. A., Fales, H. M. and Axenrod, T. (1971), *Anal. Chem.*, **43**, 1815.
Mitscher, L. A. and Showalter, H. D. H. (1972), *Chem. Commun.*, 796.
Morfin, R. F., Lear, I., Ofner, P. and Orr, J. C. (1970), *Fed. Proc.*, **29**, 247.
Munson, M. S. B. (1971), *Anal. Chem.*, **43**, 28R.
Munson, M. S. B. and Field, F. H. (1966), *J. Amer. Chem. Soc.*, **88**, 2621.
Narasimhachari, N. and Vouros, P. (1972), *Anal. Biochem.*, **45**, 154.
Parker, R. B., Snedden, W. and Watts, R. W. E. (1969), *Biochem. J.*, **115**, 103.
Parker, R. B., Snedden, W. and Watts, R. W. E. (1970), *Biochem. J.*, **116**, 317.
Petersson, B. and Ryhage, R. (1967), *Arkiv. Kemi*, **26**, 293.
Pomerantz, S. H. and Ward, H. G. (1958), *J. Biol. Chem.*, **231**, 514.
Popjak, G., Cornforth, J. W., Cornforth, R. H., Ryhage, R. and Goodman, D. S. (1962), *J. Biol. Chem.*, **237**, 56.
Prox, A., Zimmer, A. and Machleidt, H. (1973), *Xenobiotica*, **3**, 103.
Reed, R. I. (1966), *Applications of mass spectrometry to organic chemistry*, Academic Press, London and New York.
Reed, R. I. (1968), *Modern aspects of mass spectrometry*, Plenum Press, New York.

Robertson, A. J. B. and Viney, B. W. (1966), *J. Chem. Soc. (A)*, 1843.
Ryhage, R. (1964), *Anal. Chem.*, **36**, 759.
Samuelsson, B., Hamberg, M. and Sweeley, C. C. (1970), *Anal. Biochem.*, **38**, 301.
Schomberg, G. and Henneberg, D. (1968), *Chromatographia*, **1**, 23.
Shemin, D. M. and Henbergh, D. R. (1946), *J. Biol. Chem.*, **166**, 627.
Snedden, W. and Parker, R. B. (1971), *Anal. Chem.*, **43**, 1651.
Spiteller, G. (1966), *Massenspektrometrische Strukturanalyse organischer Verbindungen: ein Einführung*, Verlag Chemie, Heidelberg.
Stallberg-Stenhagen, S. and Stenhagen, E. (1970), *Adv. Anal. Chem. Instrum.*, **8**, 167.
Stenhagen, E. (1966), *Chimia*, **20**, 346.
Strong, J. M. and Atkinson, A. J. (1972), *Anal. Chem.*, **44**, 2287.
Sweeley, C. C., Elliot, W. H., Fries, I. and Ryhage, R. (1966), *Anal. Chem.*, **38**, 1549.
Talroze, V. C., Raznikov, V. V. and Tantsyrev, G. D. (1964), *Dokl. Akad. Nauk SSSR*, **159**, 182.
van Heijenoort, J., Bricas, E., Das, B. C., Lederer, E. and Wolstenholme, W. A. (1967), *Tetrahedron*, **23**, 3403.
van Lear, G. E. and McLafferty, F. W. (1969), *Ann. Rev. Biochem.*, **38**, 289.
Venkataraghavan, R., McLafferty, F. W. and van Lear, G. E. (1969), *Org. Mass Spectrom.*, **2**, 1.
Vore, M., Gerber, N. and Bush, M. T. (1971), *Pharmacologist*, **13**, 220.
Vree, T. B., Gorgels, J. P. M. C., Muskens, A. Th. J. M. and van Rossum, J. M. (1971), *Clin. Chim. Acta*, **34**, 333.
Walle, T., Ishizaki, T. and Gaffney, T. E. (1972), *J. Pharmacol. Exp. Ther.*, **183**, 508.
Waller, G. R. (1972), *Biochemical applications of mass spectrometry*, Wiley, New York.
Waller, G. R., Sastry, S. D. and Kinneberg, K. (1969), *J. Chromatogr.*, **7**, 577.
Wanless, G. G. and Glock, G. A. (1967), *Anal. Chem.*, **39**, 2.
Watson, J. T. and Biemann, K. (1964), *Anal. Chem.*, **36**, 1135.
Williams, D. H. and Howe, I. (1972), *Principles of organic mass spectrometry*, McGraw-Hill, London and New York.
Zimmer, A., Prox, A., Pelzer, H. and Hankwitz, R. (1973), *Biochem. Pharmacol.*, **22**, 2213.

CHAPTER 2

Bioactivation and cytotoxicity

T. A. Connors

INTRODUCTION

Where a chemotherapeutic agent is acting on a pathway which is essential to the target cell but not vital to host cells, there is usually no advantage in the administration of an inert agent which can be metabolized *in vivo* to the active form. Sulphonamides with antifolate activity *per se* have good antibacterial properties and high therapeutic indices, and no advantage is gained by the use of, for example, diazo derivatives which must be activated *in vivo* by reduction.

However, many chemicals have useful pharmacological properties but do not have the same high selectivity as the antibacterial antibiotics, with the result that their use is often associated with unwanted effects on other tissues. In this situation a pharmacologically inactive precursor may be used which, by being activated *in vivo*, may well have a higher therapeutic index if the activation process takes place predominantly in the target cells.

The cytotoxic agents were developed initially for the treatment of cancer but many are now used in the treatment of nonlethal infections such as psoriasis, as immunosuppressants, as epilating agents and as laboratory tools to study the mechanisms of carcinogenesis, mutagenesis and teratogenesis. These agents have a broad range of biological activities, and it is obvious they can affect many types of cell. This is a great disadvantage when they are used as anticancer agents since it means that they will have many side effects, and that the margin between complete tumour-cell eradication and unacceptable toxicity will be small. Patients with certain types of cancer may be cured with these agents but the treatment is intensive using many different drugs in combination, and the side effects (although usually reversible) are serious. The use of inert and nontoxic derivatives of these agents, which can be activated *in vivo* is a major approach in the attempts to obtain more selective compounds.

Studies on the mechanism of action of the dozen or so different classes of chemicals with cytotoxic properties have shown that they act mainly on *de novo* purine and pyrimidine biosynthesis, as antifolates, as inhibitors of DNA replication and transcription and as inhibitors of RNA and protein synthesis. With the exception of asparaginase, which kills cells unable to synthesize asparagine and which is effective in the treatment of the few cancers that lack the synthetase enzyme, cytotoxic agents have no basic selectivity for cancer cells. The biochemical pathways they inhibit are as essential for nonmalignant cells as for cancer cells. Cells in cycle are less able to recover from specific inhibition of one pathway of nucleic acid or protein synthesis, and they are more susceptible to cytotoxic agents than nonproliferating cells. Thus the administration of cytotoxic agents is characterized by effects on certain tissues including bone marrow, lymphocytes, mucosal surfaces, hair-forming cells and testicular and ovarian tissues. As anticancer agents, their best effects are against rapidly growing tumours, but even in these cases treatment may have to be stopped because of side effects, before every cancer cell has been destroyed.

This is not surprising since some normal tissues consist of cells which are dividing more rapidly than the fastest growing cancers. Nevertheless, highly selective antitumour effects can be occasionally obtained and this can sometimes be due to either an activation of the cytotoxic agent in the malignant tissue or conversely to a detoxication in normal sensitive cells. In both cases the cytotoxic action of the drug is more pronounced in the tumour and some selectivity occurs. Until such time as qualitative differences in biochemical pathways are found between normal and cancer cells, it is probable that the main way in which greater selectivity will be achieved is by designing cytotoxic agents which can be activated or deactivated *in vivo*, such that there is a greater cytotoxic reaction in the malignant cell.

ALKYLATING AGENTS

The chemical reactivity of alkylating agents of the nitrogen-mustard type is dependent on the basicity of the nitrogen atom (Ross, 1962). This basicity is influenced by the presence of electron-attracting or releasing groups in the rest of the molecule, and examples are known of nitrogen mustards that react within seconds of being dissolved in a polar medium and of others that only react over a period of days or even weeks. There is, in general, a good correlation between alkylating activity and cytotoxicity (Ross, 1962; Bardos *et al*, 1969). Table 1 shows that in a series of closely related nitrogen mustards, as the basicity of the nitrogen is increased (by addition of

Table 1 Relationship between alkylating activity and toxicity of a series of closely related agents. As the basicity of the nitrogen is increased so is the alkylating activity, and the LD_{50} falls (data from Bardos *et al*, 1969)

Compound	Alkylating activity ($K'_{80} \times 10^3$)	Toxicity (LD_{50}, μmole/kg)
$C_6H_5-N(CH_3)(CH_2CH_2Cl)$	4·9	3000
$HOOC-C_6H_4-N(CH_2CH_2Cl)_2$	4·6	915
$C_6H_5-N(CH_2CH_2Cl)_2$	13·0	367
$HO-C_6H_4-N(CH_2CH_2Cl)_2$	48·6	74
$C_6H_5-N(CH_2CH_2Br)_2$	123·0	39

electron-releasing groups or removal of electron-attracting ones) so the alkylating activity increases and the compounds become more toxic. The correlation does not always hold since toxicity may also depend on the distribution and rate of excretion of the drug and whether or not it is metabolized, but in general the more chemically reactive an alkylating agent, the more toxic it is likely to be *in vivo*.

This property of nitrogen mustards makes them ideal for the preparation of cytotoxic agents to be activated *in vivo*. The general approach is to design a nitrogen mustard inactivated by electron-attracting groups, but which can be converted enzymically (e.g. by hydrolysis or by reduction) into a chemically reactive agent. Chemicals which are selectively transformed in tumour cells might be expected to be useful antitumour agents. Obviously, good selectivity would only be obtained if the activating enzymes were present in the malignant cell at much higher concentrations than in other normal tissues. A further useful property would be if the metabolite formed in the tumour had only a very short half-life so that the majority of the cytotoxic alkylation took place in the cell with little of the active material being allowed to diffuse into the general circulation.

Activation by Reduction

While many ingenious 'latent' nitrogen mustards have been synthesized, they have often not had the desired selective antitumour properties. Measurement of the concentrations of activating enzymes in tumour and normal tissues were not usually made, and the compounds may therefore have been tested under disadvantageous conditions where the tumour selected as the test model had a low level of the appropriate enzymes compared to normal tissues, especially liver. One of the earlier examples of this approach was the azo-mustard CB 1414 (**1**), which was designed to be selectively reduced by tumours to the *para*-amino derivative (**2**) (Ross and Warwick, 1955; Ross, 1962). The former (**1**) is an unreactive alkylating agent

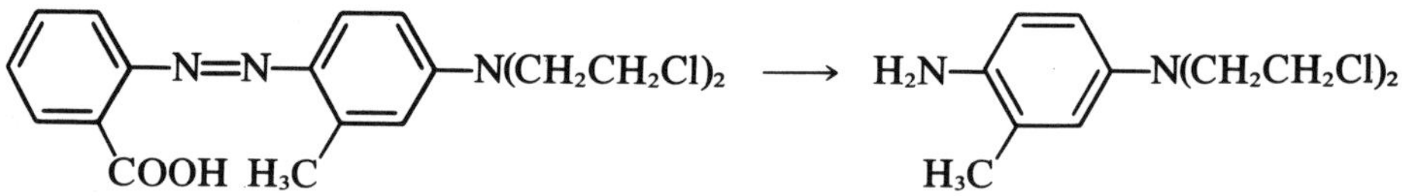

—N=N— —$N(CH_2CH_2Cl)_2$ ⟶ H_2N— —$N(CH_2CH_2Cl)_2$

COOH H_3C H_3C

(**1**) (**2**)

because of the electron-attracting properties of the conjugated ring system while the latter (**2**) is extremely reactive and toxic. Although CB 1414 (**1**) has had a limited clinical trial (Israels and Ritzmann, 1960), there was no evidence that it was any better than other alkylating agents in use at that time, as might have been expected had there been a greater activation in the malignant cells. The tumour used in animal tests was the Walker 256 carcinoma, and no measurements were made of the level of azo-reductase enzymes in this tumour. Subsequent measurements (Connors *et al*, 1973a) have shown that the compound would not be expected to be particularly selective against the Walker tumour where azo-reductase concentration is only one fifth the concentration in the liver and less than in other tissues. Because of the high level of activating enzyme in the liver, most of the agent would be biotransformed to the amine during its passage through the liver, and therefore no selective accumulation of the active metabolite in the tumour would occur.

A related approach has been described by Tsou and Su (1963). Based on the observation that Ehrlich ascites cells could reduce tetrazolium salts to formazans and further (Siegert *et al*, 1951), they prepared a series of nitrogen mustards which, as tetrazolium derivatives such as **3**, would be quite inactive because of the conjugated ring system. On reduction to the formazan (**4**), the reactivity of the alkylating moieties would be increased and further reduction to the amine (**5**) would result in a highly reactive and very toxic compound.

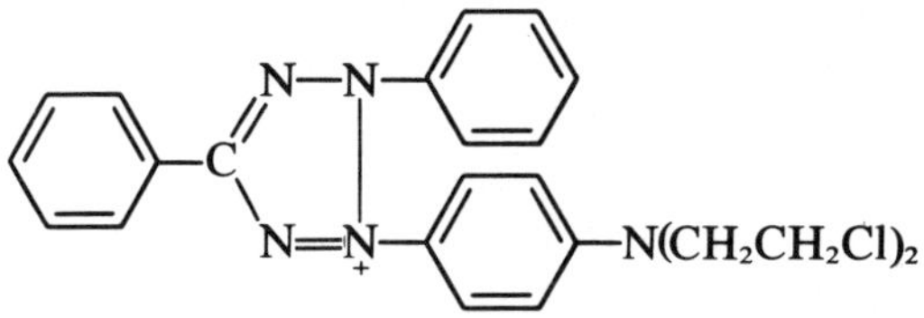

(3)

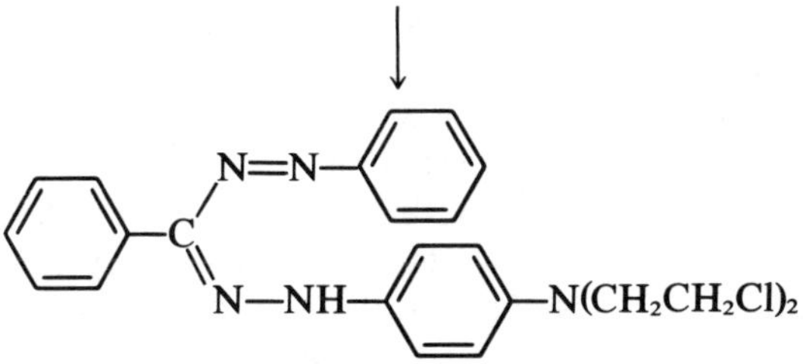

↓

(4)

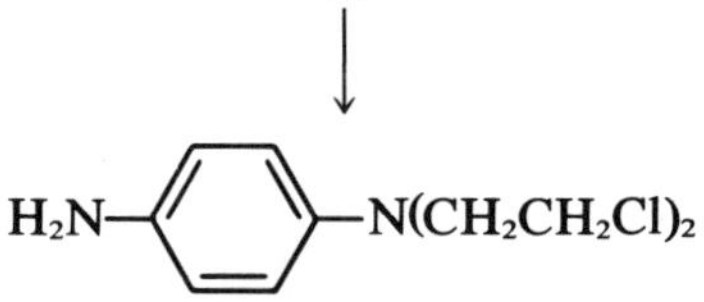

↓

(5)

Once again selectivity of antitumour action is dependent on the reducing ability of the tumour compared to normal tissues. Although Tsou and Su (1963) refer to the high dehydrogenase activity of uterine carcinoma and other types of cancer and to the ability of Ehrlich ascites cells to reduce tetrazolium salts, the actual nitrogen mustard derivatives were only shown to be reduced by kidney and liver succinic dehydrogenase preparations. The tumours used in the screening tests were not assayed for their ability to reduce the tetrazolium mustards so it is possible that these agents may still be useful if employed in the treatment of cancers which are known to be efficient in the reduction of the administered agent.

A recent adaptation of the early work on azo-benzene derivatives activated by reductases has led to the synthesis of agents specifically designed for the treatment of primary hepatocytic cancer of the liver (Bukhari *et al*, 1973). Following the initial observation of Warwick (1972) that hepatocellular carcinoma in man had azo-reductase levels almost as high as normal hepatocytes, a series of agents was designed to be activated by this enzyme. A modification of the early approach was to prepare a compound which would on reduction produce an alkylating agent of extremely short half-life, thus confining cytotoxic alkylations to liver cells. Theoretically, such an agent should be highly selective since, from past experience with nitrogen mustards in the treatment of cancer, it is known that little damage is caused to liver, presumably because of its low mitotic index. An azo-benzene given orally might be completely activated on its first passage through the liver. Because of the short half-life of the metabolite, only normal and malignant liver cells would be alkylated. The latter, which are rapidly dividing, might be highly sensitive to alkylation, while the former are known to be resistant. Even if the active metabolite escaped from the liver, since its half-life is short, it would be hydrolysed to nontoxic products before reaching the bone marrow which is easily damaged by alkylation. Table 2 shows some of the derivatives that were studied for their ability to be rapidly reduced by rat-liver azo-reductase. Confirming the earlier results of Ross and Warwick (1955) and Ross (1962), it was shown that substitution on the aromatic ring *ortho* to the azo linkage greatly increased the rate of reduction of the azo group. In particular, a carboxyl group in the *ortho* position increased the rate of reduction by more than a thousandfold. The rate could be further increased by attachment of a methyl group to the *ortho* position in the other ring. These substitutions probably increase reducibility by making the azo linkage more available to the active site of the reductase enzyme.

It was also necessary that the metabolite formed on reduction should be

Table 2 Rate of reduction of some azo-benzene mustards by rat liver 9000 g supernatant. Compounds which are not reduced are nontoxic since no alkylating products are formed. M = —$N(CH_2CH_2Br)_2$ (data from Connors *et al*, 1973a)

Compound	LD_{50} (mg/kg)	Metabolism (nmol/g/15′)
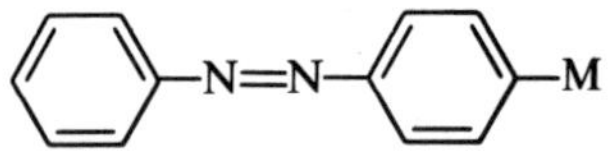 C_6H_5—N=N—C_6H_4—M	951	0
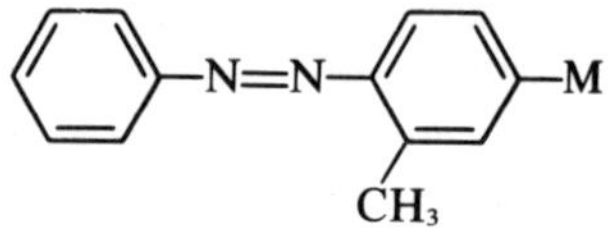 C_6H_5—N=N—$C_6H_3(CH_3)$—M	1600	0
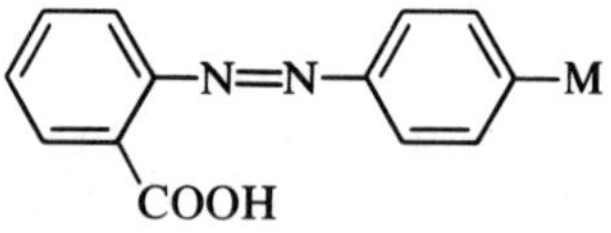 $C_6H_4(COOH)$—N=N—C_6H_4—M	57	1350
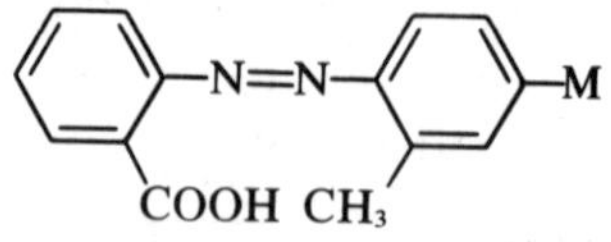 $C_6H_4(COOH)$—N=N—$C_6H_3(CH_3)$—M	18	2383

very reactive, having a half-life for hydrolysis of only a few seconds. The metabolite formed on complete reduction of the unsubstituted derivative (Table 3) has a half-life in water of 4·8 min at pH 7·0 and 37°C. Compared with the blood circulation time, this is quite long and would allow the metabolite to escape from liver cells and reach sensitive tissues, such as bone marrow, while still in an active form. The reactivity of nitrogen

Table 3 Rate of hydrolysis of alkylating agents produced on complete reduction of various azo-mustards (data from Connors *et al*, 1973a)

Compound	$t_{\frac{1}{2}}$* (min)
H_2N–$C_6H_3(CH_3)$–$N(CH_2CH_2Cl)_2$	8·5
H_2N–C_6H_4–$N(CH_2CH_2Cl)_2$	4·8
H_2N–$C_6H_3(CH_3)$–$N(CH_2CH_2Br)_2$	4·8
H_2N–$C_6H_3(CH_3)$–$N(CH_2CH(CH_3)Br)_2$	0·68

*$t_{\frac{1}{2}}$ = half-life in water at 37°C and pH 7.0.

mustards can be enhanced by replacing the chlorine atoms of the bis-2-chloroethylamino group by bromine (or by iodine) and also by inserting a methyl group on the carbon atom carrying the halogen. All these modifications led to enhanced activity (Table 3) and the compound selected for clinical trial was the 2-bromopropyl derivative (**6**) which is rapidly reduced by liver azo-reductase to the alkylating metabolite (**7**). This, in turn has a half-life of only 41 s (Table 3) and will be rapidly hydrolysed to the innocuous hydroxypropyl derivative (**8**).

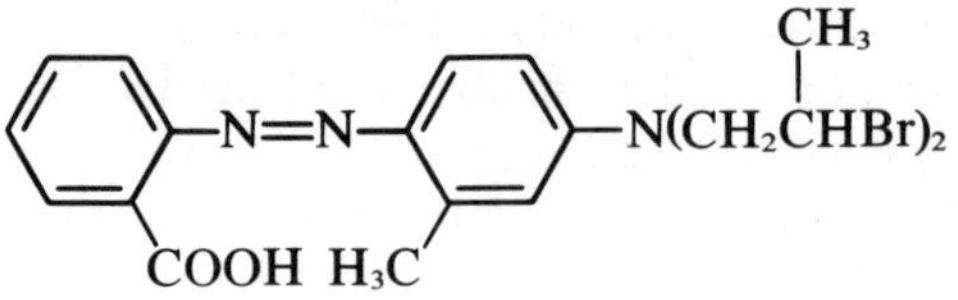

$$\text{Azomustard (6)} \longrightarrow \text{Active metabolite (7)} \longrightarrow \text{Inactive hydrolysis product (8)}$$

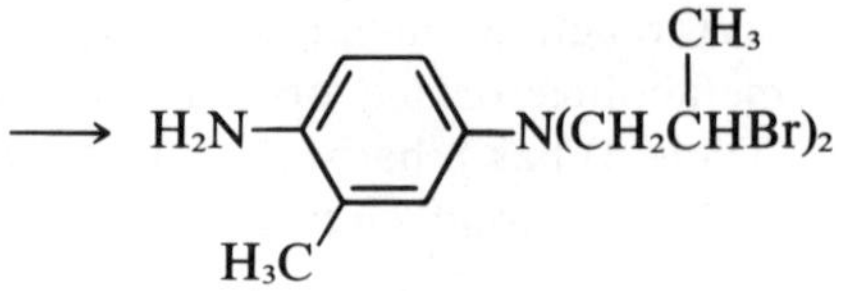

(6): $C_6H_4(COOH)-N{=}N-C_6H_3(CH_3)-N(CH_2CH(CH_3)Br)_2$

Azomustard

(6)

(7): $H_2N-C_6H_3(CH_3)-N(CH_2CH(CH_3)Br)_2$

Active metabolite

(7)

(8): $H_2N-C_6H_3(CH_3)-N(CH_2CH(CH_3)OH)_2$

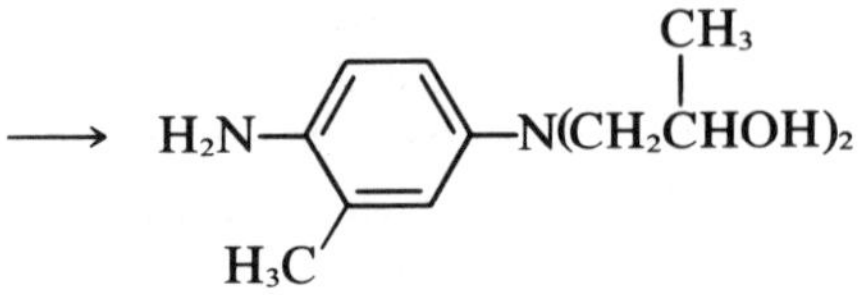

Inactive
hydrolysis product

(8)

Activation by Esterases

An early histochemical study (Seligman *et al*, 1949), using β-naphthylacetate as substrate, showed that normal gastric glands had a high level of nonspecific esterase activity, whereas none was detectable in the cells of a bordering undifferentiated carcinoma. An extension of this work (Cohen *et al*, 1951) revealed that many human carcinomas (with the exception of carcinoma of the thyroid) were generally much lower in nonspecific esterase activity than the corresponding normal tissue. This confirmed the results of Greenstein (1944) who showed that cancers in rodents were low in esterase activity when butyric esters were used as substrate, and the results of Gomori (1946) who showed using *Tween* as a substrate, that neoplasms were generally much lower in lipases than normal tissues. These studies were the rationale for the design of cytotoxic esters whose split products were much less toxic than the ester itself. Selectivity would arise from detoxication in normal tissues by hydrolysis, with destruction of tumours low in esterase activity (Tsou *et al*, 1961; Su *et al*, 1961; Tsou *et al*, 1963). One example of this approach was the synthesis of difunctional aziridines, e.g. **9**, which could be converted to the less-toxic monofunctional derivatives (**10**) by esterase enzymes. Although agents of this type have been

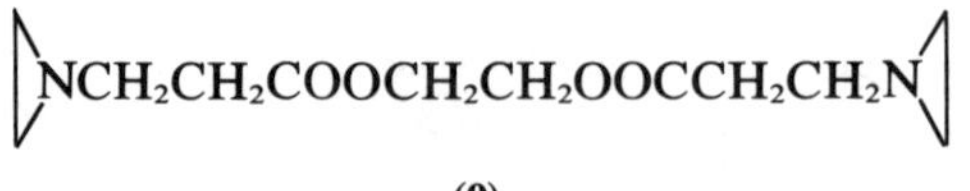

$$\text{(aziridinyl)}NCH_2CH_2COOCH_2CH_2OOCCH_2CH_2N\text{(aziridinyl)} \longrightarrow \text{(aziridinyl)}NCH_2CH_2COOH$$

(9) 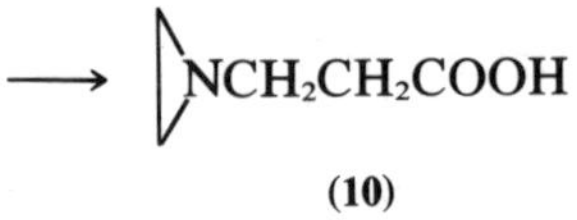 **(10)**

shown to have activity against a number of transplanted animal tumours, no correlation has been made between therapeutic index and esterase level of the various tumours.

The report of Ross *et al* (1955) that the benzoate and acetate of 4-[N,N-

HO–C_6H_4–$N(CH_2CH_2Cl)_2$ **(11)**

H_2N–C_6H_4–$N(CH_2CH_2Cl)_2$ **(5)**

bis(2-chloroethyl)amino] phenol (**11**) were more effective against the Walker 256 carcinoma than the parent compound, was the starting point for the synthesis of a number of latent alkylating agents designed to release the parent phenol selectively in malignant tissue. A series of benzoate esters of the phenol (**11**) were synthesized by Vickers *et al* (1969), and evidence was obtained that the esters were not good antitumour agents *per se*, but required enzymic hydrolysis to the cytotoxic phenol (Table 4). The 2-methylbenzoate, for example, (**12**; Table 4) was readily hydrolysed to the phenol by rat-liver homogenates and was a good antitumour agent, whereas the 2,6-dimethyl analogue (**12a**; Table 4) was only slowly hydrolysed and had no anticancer activity. No similar measurements of enzyme activity were made with Walker-tumour homogenates but the ester is definitely more selective than the parent phenol, with a therapeutic index three times greater, implying that more of the toxic phenol is being formed in the tumour than in sensitive normal tissues.

Hebborn and Danielli (1958) had earlier prepared acyl derivatives of the phenol (**11**) and amine (**5**), and made measurements of the deacylating ability of tumour and normal tissues using acylated anilines or β-naphthols as

Table 4 The antitumour activity of two esters compared with their ease of de-esterification by rat-liver homogenates (data of Vickers *et al*, 1969)

	Compound	LD_{50} (mg/kg)	ID_{90}	T.I.*	Enzyme activity†
(11)	HO–C_6H_4–$N(CH_2CH_2Cl)_2$	20	8·5	2·3	
(12)	2-$CH_3C_6H_4$–COO–C_6H_4–$N(CH_2CH_2Cl)_2$	68	10·0	6·8	115
(12a)	2,6-$(CH_3)_2C_6H_3$–COO–C_6H_4–$N(CH_2CH_2Cl)_2$	290	180	1·6	1·0

*T.I. = Therapeutic index.
†Phenol released (μmol/25 min $\times 10^{-2}$) from the corresponding N,N-diethyl analogues.

substrates. They showed that acylation reduced the toxicity of the compounds but that the selective toxicity of these derivatives for the Walker tumour could be strikingly higher or lower than the parent compound. A rough correlation was shown between the anticancer activity of the compound and its ability to be activated by tumour extracts. Thus the benzamido derivative (**14**; Table 5) was not hydrolysed to the amine and had no antitumour activity. The acetylamino and chloracetylamino compounds, on the other hand (**13**, **15**; Table 5) were activated by tumour homogenates and were more selective antitumour agents than the parent compound. These results only show that for chemicals of this sort to have anticancer activity they must first be converted to the amine (or phenol) by an activating enzyme. Selectivity is not necessarily to be expected by this approach since the liver usually contains from 10 to 20 times the concentration of the activating enzyme seen in the tumour, and it is likely that the majority of the transformation takes place in the liver.

An extension of this work has been the preparation of N,N-bis(2-chloroethyl)-N′-glycyl-*p*-phenylenediamines (Dalton and Hebborn, 1965). Activation of these compounds is a two-stage process. In the first step an acylase converts the parent compound, e.g. **16**, to a glycinamide derivative (**17**) which can then be acted on by an aminopeptidase to release the cytotoxic amine (**5**). The starting glycyl derivatives are chemically unreactive and in their own right not likely to be antitumour agents. That the

Table 5 Correlation between the deacylating activity of the Walker tumour and antitumour effectiveness of a series of acylamino mustards (data of Hebborn and Danielli, 1958)

	Compound	LD_{50} (mg/kg)	Deacylating enzyme activity (mg amine liberated/g tissue/h) Liver	Tumour	Antitumour effect
(**5**)	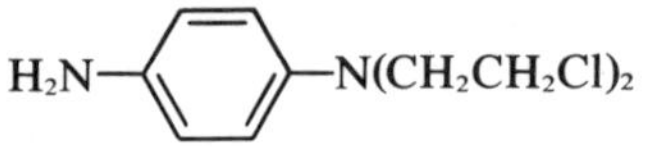 $H_2N-C_6H_4-N(CH_2CH_2Cl)_2$	6·0			+
(**13**)	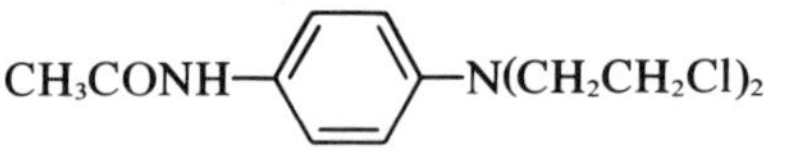 $CH_3CONH-C_6H_4-N(CH_2CH_2Cl)_2$	48	1·5	0·2	++
(**14**)	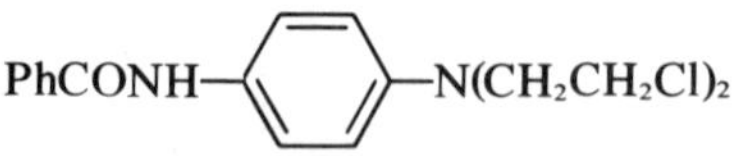 $PhCONH-C_6H_4-N(CH_2CH_2Cl)_2$	350	0·3	0·0	–
(**15**)	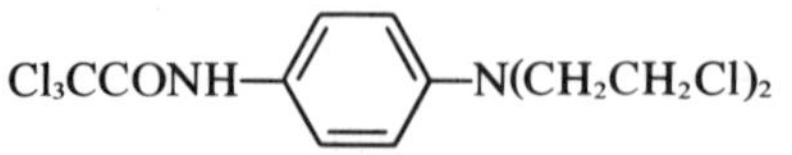 $Cl_3CCONH-C_6H_4-N(CH_2CH_2Cl)_2$	>1000	37·4	0·2	++

$$M-C_6H_4-NHCOCH_2NHCOCH_3 \xrightarrow{\text{(Acylase)}} M-C_6H_4-NHCOCH_2NH_2$$

(16) (17)

$$\xrightarrow{\text{(Aminopeptidase)}} M-C_6H_4-NH_2$$

(5)

$M = -N(CH_2CH_2Cl)_2$

cytotoxicity observed was due to the formation of the reactive amine (**5**) was clear from the direct correlation obtained between the toxicity of the various starting materials and the rate of hydrolysis of the amide bond. The nonacetylated glycyl derivatives, e.g. **17**, were rapidly hydrolysed by rat-tissue homogenates. However, there was much less of the activating enzyme in the tumour than in the liver and their therapeutic index was poor. The acetylated derivatives, such as **16**, were much more slowly hydrolysed to the amine, the rate-limiting step of the conversion therefore being the deacylation. In this case the level of the acylase enzyme in tumour and liver was similar and explains why the acetylated glycyl compounds are more effective antitumour agents than their nonacetylated analogues.

This work illustrates the important point that, as the number of variables for activation to take place is increased so the differences between tissues are likely to be greater, enabling the possible design of a highly selective anticancer agent.

The continued synthesis of latent derivatives of the phenol mustard (**11**) and amine (**5**) led to the discovery of compounds (**20**, **21**; Table 6) with therapeutic indices against the Walker tumour of greater than a hundred. These two compounds were members of a series designed to be activated by hydrolysis of the urethane linkage. It can be seen that slight alterations in the molecule, e.g. the insertion of a carboxyl or carboxymethyl group, can greatly increase the selectivity of action of the parent urethane, and make agents very much more selective than the phenol or amine which they can release (Table 6; Bardos *et al*, 1969). However, it is not absolutely clear that this high selectivity is due to conversion to the amine or phenol, especially as the compounds are themselves chemically reactive. From a consideration of the structure of the less selective and more selective carbamides, the authors have concluded that neither organic chemical nor physicochemical factors can account for the selectivity obtained and that the activity may be determined by the presence of specific tumour receptors.

Activation by other Hydrolytic Enzymes

The finding that a simple aromatic nitrogen mustard, N,N-di-2-chloroethylaniline (aniline mustard, **23**) could cure mice with terminal,

Table 6 Urethane mustards with high selectivity against the Walker carcinoma $M = -N(CH_2CH_2Cl)_2$ (data from Bardos *et al*, 1969)

	Compound	LD_{50} (μmol/kg)	ID_{90} (μmol/kg)	T.I.*
(5)	$M-C_6H_4-NH_2.HCl$	15	20	1·0
(18)	$M-C_6H_4-NHCOO-C_6H_5$	567	84	6·7
(19)	$M-C_6H_4-NHCOO-C_6H_4-COOH$	171	2·0	85
(20)	$M-C_6H_4-NHCOO-C_6H_4-COOCH_3$	278	2·2	126
(21)	$M-C_6H_4-NHCOO-C_6H_4-COOCH_3$	268	1·95	137
(11)	$M-C_6H_4-OH$	82	35	2·3
(22)	$M-C_6H_4-OCONH-C_6H_4-COOH$	151	9	17·0

*T.I. = Therapeutic index.

disseminated plasma-cell tumours was remarkable since from earlier work, it was thought that the tumour line was insensitive, even at an early stage, to most anticancer agents, including nitrogen mustards such as β-naphthylamine mustard (**24**) closely related to **23** (Connors *et al*, 1965; Whisson and Connors, 1965). This observation was of particular interest since aniline mustard, although highly effective against this tumour, does not

$N(CH_2CH_2Cl)_2$ $N(CH_2CH_2Cl)_2$

(23) **(24)**

compare favourably with other alkylating agents when tested on different tumour lines. Obviously in this case there must be some special biochemical property of the tumour which makes it particularly sensitive to **23**.

In examining the reasons for this selectivity, it was found that the *meta*-methyl derivative (**25**; Table 7) could also cause complete regression and cure of mice bearing advanced tumours. However, the isomeric *para*-methyl derivative (**26**) had no effect on established tumours despite the fact that, being less toxic, more of the chemical could be administered. From a large number of aromatic nitrogen mustards tested on the PC5 tumour, it was clear that blocking the *para* position of the benzene ring (e.g. **26, 27, 11**, Table 7) led to complete loss of activity. The *para*-hydroxy mustard was very much more toxic than other members of the series, and it was suggested that selectivity could be due to formation of this agent predominantly in the tumour. However, although many substituted anilines are *para* hydroxylated, *in vivo* this reaction takes place mainly in the liver and very little would be expected to occur in tumours which are generally very low in mixed-function oxidases. Subsequently it was shown that on injection, aniline mustard was largely converted to a metabolite which has recently been identified as the O-glucuronide (Connors *et al*, 1973b). It now seems that aniline mustard is transformed in the liver to the *para*-hydroxy

Table 7 Effect of aniline mustard and related compounds on the growth of the PC5 plasma-cell tumour (data from Whisson *et al*, 1966)

	Compound	LD_{50} (mg/kg)	Cures of established tumours (%)
(23)	C_6H_5—$N(CH_2CH_2Cl)_2$	117	100
(25)	*m*-H_3C—C_6H_4—$N(CH_2CH_2Cl)_2$	191	100
(26)	H_3C—C_6H_4—$N(CH_2CH_2Cl)_2$	450	0
(27)	F—C_6H_4—$N(CH_2CH_2Cl)_2$	415	0
(11)	HO—C_6H_4—$N(CH_2CH_2Cl)_2$	5	0

derivative and then conjugated to glucuronic acid. The plasma-cell tumour has an abnormally high level of β-glucuronidase, not only in the lysosomes but also diffusely spread in the cytoplasm (Connors and Whisson, 1966) and might be expected to convert the glucuronide (**28**) to the toxic phenol mustard. The following sequence of reactions probably leads to selective release of a cytotoxic agent in the tumour:

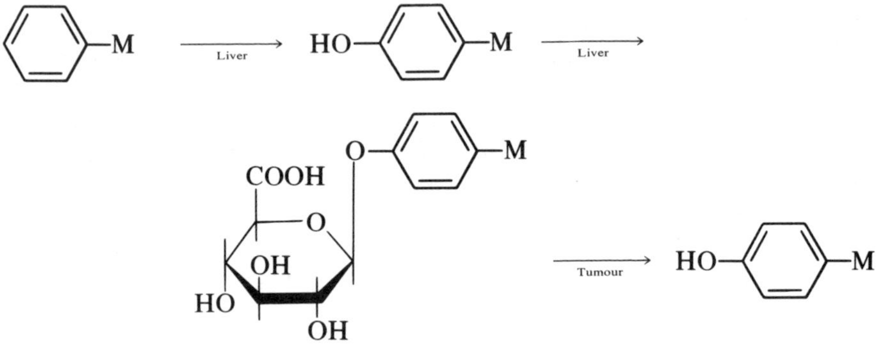

Ph—M —(Liver)→ HO—C₆H₄—M —(Liver)→ (**28**) —(Tumour)→ HO—C₆H₄—M

(**28**)

$M = —N(CH_2CH_2Cl)_2$

The glucuronide (**28**) has been synthesized and shown to be less toxic than the parent compound, so that tissues low in β-glucuronidase receive a detoxified product after injection of **23**, while tissues rich in the enzyme convert it to an agent twenty times more toxic (Bukhari *et al*, 1972). That this reaction sequence can occur under physiological conditions was confirmed by the finding that, after injection of phenolphthalein glucuronide, free phenolphthalein could only be isolated from the tumour and not from any other tissue, including liver.

This method of bioactivation is similar to the design of agents to be activated by esterases mentioned above. The same approach could be adapted to the synthesis of glucuronides of other toxic agents which might similarly be hydrolysed specifically in tumours with high β-glucuronidase activity. An analogous approach would be the use of aniline mustard sulphate (**29**) and phosphate (**30**) in the treatment of cancers high in sulphatase and phosphatase, provided these compounds are much less cytotoxic than the phenol mustard they release. The diphosphate of stilboestrol has, in fact, been used for some years in the treatment of prostatic carcinoma since this cancer is often high in acid-phosphatase activity.

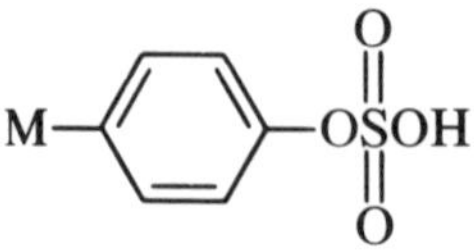

M—C₆H₄—OSO₂OH (**29**)   M—C₆H₄—OP(O)(OH)—OH (**30**)

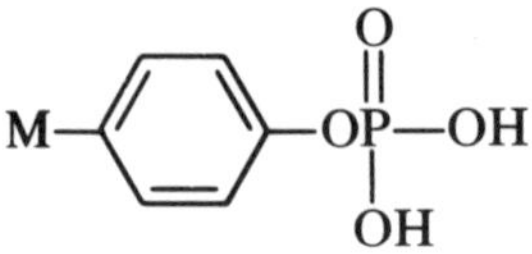

$M = —N(CH_2CH_2Cl)_2$

Having shown that in an animal model a particular biochemical characteristic can be exploited to get good antitumour selectivity with a chemical agent, its clinical application will only be of value for tumours with similar enzymic properties. Thus aniline mustard would only be expected to be useful against tumours that were not only very high in β-glucuronidase activity but which also contained the enzyme diffusely distributed and not confined to lysosomes. In a preliminary clinical trial (Young, 1973) on 71 patients with advanced cancer of different types, tumours were assayed for β-glucuronidase activity prior to receiving a course of aniline mustard. A correlation was found between intense glucuronidase staining of the biopsy specimen and tumour regression in 2/2 cases of prostate cancer and 2/2 cases of kidney cancer. Cancers with no enzyme activity did not respond to therapy. Three breast cancers were also shown to be high in β-glucuronidase, but no tumour regression was obtained. In this case, the staining for glucuronidase was particulate, presumably lysosomal, whereas in the case of prostate and renal cancer it was diffuse and more like the pattern of the mouse plasma-cell tumour. This trial indicates that the drug is likely to be of use only in the relatively small number of cancers which have a high concentration of the enzyme. It also illustrates the importance of making individual determinations of the concentration of the activating enzyme, because even though a class of cancer comprises histologically similar types, their biochemical properties may vary greatly.

The glucuronide of aniline mustard may be even more selective against tumours high in β-glucuronidase since the initial *para*-hydroxylation step may not be the same in man as in rodents.

Microsomal Activation

The early attempts of Seligman and his colleagues (Seligman *et al*, 1949) to prepare latent alkylating agents activated by acid phosphatase culminated in the synthesis of cyclophosphamide (**31**) by Arnold *et al*, (1958; 1961). This nitrogen mustard has proved to be onc of the best and safest of alkylating agents in the chemotherapy of cancer.

$$_2(ClCH_2CH_2)N\overset{O}{\overset{\|}{P}}\begin{matrix} O-CH_2 \\ NH-CH_2 \end{matrix}\!\!>CH_2 \longrightarrow {}_2(ClCH_2CH_2)NH$$

(**31**) (**32**)

Seligman and his colleagues at first prepared phosphoric esters such as (**33**) which would be converted by acid phosphatase to the hemisulphur mustard (**34**), in the hope that the latter would be more toxic than the former and selectively formed in tumour cells. The approach was not followed up since there was no evidence that increased chemical reactivity and therefore

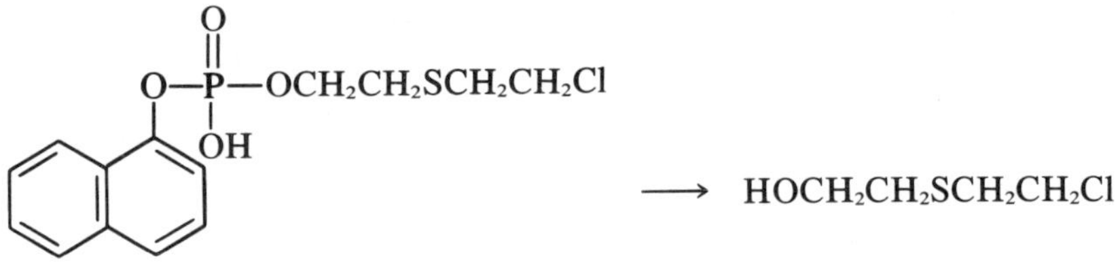

$$\text{(1-naphthyl)O}-\overset{\overset{\displaystyle O}{\|}}{\underset{\underset{\displaystyle OH}{|}}{P}}-OCH_2CH_2SCH_2CH_2Cl \longrightarrow HOCH_2CH_2SCH_2CH_2Cl$$

(33) (34)

increased toxicity would result from hydrolysis of the phosphate-ester linkage.

A similar approach was based on reports that many tumours had high levels of phosphamidase (Ichihara, 1933; Gomori, 1948). Although there is now some doubt about the specificity of these measurements (Montgomery and Struck, 1973), Friedman and Seligman (1954) made a variety of phosphamide alkylating agents to be activated by phosphamidase, such as **35** which could be converted to di-2-chloroethylamine (**32**).

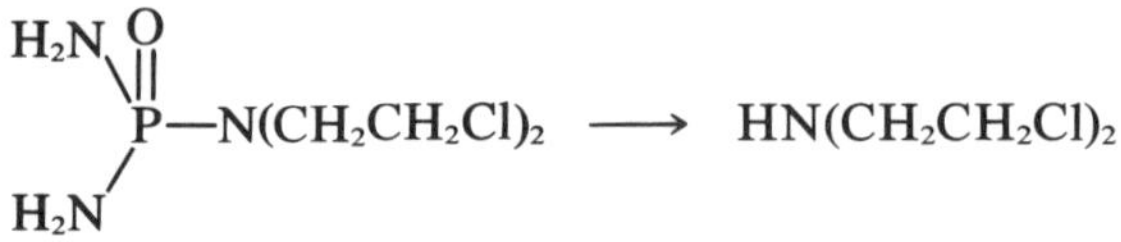

$$(H_2N)_2P(=O)-N(CH_2CH_2Cl)_2 \longrightarrow HN(CH_2CH_2Cl)_2$$

(35) (32)

Some time later, Arnold *et al*, (1958) working on similar lines synthesized many hundreds of phosphorus-containing compounds with alkylating function. Cyclophosphamide (**31**) was among these, and it was found to be very selective against the Yoshida sarcoma (Brock, 1967). Similar to the derivatives prepared by Seligman and his colleagues, it was designed to release nor-HN2 (**32**) in tumours rich in the appropriate enzyme. Clinically, cyclophosphamide is superior to other alkylating agents in the treatment of most cancers, but it soon became apparent that its activity was not due to the release of nor-HN2, but was the result of a preliminary activation step which occurred in liver microsomes (Foley *et al*, 1961). Thus from experiments of the type shown in Table 8, it can be seen that the concentration of cyclophosphamide, or its metabolites, required to cause regression of the Walker carcinoma *in vivo* is far less than that required to kill the same cells *in vitro*. The *in vivo* situation can be simulated *in vitro* by the addition of liver microsomes and an NADPH generating system. Detailed investigations on the metabolism of cyclophosphamide (Montgomery and Struck, 1973) led to the identification of a number of metabolites isolated from the urine after injection, or from microsomal incubations. The major urinary metabolite was carboxycyclophosphamide (**39**; Struck, 1971) with lesser amounts of 4-ketocyclophosphamide (**38**; Struck *et al*, 1971). However, both are ineffective antitumour agents *in vivo* and this indicates that a metabolite produced at an early stage in the metabolic pathway is the active agent. This metabolite

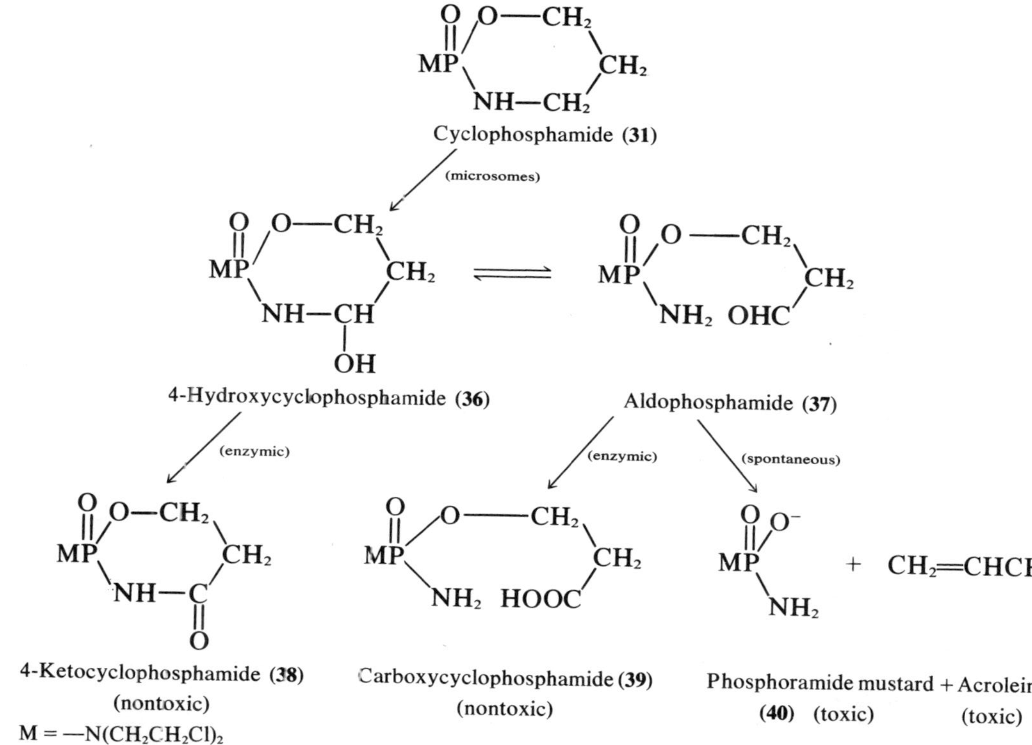

Figure 1 Metabolism of cyclophosphamide *in vivo*. The primary metabolite, 4-hydroxycyclophosphamide, is not a cytotoxic agent and may be coverted to the stable and nontoxic keto and carboxylic-acid derivatives by soluble enzymes. In the absence of these enzymes the tautomer of 4-hydroxycyclophosphamide, aldophosphamide may break down chemically to the toxic phosphoramide mustard and acrolein

Table 8 Activation of cyclophosphamide by liver microsomes (data from Connors *et al*, 1972; Phillips, 1974)

Walker carcinoma	Dose to kill 50% of cells (μg/ml)
Solid tumour *in vivo*	20
Ascites tumour cells in culture	6000
Ascites tumour cells in culture + liver microsomes + NADPH	10
Freshly removed ascites tumour cells incubated *in vitro*	800
Freshly removed ascites tumour cells incubated *in vitro* with liver microsomes and NADPH	20

has been predicted to be the primary oxidation product of the 4-carbon atom, namely the 4-hydroxy derivative (**36**; Norpoth, 1969 quoted in Montgomery and Struck, 1973), and a derivative of it has recently been isolated from microsomal incubations (Connors *et al*, 1974). Also isolated from microsomal preparations have been acrolein (**41**; Alarcon and Meienhoffer, 1971) and phosphoramide mustard (**40**; Colvin *et al*, 1973) both of which could arise from the primary C-4 oxidation product or from its ring-opened isomer, aldophosphamide (**37**; Hill, 1971). The 4-hydroxy derivative (**36**) has also been synthesized (Takamizawa *et al*, 1973) and has antitumour properties. Taking all these facts, which are supported by many chemical studies, cyclophosphamide is probably metabolized by the scheme shown in Figure 1.

In the scheme, 4-hydroxycyclophosphamide, the primary metabolite of microsomal oxidation and its equilibrium product, aldophosphamide, can both be converted enzymically to products (4-ketocyclophosphamide, carboxycyclophosphamide) which have been proven to be less toxic and to be without antitumour effects *in vivo*. There is also some evidence that enzymes in the soluble fraction of liver cells can convert the primary metabolite into these end-products (Hill, 1971). However, in the absence of these soluble enzymes, that is in washed microsomal preparations, the highly cytotoxic acrolein (**41**) and phosphoramide mustard (**40**) are produced by spontaneous breakdown of aldophosphamide (**37**). Since both nontoxic and highly toxic products can arise from the primary metabolite, it is apparent that selectivity can be explained by a greater formation of the more cytotoxic materials in the tumour. Thus if tumour cells had far less of the enzymes required to convert 4-hydroxycyclophosphamide to its inactive metabolites, then a larger amount of the primary metabolite that entered malignant cells might break down to toxic products than in normal cells which contained higher concentrations of the detoxifying enzymes. If this is the mechanism by which cyclophosphamide acts, it is an example where selectivity is achieved by detoxication of a compound in host tissues and is an important pathway since tumour cells tend to lose rather than acquire enzymes.

Activation by Differences in pH

A number of tumours, including human tumours, are more acidic than normal tissues (Papanastassiou *et al*, 1966; Ashby, 1966). This is a result of their high anaerobic-glycolysis rate and the absence of sufficient levels of 'shunt' enzymes to transfer the NADH formed to the mitochondrial electron-transport system. The excess NADH is oxidized in the conversion of pyruvate to lactate, which cannot be completely neutralized by cell buffers, or by diffusion, with the result that the pH may be lowered to a limiting value of about 6. Attempts have been made to exploit what may be a general property of rapidly growing cancers by designing cytotoxic agents that should concentrate in regions of low pH (Ross, 1961) or be selectively precipitated by virtue of the insolubility of the un-ionized form (Calvert *et al*, 1968). Alkylating agents have also been used which are acid catalysed so that they react to a greater extent, and therefore are more cytotoxic in acidic tumour cells. In order to further increase the pH differential, glucose has often been administered simultaneously to stimulate the rate of anaerobic glycolysis and increase the accumulation of lactic acid. Antitumour agents of the aziridine (ethyleneimine) and epoxide type are acid catalysed and the antitumour activity of triethylenemelamine (TEM; **42**) can be increased fourfold by the administration of large doses of glucose, presumably by the increased activation of the compound in the tumour (Connors *et al*, 1964).

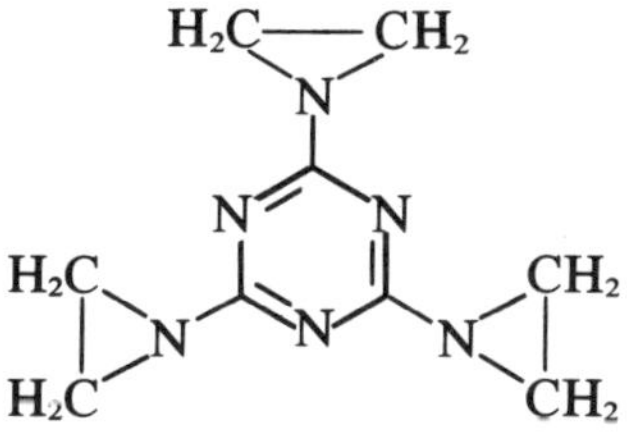

H_2C—CH_2 N N N N H_2C CH_2 N N H_2C CH_2

(42)

Activation of other Agents with Alkylating Activity

3,3-Dimethyltriazenes were known to be active against some animal tumours twenty years ago (Clark *et al*, 1955), but their clinical use originated from attempts to design antagonists of 5-aminoimidazole-4-carboxamide (**43**) whose ribotide is a precursor in purine biosynthesis. 5-(3,3-Dimethyl-1-triazeno) imidazole-4-carboxamide (DIC, **44**) is of particular use in the treatment of melanoma (Carter and Friedman, 1972).

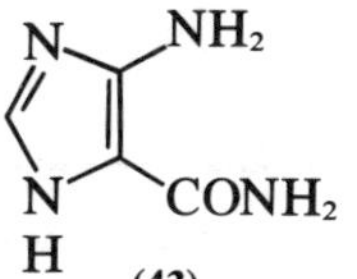

N NH_2 N $CONH_2$ H

(43)

N $N{=}N{-}N(CH_3)_2$ N $CONH_2$ H

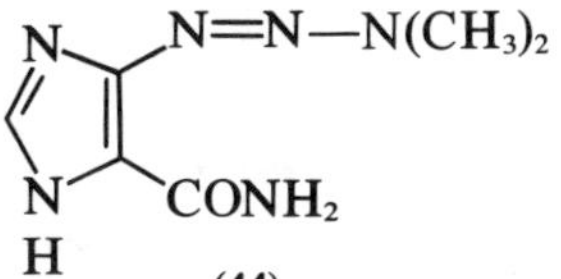

(44)

From a series of triazenes synthesized since that time, it is quite clear that the sole structural requirement for activity against animal tumours is the presence of an N-3-methyltriazeno group. It can be seen from Table 9 that the cyclic structure carrying the triazeno substituent can be either a heterocyclic imidazole or phenyl without significantly altering the antitumour properties of the compound. Their activity is also not changed

Table 9 Effect of a number of triazenes on the growth of the TLX5 lymphoma. Compound **50** is dealkylated considerably and compound **49** is de-ethylated at a faster rate than it is demethylated (data from Audette *et al*, 1973).

	Compound	IST (%)*	Toxic dose	Substrate demethylation (%)
(44)†	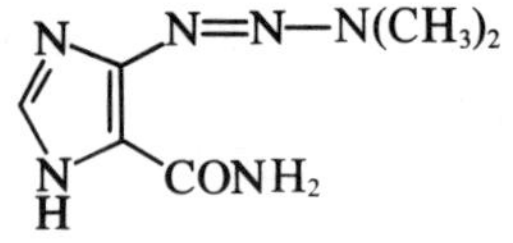 N, N H; N=N—N$(CH_3)_2$; $CONH_2$	69	200	
(45)	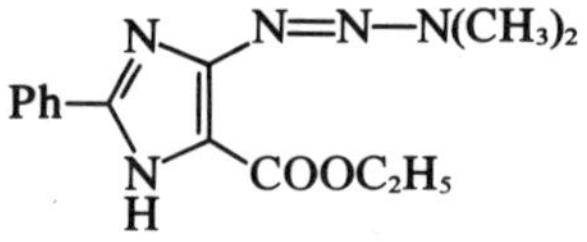 Ph—, N, N H; N=N—N$(CH_3)_2$; $COOC_2H_5$	56	200	11·3
(46)	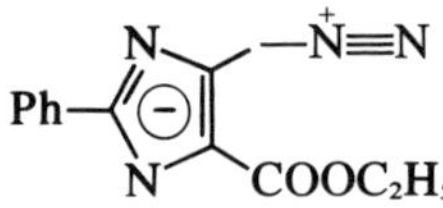 Ph—, N, N, (−); —$\overset{+}{N}\equiv N$; $COOC_2H_5$	inactive	16	—
(47)	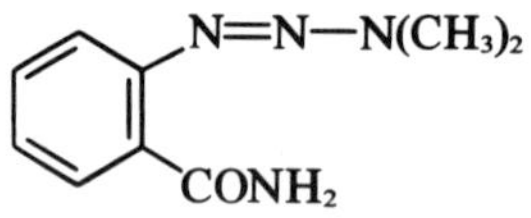 N=N—N$(CH_3)_2$; $CONH_2$	79	128	21·4
(48)	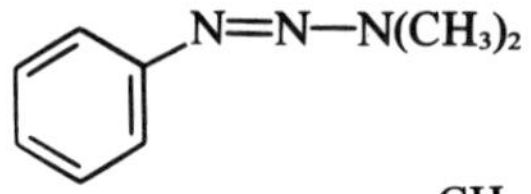 N=N—N$(CH_3)_2$	53	128	41·6
(49)	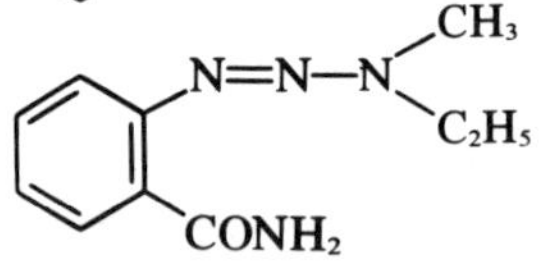 N=N—N(CH_3)(C_2H_5); $CONH_2$	63	200	10
(50)	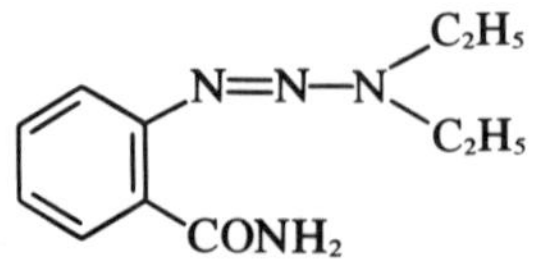 N=N—N(C_2H_5)(C_2H_5); $CONH_2$	inactive	200	—

*IST (%) = increase in survival time: a measure of antitumour effectiveness.
†R1 lymphoma.

markedly by substitution on the cyclic nucleus or by alteration of the 4-carboxamide group (**45**; Table 9). However, loss of the dimethyltriazeno group leads to inactive compounds since the diazonium analogues, e.g. **46**, although highly toxic, have no antitumour activity *in vivo*. Substitution of one of the two N-3 methyl groups does not alter the properties of the compound (**49**) but disubstitution by diethyl, gives agents that are just as toxic as the dimethyltriazenes but which are lacking in antitumour activity (**50**).

The dimethyltriazenes are also carcinogenic, and it has been suggested that they act *in vivo* only after they have been converted to electrophilic reactants. Two pathways have been proposed (figure 2). In one scheme there is enzymic monodemethylation by mixed-function oxidases to a

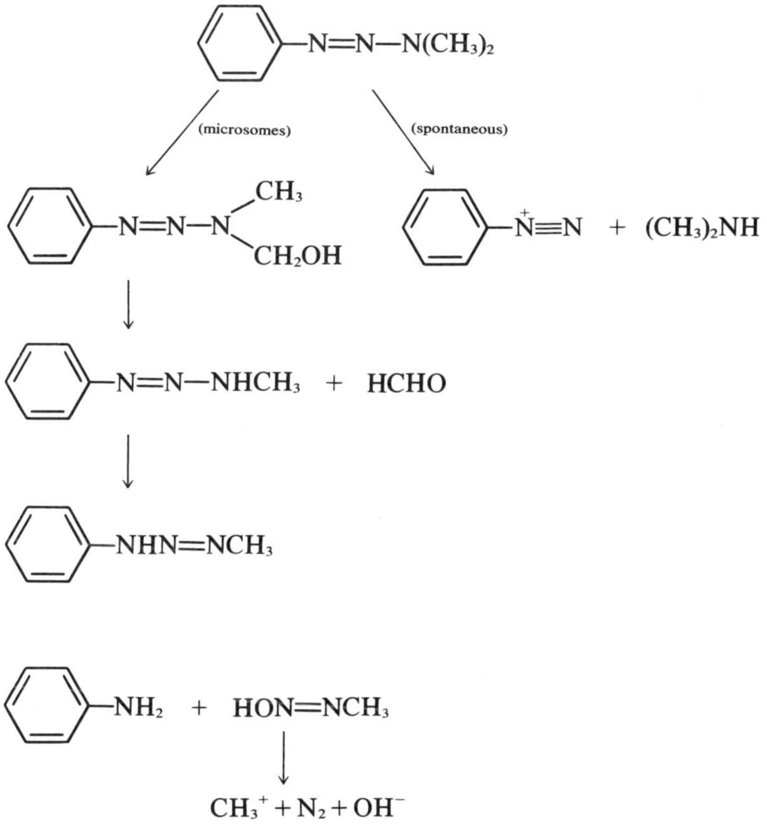

$C_6H_5-N{=}N-N(CH_3)_2$

(microsomes) (spontaneous)

$C_6H_5-N{=}N-N(CH_3)(CH_2OH)$ $\quad\quad$ $C_6H_5-\overset{+}{N}{\equiv}N + (CH_3)_2NH$

$\downarrow$

$C_6H_5-N{=}N-NHCH_3 + HCHO$

$\downarrow$

$C_6H_5-NHN{=}NCH_3$

$C_6H_5-NH_2 + HON{=}NCH_3$

$\downarrow$

$CH_3^+ + N_2 + OH^-$

Figure 2 Proposed mechanism of action of the cytotoxic triazenes. Enzymically, triazenes may be dealkylated to form the monoalkyl derivatives which are unstable and break down to form the aromatic or heterocyclic amine and the alkyl diazonium hydroxide which may break down further to release alkyl carbonium ions. Alternatively, under the influence of light or acid, the triazenes may break down to diazonium compounds

monomethyltriazene which, after rearrangement, breaks down to release an aromatic or heterocyclic amine and methyl carbonium ions which can react with nucleophilic centres (Preussmann *et al*, 1969; Skibba *et al*, 1970). Alternatively it has been proposed that the triazenes decompose *in vivo* to form aryl or heterocyclic diazo compounds (Shealy *et al*, 1962; Yamamoto, 1969).

Diethyl and other dialkyltriazenes are also carcinogenic and teratogenic (Druckrey, 1973) and either of these metabolic pathways (figure 2) may account for their biological effects. However, it is difficult to see how this scheme can explain the antitumour effect of the triazenes since there seems to be an absolute requirement for at least one N-3 methyl group, yet diethyltriazenes are readily dealkylated and presumably follow the same pathway as dimethyltriazenes to form ethyl carbonium ions. Similarly the conditions for chemical breakdown of the dimethyl compounds to form diazo derivatives would be the same for breakdown of the diethyltriazenes.

Some diazo derivatives of the triazenes are stable enough to be isolated and they have been shown to be extremely toxic to tumour cells *in vitro*. However, they are not good antitumour agents because they are toxic to whole animals and so no selectivity is obtained. This diazo-forming pathway would be responsible for the antitumour effects observed only if there were greater conversion, e.g. by acid catalysis, to the diazo compound in cancer cells.

If the demethylation pathway is required for activation, it must be assumed that the methyl carbonium ions produced have greater antitumour effects than ethyl or other carbonium ions, or alternatively that the formaldehyde released plays an essential role. Nevertheless, many other methylating agents, or agents that release formaldehyde, are without antitumour activity.

The situation is more complicated since, although the liver microsomes of animals bearing sensitive tumours have good demethylating ability, no activity has been detected in the tumour cells themselves. It is difficult to see how methyl carbonium ions, formed in the liver, and with short half-lives, can affect a distant tumour. The monodemethylated product could act as a more-stable transport form, but if produced in the liver there is no reason why it should have antitumour selectivity. An alternative explanation is that some liver products are methylated to produce compounds with specific tumour-inhibitory properties. In this connection, it is of interest that Alderson (1973) has shown that the reaction product of formaldehyde and the adenine of RNA is a selective antitumour agent *in vivo* and *in vitro*. The postulated product is the N-6 methylol of adenine which can arise by direct reaction with formaldehyde or, conceivably, from initial N-6 methylation followed by microsomal hydroxylation. The bioactivation of two other clinically useful antitumour agents, natulan (**51**; procarbazine) and hexamethylmelamine (**52**) may occur by pathways similar to that proposed for the dimethyltriazenes.

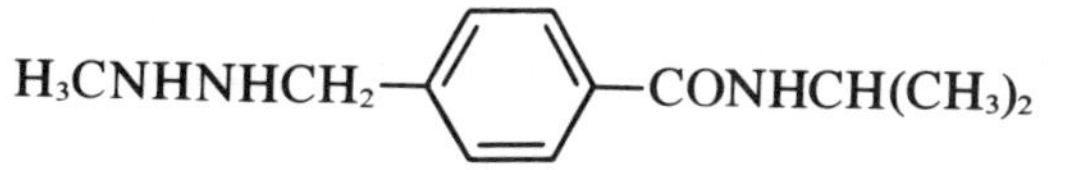

$H_3CNHNHCH_2-C_6H_4-CONHCH(CH_3)_2$

(51)

$N(CH_3)_2$

$(H_3C)_2N$ $N(CH_3)_2$

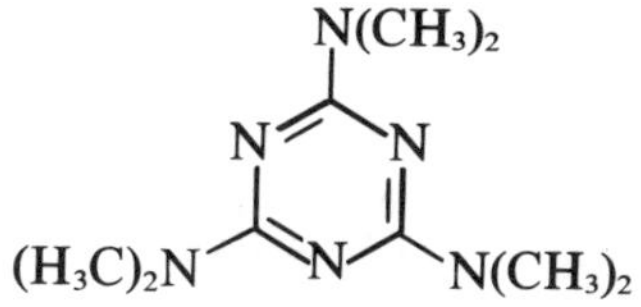

(52)

The finding that natulan released formaldehyde *in vitro* and that the N-demethylated analogue was inactive led to an early suggestion that this compound acted by release of formaldehyde *in vivo* (Weitzel *et al*, 1964). That this compound is enzymically activated *in vivo* was confirmed by the finding that freshly prepared solutions had no activity against cells *in vitro* (Gale *et al*, 1967; Huang and Kremer, 1969). Further studies on the mechanism of action of natulan obtained evidence for at least two metabolic pathways, and indicated that the N-methyl group contributed not only to the formate pool but could also be transferred by a direct transmethylation to the guanine of RNA (Kreis *et al*, 1966). A metabolic scheme by which natulan could both contribute to and by-pass the formate pool has been proposed by Baggiolini *et al* (1969) and is in agreement with the observations of Kreis *et al* (1966). Natulan is thus similar to the dimethyltriazenes in that it can both release formaldehyde and act as a methylating agent.

Hexamethylmelamine has been known to be an inhibitor of a number of animal tumours for many years (Buckley *et al*, 1950), but it has only recently had a successful clinical trial against carcinoma of the lung (Weiss and Wilson, 1971; Takita, 1972). Like the tumour-inhibitory triazenes and natulan, it is metabolized by liver microsomes with the release of formaldehyde (Worzalla *et al*, 1972); metabolism is a sequence of demethylations, finally resulting in the formation of melamine (**53**) which is not a tumour inhibitor. The activity of the trimethylolmelamine (**54**; Hendry *et al*, 1951) suggests that this is the active metabolite and causes toxicity either by releasing formaldehyde, by acting in its own right or by further reacting with other compounds, e.g. amines, analogous to the N-6 methylol of adenine described by Alderson (1973).

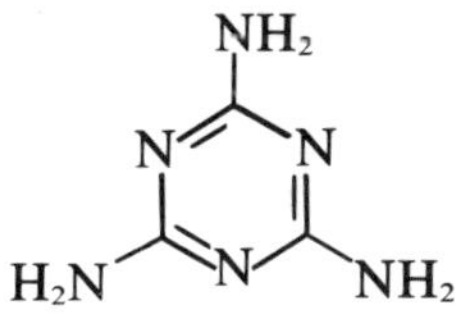

NH_2

H_2N NH_2

(53)

$NHCH_2OH$

$HOCH_2HN$ $NHCH_2OH$

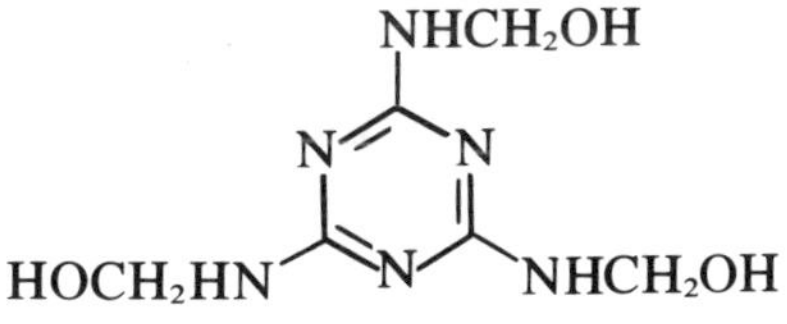

(54)

ACTIVATION OF ANTITUMOUR ANTIBIOTICS

Most antitumour antibiotics whose mechanism of action is known, kill cells by binding strongly to DNA and subsequently interfering with DNA synthesis and function. In most cases, binding is achieved by intercalation and requires planarity of the antibiotic and a precise molecular size. The antibiotic reacts with the double helix and causes it to unwind so that a space large enough for the insertion of one molecule between the stacked base pairs occurs. The molecule intercalated in this way is held in position by electronic interaction with the base pairs above and below. The resulting distortion of the structure of DNA is responsible for the disturbance of its function (figure 3). Some antitumour antibiotics, such as the actinomycins, also interact strongly with DNA but not by a process of intercalation (Newton, 1970).

Daunorubicin and adriamycin are two antibiotics useful in the treatment of certain leukaemias and solid tumours. Clinically the compounds have the undesirable property of being rapidly excreted, have toxic effects on rapidly dividing cells such as bone marrow, and cause damage to cardiac muscle. It has been known for some time that molecules intercalated with DNA are protected from enzymic and chemical breakdown. The amino groups of proflavine, for instance, are protected from diazotization when intercalated with DNA. Making use of this stability of intercalated complexes, Trouet *et al* (1972) have prepared complexes of DNA and daunorubicin as latent carrier forms which might show greater specificity for tumour cells. Renal excretion of the complex would be less because of its high molecular weight, and cardiac toxicity might be avoided since there is no evidence that this tissue can take up the complex, whereas many tumours have been reported to concentrate large molecules by endocytosis. The daunorubicin complex with DNA is in inert form since it exerts no antibacterial activity, but can be

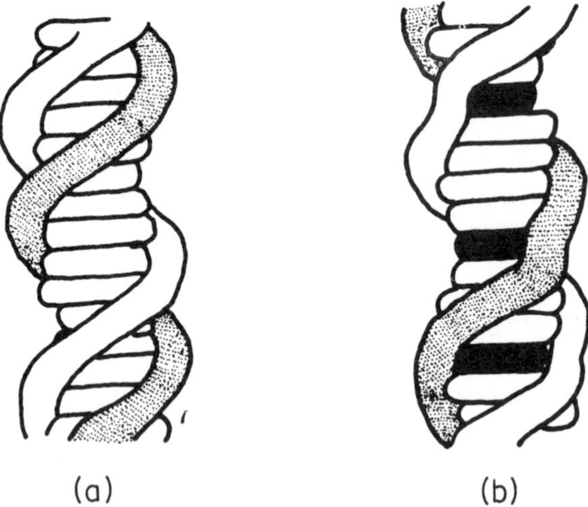

Figure 3 A normal section of double stranded DNA (a), and after reaction with an intercalating compound (b). The insertion of a number of molecules of the intercalating agent between the base pairs distorts the double helical structure. From Newton (1970) and Lerman (1964)

degraded by lysosomal DNAase preparations to release the active antibiotic. Against a variety of tumour cells in culture the DNA–daunorubicin complex was as potent as free daunorubicin and was shown to be activated by the scheme of figure 4. The complex is too large to enter cells by diffusion or active transport, but is endocytosed, forming an intracellular phagosome which fuses with a lysosome. Under the influence of the lysosomal enzymes, the DNA is broken down, the antibiotic is released and causes cytotoxicity by entering the nucleus and binding to DNA. Experiments comparing free daunorubicin with the DNA complex have shown that the latter is less toxic and a more selective inhibitor of animal tumours (Trouet *et al*, 1972) than the

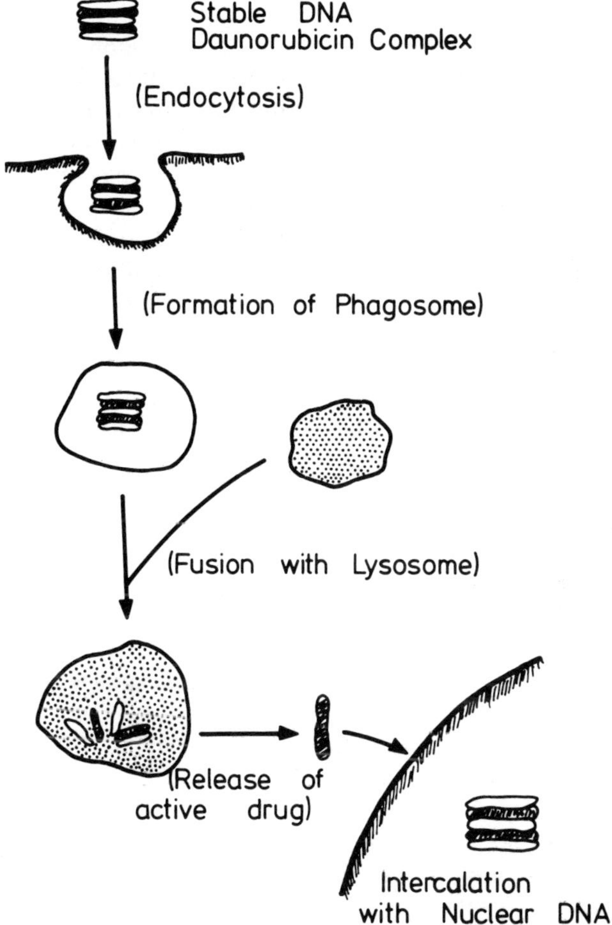

Figure 4 Selective uptake of daunorubicin by tumour cells. The DNA–daunorubicin intercalated complex stimulates endocytosis in tumour cells. After condensation with a lysosome, the intercalated antibiotic is released and can react with nuclear DNA. Adapted from Trouet *et al* (1972)

former. In preliminary clinical trials, the complex has also been shown to have good antileukaemic activity (Sokal *et al*, 1973). A general criterion for the use of such complexes is that there should not be a high level of the activating enzyme in the extracellular fluid, otherwise the drug would be released before being taken up by tumour cells. Furthermore, the antibiotic must be able to survive the lysosomal environment until it can diffuse into the cytoplasm. Actinomycin D, for instance, could be similarly complexed to DNA but might well be degraded by proteases in the lysosomes.

A number of related approaches have also been suggested as a means for increasing selectivity by carrying the agent to the target cell in an inert form, including the use of the drug sequestered in liposomes (Gregoriadis and Buckland, 1973) or attached to tissue specific antibodies (Ghose and Nigam, 1972).

Mitomycins and the related porfiromycin antibiotics do not act by complexing with DNA, but by alkylation. Many of their biological properties are similar to the tumour-inhibitory difunctional alkylating agents and like them they have been shown to crosslink complementary strands of DNA (Iyer and Szybalski, 1964). However, crosslinking does not occur between mitomycin and purified DNA, and activation by bacterial lysates or liver homogenates is necessary (Schwartz *et al*, 1963; Iyer and Szybalski, 1963). That the activation which required anaerobic conditions, was an enzymic reduction was confirmed by the finding that mitomycin could also be activated chemically by reducing agents such as ascorbic esters, sodium hydrogen sulfite and hydrogen and palladium charcoal. Like many chemically reactive alkylating agents, the activated form of mitomycin C is unstable and under polar conditions rapidly loses its ability to crosslink purified DNA.

The preliminary activation step is most probably reduction of the quinone of mitomycin C (**55**) followed by rearrangement with loss of methanol to form the alkylating agent (**56**; Iyer and Szybalski, 1964). This is likely to be a difunctional alkylating agent since the carbamate anion is a good leaving-group and the aziridine, deactivated in the mitomycin structure by withdrawal of electrons from the N-4 into the quinone ring, is much more reactive. In polar solvents the likely alkylating species is **57**.

Mitomycin C might have some antitumour selectivity if the primary activation process were a reduction, since the lower oxidation–reduction potential of a number of tumours relative to normal tissue has been established (Cater and Phillips, 1954). However, there is no doubt that the antibiotic can also be reduced by liver extracts under anaerobic conditions so no great selectivity would be experienced, which is consistent with clinical experience in the use of this compound.

The pyrrolizidine alkaloids isolated from several genera of plants, are hepatotoxins and cause liver cancer in a number of animal species. In structure they are closely related to the mitomycins, both having two fused

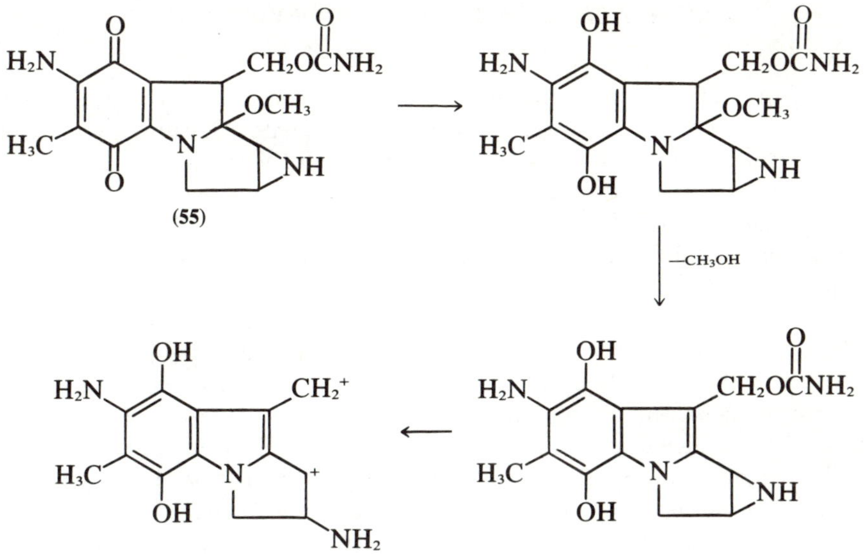

(55)

$-CH_3OH$

(57) (56)

five-membered rings with a nitrogen backbone. In many of their biological effects, they are reminiscent of the alkylating agents, although since many are only activated to monofunctional agents they are not good tumour inhibitors (Culvenor *et al*, 1962; Culvenor *et al*, 1969). The minimal structural requirements for biological activity (carcinogenicity and hepatotoxicity) are shown in the general formula **58** (where R = branched-chain alkyl, R′ = H, OH or O-acyl) which has a 1, 2 double bond in the pyrrolidine ring and the primary hydroxyl esterified with a branched chain acid. Activation has been demonstrated *in vitro* by rat-liver microsomes and, analogous to mitomycin C, involves a reduction, in this case to the corresponding pyrrole (**59**). These

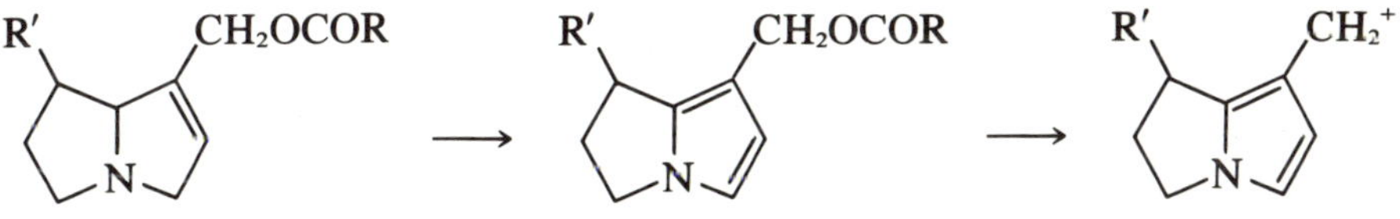

(58) (59) (60)

are the biologically active metabolites, since they can lose the O-acyl group to give the alkylating species (**60**). Pyrrolizidine alkaloids are predominantly hepatotoxic because the major site of activation is in the liver, and most alkylation takes place in this organ. However, some activated material diffuses out which probably accounts for the systemic toxicity of these compounds.

ACTIVATION OF PURINE AND PYRIMIDINE ANTIMETABOLITES

A large number of analogues of naturally occurring purine and pyrimidine bases are effective antibacterial and anticancer agents and cause a variety of cytotoxic side effects. Examples are the fluoro- and azapyrimidines, the thio- and azapurines and the ring analogues of adenine and adenosine. Most have more than one mechanism of action causing cytotoxicity by inhibition of purine or pyrimidine *de novo* synthesis or by interfering with nucleic-acid synthesis and function.

The base analogues are not active *per se* but must be transformed to the appropriate nucleotide because the important pathways they interfere with operate at the nucleotide and di- and triphosphate levels. Conversion to a nucleotide is clearly an essential activation process since tumour cells can acquire resistance to purine and pyrimidine analogues by loss of the relevant activating enzyme. Bases are converted to their nucleotides in one step by specific purine (or pyrimidine) nucleotide pyrophosphate phosphoribosyl-transferases, and analogues, such as 8-azaxanthine (**61**) have no antitumour activity because mammalian cells have only low levels of the activating enzyme xanthine phosphoribosyltransferase.

Alternatively a base may be converted to its riboside by a nucleoside phosphorylase and then phosphorylated by a kinase. The sensitivity of cells depends on the ability of the analogue to act as substrate for the various transferases and kinases, and differences in response between cells is often the result of a difference in the level of activating enzyme. Thus a correlation has been observed between the response of a series of mouse leukaemias to 5-fluorouracil (**62**) and their ability to convert it to its active nucleotides (Kessel *et al*, 1966) implying that this property of the cell is the major determinant of drug sensitivity. Similarly the response of a number of animal tumours to cytosine arabinoside (**63**) has been correlated with their ability to form nucleotides (Kessel *et al*, 1967), and the development of resistance to this antimetabolite is frequently associated with the loss of the phosphorylating enzyme (Chu and Fischer, 1965).

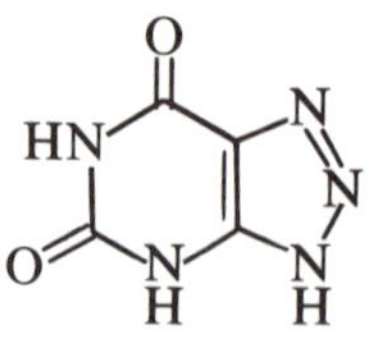

(**61**) 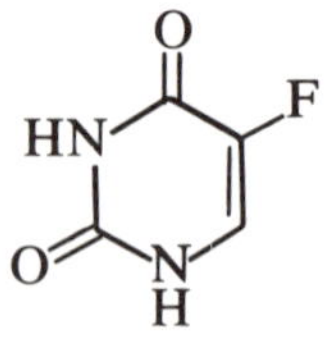 (**62**) 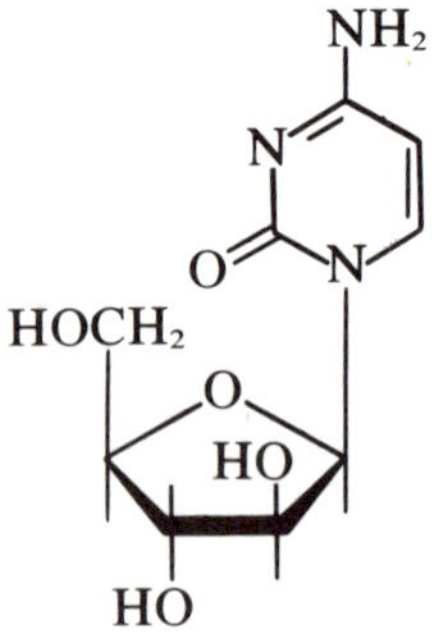 (**63**)

Antimetabolites act mainly on cells in cycle so, besides the level of activating enzymes, the rate of proliferation of the tumour and the number of cells in cycle is of obvious importance in determining sensitivity. A further factor that can alter the response of a cell, is the level of purine and pyrimidine catabolizing enzymes if the antimetabolite can be degraded by these.

Thus, although the sensitivity of tumours to cytosine arabinoside has been correlated with the levels of the activating enzyme, the response of patients with leukaemia has also been correlated with the level of the catabolic enzyme, cytidine deaminase (Steuart and Burke, 1971). Patients who responded well when treated with a combination of drugs containing cytosine arabinoside had six times less cytidine deaminase than patients who did not show a good response. Furthermore, some patients who responded to initial therapy but did less well on subsequent courses, showed a significant rise in the level of the deactivating enzyme in the bone marrow.

Since response may thus be related to both the level of activating and deactivating enzymes, it has been suggested that the ratio of the two is a more reliable indicator of sensitivity (Hart *et al*, 1972).

8-Azaguanine (**64**), a tumour inhibitor after conversion to its nucleotides, can also be deaminated in this case by guanase to 8-azaxanthine (**61**) which is

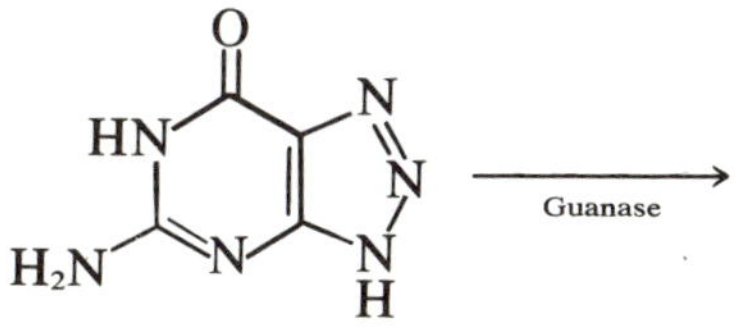

Guanase

(64) **(61)**

nontoxic because of its failure to be transformed to its nucleotide. Tumours with low guanase activity might therefore be particularly susceptible to 8-azaguanine (Hirschberg *et al*, 1952).

5-Fluorouracil (**62**) is degraded to a variety of products by most normal tissues (Chaudhuri *et al*, 1958), such as α-fluoro-β-ureidopropionic acid (**65**) and α-fluoro-β-alanine (**66**), neither of which are cytotoxic. Little breakdown of 5-fluorouracil takes place in cancer cells, however, and it is thought that this may be one reason why the compound is such a good antitumour agent (Mukherjee and Heidelberger, 1960).

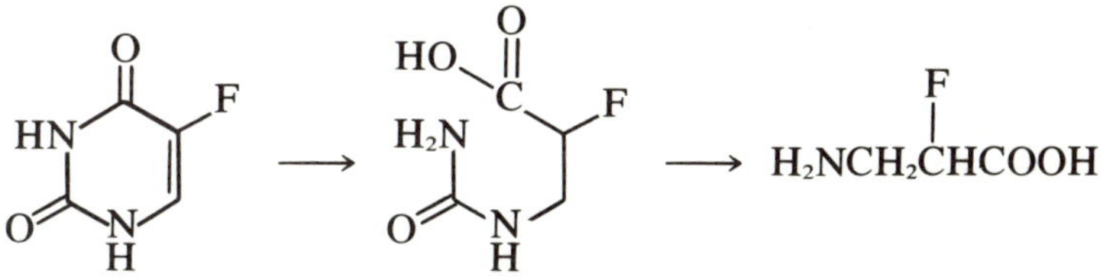

$H_2NCH_2CH(F)COOH$

(62) **(65)** **(66)**

Differences in esterase activity between tumours and normal tissue that provided the rationale for the design of alkylating agents with latent activity, have also been used in attempts to increase the selectivity of 5-fluorouracil (Birnie *et al*, 1963).

The 3′, 5′-di-O-acetyl derivative of 2′-deoxy-5-fluorouridine (**67**), for example, would release the active antimetabolite under the influence of

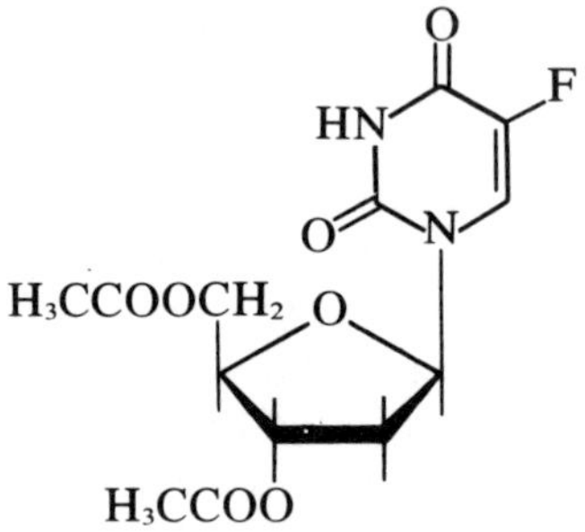

(67) 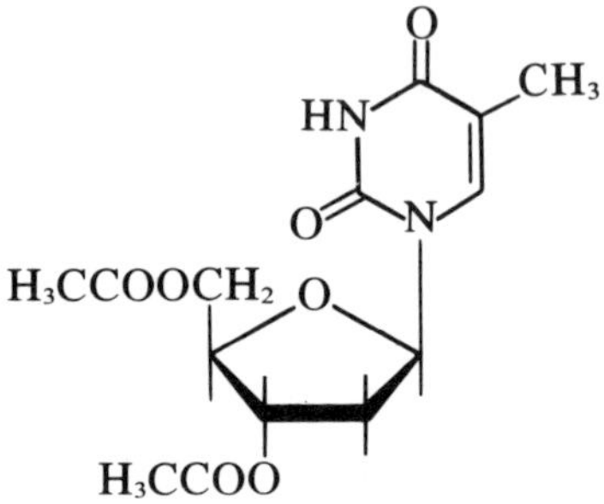 **(68)**

esterase enzymes and might be effective against tumours with high levels of the enzyme. Conversely, tumours very low in esterase activity might be selectively killed by concomitant administration of deoxyfluorouridine and the 3′,5′-di-O-acetyl derivative of thymidine (**68**). Thymidine protects against the cytotoxicity of deoxyfluorouridine, and in cells possessing good esterase activity the toxicity of the antimetabolite would be reversed by the thymidine released.

Tumour cells, unlike normal cells, can readily acquire resistance to antimetabolites. This is usually from the loss of the activating enzyme or by an increase in the catabolizing enzyme. Alternatively there is sometimes a large increase in the level of the essential enzyme inhibited by the antimetabolite so that there is still an excess of the enzyme for converting the normal metabolite, even in the presence of a strongly binding antimetabolite. Resistant cells, by these adaptations, can survive high levels of normally toxic antimetabolites, but it has been suggested that at the same time, they may now be more susceptible to other forms of treatment (Goodman *et al*, 1964; Tattersall, 1973).

Cells in culture, for instance, that have acquired resistance to azaguanine by loss of the hypoxanthine, guanine phosphoribosyltransferase enzyme, are selectively killed by the addition of methotrexate, thymidine and hypoxanthine, to the culture. Normal cells overcome the toxicity of methotrexate by using hypoxanthine as a source of purines but the resistant cells are unable to do this because they lack the enzyme necessary to convert hypoxanthine to inosinic acid.

Tumour cells may acquire resistance to methotrexate by an excessive increase in the levels of di- and tetrahydrofolate reductase, the enzyme essential for the activation of folic acid and which binds methotrexate essentially irreversibly. A related antimetabolite homofolate is also a good growth inhibitor but only after reduction to tetrahydrohomofolate. It is a good substrate for the folate reductase enzyme and is particularly effective against tumour cells which are resistant to methotrexate by virtue of a high level of folate reductase (Mishra and Mead, 1972).

5-Fluorocytosine (**69**) is used as an antifungal agent because it is deaminated by these organisms to 5-fluorouracil (**62**) which, as its deoxyribonucleotide, inhibits the synthesis of thymidylic acid. It is nontoxic to mammalian cells because they have low levels of the activating enzyme cytidine

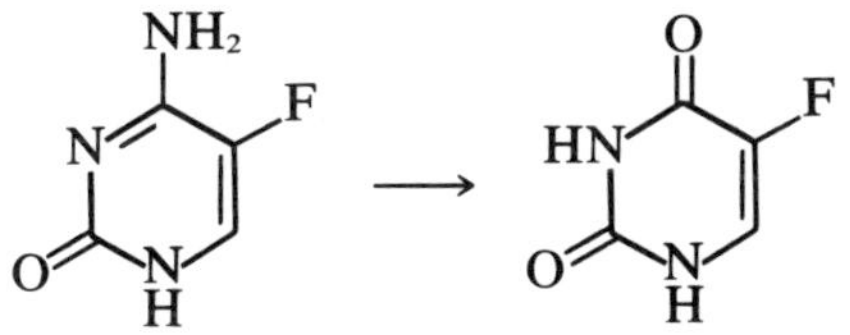

(**69**) → (**62**)

deaminase. However, it has been shown that resistance to cytosine arabinoside may be due to an increase in the levels of cytidine deaminase (Steuart and Burke, 1971), and in a preliminary clinical trial, patients who have been treated with cytosine arabinoside and who subsequently show a high cytidine deaminase activity in their leukaemic cells, are then given 5-fluorocytosine or its riboside in the hope that selective conversion to the cytotoxic agent will take place in the malignant cell.

CONCLUSIONS

Clearly the best way to obtain true selectivity of action is to use a chemical which inhibits a biochemical pathway essential to the target cell but unimportant to all other cells. Drugs that act in this way are known in some areas of pharmacology, and it is of interest that their unique biological properties are usually discovered first and their mechanism of action worked out later. It is possible that each cell type is unique in some aspect of its biochemistry, and that in due course these features will be elucidated and pave the way for the development of agents effective in the treatment of many diseases, including cancer.

In the meantime, the selectivity of action of the cytotoxic agents can be improved by various procedures, such as using each drug at its optimal dose schedule, and as part of a multiple-drug combination. The design of agents to be bioactivated by the target tissue is also an important approach, which has had some success in the past, and is still of potential value for the future.

The failure of many attempts to utilize the principle of latent activity has been due largely to neglecting the necessary biochemical measurements. Thus the statement that a 'cancer' has a high level of a particular enzyme has often been taken to mean that this is a property common to all malignancies.

As a result, elegantly designed chemicals have often been tested on a tumour line completely lacking the enzymic pathway they were intended to exploit.

Another major drawback has been the failure to compare the level of the activating enzyme in target tissues and normal tissues. A high level of a particular enzyme in a tumour is not very important if the level of the enzyme in the liver is very much higher, since most of the activation will take place in the latter and the active metabolite will be distributed systemically. In these circumstances, selectivity may be achieved if the half-life of the active metabolite is short, so that its effects are only exerted in the tissue in which it is activated, and if there are only low levels of the activating enzyme in normal sensitive tissues.

There are therefore a number of conditions that must be met if a drug is to have any possibility of acting as a latent agent with selectivity for a particular tissue:

1. The model system used to test the hypothesis must contain target cells in which the level of the activating enzyme has been measured and shown to be high.
2. The concentration of the enzyme in the target tissue must be high compared with all other tissues.
3. The latent agent must be shown to be a substrate for the activating enzyme *in vitro* and preferably *in vivo*.
4. The half-life of the active metabolite must preferably be very short so that cytotoxicity is confined to the activating tissue.
5. The agent must be used in man against human target cells which have been shown by direct measurement to contain a high level of the activating enzyme.

Even if these criteria are fulfilled, the desired selectivity may not be obtained because of a variety of factors such as detoxication of the active metabolite, very rapid excretion or failure to reach the target tissue.

Exploitable differences between tissues have occasionally been discovered as a result of comparative biochemical studies on different cell types, but more often from the examination of the mechanism or action of a drug found by chance to have high selectivity, e.g. in a screening test. Using this as a starting point, quantitative or even qualitative biochemical differences between cells have been demonstrated. Undoubtedly other quantitative differences exist between cells which remain to be discovered and which, when known, will be utilized to greatly improve upon the selectivity of present-day pharmacological agents.

REFERENCES

Alarcon, R. A. and Meienhofer, J. (1971), *Nature*, **233**, 250.
Alderson, T. (1973), *Nature*, **244**, 3.
Arnold, H., Bourseaux F. and Brock, N. (1958), *Naturwissenschaften*, **45**, 64.
Arnold, H., Bourseaux, F. and Brock N. (1961), *Arzneim.-Forsch.*, **11**, 143.

Ashby, B. S. (1966), *Lancet*, **2**, 312.
Audette, R. C. S., Connors, T. A., Mandel, H. G., Merai, K. and Ross, W. C. J. (1973), *Biochem. Pharmacol.*, **22**, 1855.
Baggiolini, M., Dewald, B. and Aebi, H. (1969), *Biochem. Pharmacol.*, **18**, 2187.
Bardos, T. J., Chmielewicz, Z. F. and Hebborn P. (1969), *Ann. NY Acad. Sci.*, **163**, 1006.
Birnie, G. D., Kroeger, H. and Heidelberger, C. (1963), *Biochemistry*, **2**, 566.
Brock, N. (1967), *Cancer Chemother. Rep.*, **51**, 315.
Buckley, S. M., Stock, C. C., Crossley, M. L. and Rhodes, C. P. (1950), *Cancer Res.*, **10**, 207.
Bukhari, A., Connors, T. A., Gilsenan, A. M., Ross, W. C. J., Tisdale, M. J., Warwick, G. P. and Wilman, D. E. V. (1973), *J. Nat. Cancer Inst.*, **50**, 243.
Bukhari, M. A., Everett, J. L. and Ross, W. C. J. (1972), *Biochem. Pharmacol.*, **21**, 963.
Calvert, N., Connors, T. A. and Ross, W. C. J. (1968), *Eur. J. Cancer*, **4**, 627.
Carter, S. K. and Friedman, M. A. (1972), *Eur. J. Cancer*, **8**, 85.
Cater, D. B. and Phillips, A. F. (1954), *Nature*, **174**, 121.
Chaudhuri, N. K., Mukherjee, K. L. and Heidelberger, C. (1958), *Biochem. Pharmacol.*, **1**, 328.
Chu, M. Y. and Fischer G. A. (1965), *Biochem. Pharmacol.*, **14**, 333.
Clark, D. A., Barclay, R. K. Stock, C. C. and Rondestvedt, C. S. (1955), *Proc. Soc. Exp. Biol. Med.*, **90**, 484.
Cohen, R. B., Nachlas, M. M. and Seligman, A. M. (1951), *Cancer Res.*, **11**, 709.
Colvin, M., Padgett, C. A. and Fenselau, C. (1973), *Cancer Res.*, **33**, 915.
Connors, T. A., Cox, P. J., Farmer, P. B., Foster, A. B. and Jarman, M. (1974), *Biochem. Pharmacol.*, **23**, 115.
Connors, T. A., Gilsenan, A. M., Ross, W. C. J., Bukhari, A., Tisdale, M. J. and Warwick, G. P. (1973a), in Garattini, S. and Franchi, G. (ed.), *Chemotherapy of cancer dissemination and metastasis*, p. 367, Raven Press, New York.
Connors, T. A., Farmer, P. B., Foster, A. B., Gilsenan, A. M., Jarman, M. and Tisdale, M. J. (1973b), *Biochem. Pharmacol.*, **22**, 1971.
Connors, T. A., Grover, P. L. and McLoughlin, A. M. (1970), *Biochem. Pharmacol.*, **19**, 1533.
Connors, T. A., Jeney, A., Warwick, G. P. and Whisson, M. E. (1965), in Roth, L. J., (ed.), *Isotopes in experimental pharmacology*, p. 433, Univ. Chicago Press, Chicago.
Connors, T. A., Mitchley, B. C. V., Rosenoer, V. M. and Ross, W. C. J. (1964), *Biochem. Pharmacol.*, **13**, 395.
Connors, T. A. and Whisson, M. (1966), *Nature*, **210**, 866.
Culvenor, C. C. J., Dann, A. T. and Dick, A. T. (1962), *Nature*, **195**, 570.
Culvenor, C. C. J., Downing, D. T. and Edgar, J. A. (1969), *Ann. NY Acad. Sci.*, **163**, 837.
Dalton, C. and Hebborn, P. (1965), *Biochem. Pharmacol.*, **14**, 1567.
Druckrey, H. (1973), in Tomatis, L. and Mohr, U. (ed.), *Transplacental carcinogenesis*, p. 45, IACR Scientific Publication No. 4, Lyon, 1973.
Foley, G. E., Friedman, O. M. and Drolet, B. P. (1961), *Cancer Res.*, **21**, 57.
Friedman, O. M. and Seligman, A. M. (1954), *J. Amer. Chem. Soc.*, **76**, 655.
Gale, G. R., Simpson, J. G. and Smith, A. B. (1967), *Cancer Res.*, **27**, 1186.
Ghose, T. and Nigam, S. P. (1972), *Cancer*, **29**, 1398.
Gomori, G. (1946), *Arch. Pathol.*, **41**, 121.
Gomori, G. (1948), *Proc. Soc. Exp. Biol. Med.*, **69**, 407.
Goodman, L., DeGraw, J., Kisliuk, R. L., Friedkin, M., Pastore, E. J., Crawford, E. J., Plante, L. T., Al-Nahas, A., Morningstar, J. F., Kwok, G., Wilson, L., Donovan, E. F. and Ratzan, J. (1964), *J. Amer. Chem. Soc.*, **86**, 308.

Greenstein, J. P. (1944), *J. Nat. Cancer Inst.*, **5**, 31.
Gregoriadis, G. and Buckland, R. A. (1973), *Nature*, **244**, 170.
Hart, J. S., Ho, D. H., George, S. L., Salem, P., Gottlieb, J. A. and Frei, E. (1972), *Cancer Res.*, **32**, 2711.
Hebborn, P. and Danielli, J. F. (1958), *Biochem. Pharmacol.*, **1**, 19.
Hendry, J. A., Rose, F. L. and Walpole, A. L. (1951), *Br. J. Pharmacol.*, **6**, 201.
Hill, D. L. (1971), *Proc. Amer. Assoc. Cancer Res.*, **12**, 67.
Hirschberg, E., Kream, J. and Gellhorn, A. (1952), *Cancer Res.*, **12**, 524.
Huang, A. T. and Kremer, W. B. (1969), *Proc. Amer. Assoc. Cancer Res.*, **10**, 41.
Ichihara, M. (1933), *J. Biochem. Tokyo*, **18**, 87.
Israels, L. G. and Ritzmann, S. E. (1960), *Acta Un. Intern. contra. Cancrum*, **16**, 665.
Iyer, V. N. and Szybalski, W. (1963), *Proc. Nat. Acad. Sci.*, **50**, 355.
Iyer, V. N. and Szybalski, W. (1964), *Science*, **145**, 55.
Kessel, D., Hall, T. C. and Wodinsky, I. (1966), *Science*, **154**, 913.
Kessel, D., Hall, T. C. and Wodinsky, I. (1967), *Science*, **156**, 1240.
Kreis, W., Piepho, S. B. and Bernhard, H. V. (1966), *Experientia*, **22**, 431.
Lerman, L. S. (1964), *J. Mol. Biol.*, **10**, 367.
Mishra, L. C. and Mead, J. A. R. (1972), *Chemotherapy*, **17**, 283.
Montgomery, J. A. and Struck, R. F. (1973), *Progr. Drug Res.*, **17**, 320.
Mukherjee, K. L. and Heidelberger, C. (1960), *J. Biol. Chem.*, **235**, 433.
Newton, B. A. (1970), *Adv. Pharmacol. Chemother.*, **8**, 149.
Papanastassiou, Z. B., Bruni, R. J., White, E. and Levins, P. L. (1966), *J. Med. Chem.*, **9**, 725.
Phillips, B. J. (1974), *Biochem. Pharmacol.*, **23**, 131.
Preussmann, R., Druckrey, H., Ivankovic, S. and Hodenberg, A. (1969), *Ann. NY Acad. Sci.*, **163**, 697.
Ross, W. C. J. (1961), *Biochem. Pharmacol.*, **8**, 235.
Ross, W. C. J. (1962), *Biological alkylating agents*, Butterworth, London.
Ross, W. C. J. and Warwick, G. P. (1955), *Nature*, **176**, 298.
Ross, W. C. J., Warwick, G. P. and Roberts, J. J. (1955), *J. Chem. Soc.*, 3110.
Schwartz, H. S., Sodergren, J. E. and Philips, F. S. (1963), *Science*, **142**, 1181.
Seligman, A. M., Nachlas, M. M., Manheimer, L. H., Friedman, O. M. and Wolf, G. (1949), *Ann. Surg.*, **130**, 333.
Shealy, Y. F., Krauth, C. A. and Montgomery, J. A. (1962), *J. Org. Chem.*, **27**, 2150.
Siegert, R. S., Bruckel, K. W. and Reid, W. (1951), *Z. Ges. Exp. Med.*, **117**, 626.
Skibba, J. L., Beal, D. D., Ramirez, G. and Bryan, G. P. (1970), *Cancer Res.*, **30**, 147.
Sokal, G., Trouet, A., Michaux, J. L. and Cornu, G. (1973), *Eur. J. Cancer*, **9**, 391.
Steuart, C. D. and Burke, P. J. (1971), *Nature New Biol.*, **233**, 109.
Struck, R. F. (1971), *Proc. Amer. Assoc. Cancer Res.*, **12**, 68.
Struck, R. F., Kirk, M. C., Mellett, L. B., El Dareer, S. and Hill, D. L. (1971), *Molec. Pharmacol.*, **7**, 519.
Su, H. C. F., Segebarth, C. and Tsou, K. C. (1961), *J. Org. Chem.*, **26**, 4990.
Takamizawa, A., Matsumoto, S., Iwata, T., Katagiri, K., Tochino, Y. and Yamaguchi, K. (1973), *J. Amer. Chem. Soc.*, **95**, 985.
Takita, H. (1972), *Proc. Amer. Ass. Cancer Res.*, **13**, 88.
Tattersall, M. H. N. (1973), *Brit. J. Cancer*, **27**, 406.
Trouet, A., Deprez de Campeneere, D. and de Duve, C. (1972), *Nature New Biol.*, **239**, 110.
Tsou, K. C., Hoergerle, K. and Su, H. C. F. (1963), *J. Med. Chem.*, **6**, 435.
Tsou, K. C. and Su, H. C. F. (1963), *J. Med. Chem.*, **6**, 693.
Tsou, K. C., Su, H. C. F., Segebarth, C. and Mirachi, U. (1961), *J. Org. Chem.*, **26**, 4987.
Vickers, S., Hebborn, P., Moran, J. F. and Triggle, D. J. (1969), *J. Med. Chem.*, **12**, 491.

Warwick, G. P. (1972), unpublished results.
Weiss, A. J. and Wilson, W. L. (1971), *Cancer Chemother. Rep.*, **55**, 299.
Weitzel, G., Schneider, F. and Fretzdorf, A. M. (1964), *Experientia*, **20**, 38.
Whisson, M. and Connors, T. A. (1965), *Nature*, **206**, 689.
Whisson, M. E., Connors, T. A. and Jeney, A. (1966), *Arch. Immun. Ther. Exp.* **14**, 825.
Worzalla, J. F., Lee, D. M., Johnson, R. O. and Bryan, G. T. (1972), *Proc. Amer. Ass. Cancer Res.*, **13**, 41.
Yamamoto, I. (1969), *Biochem. Pharmacol.*, **18**, 1463.
Young, C. (1973), personal communication.

CHAPTER 3

The role of epoxides in bioactivation and carcinogenesis

R. C. Garner

INTRODUCTION

Epoxides (oxides, oxiranes) are three-membered cyclic ethers of which the simplest, ethylene oxide, was first prepared by Wurtz (1859) by the reaction of potassium hydroxide with ethylene chlorohydrin. Most epoxides are highly strained molecules and are extremely reactive because of the ease with which the ring can be opened. Although much was known about the chemistry of epoxides, it was probably not until 1950 that it was suggested that they might be formed during the metabolism of foreign compounds by animals (Boyland, 1950).

Although Boyland's group continued during this time to amass considerable data which all pointed to epoxide formation during the metabolism of aromatic polycyclic hydrocarbons, it took fifteen years for intensive study of epoxide formation to be started. Perhaps it was the fact that metabolic transformations were thought always to produce less toxic compounds than the parent which inhibited the consideration that such intermediates might be formed. Nevertheless, it is now clearly established that epoxides are generated during the metabolism of a large number of compounds in the body, both of exogenous and endogenous origin.

As much of the work concerning epoxide formation has centred around aromatic polycyclic hydrocarbon metabolism, this will be discussed in some detail. However, examples will also be cited of other compounds for which there is evidence of epoxide formation or for which epoxide formation might occur.

It should be emphasized from the outset that because epoxides are reactive compounds their formation must always be considered to be a bioactivation process. However, further reactions of epoxides, such as rearrangement to a phenol in the case of arene oxides, conversion to a dihydroxy compound or conjugation with glutathione may modify possible toxic effects produced by the intermediate epoxide. Epoxide formation therefore cannot be discussed in isolation without considering the relative rates of these other reactions, which for this reason will also be outlined.

CHEMICAL SYNTHESIS OF EPOXIDES

Elimination

Epoxides can be synthesized by dehydrohalogenation of halohydrins by alkali. This procedure has been used for the preparation of a number of hydrocarbon epoxides (Sims, 1971).

Br OH —KOH→ O

Another procedure, again starting with the bromohydrin, involves blocking the hydroxyl group by esterification and reacting with N-bromosuccinimide followed by strong base (Yagi and Jerina, 1973), as in Scheme A.

An alternative approach is the removal of oxygen from a dialdehyde, and this can be done by using the reagent tris(dimethylamino)phosphine (Newman and Blum, 1964), as in Scheme B.

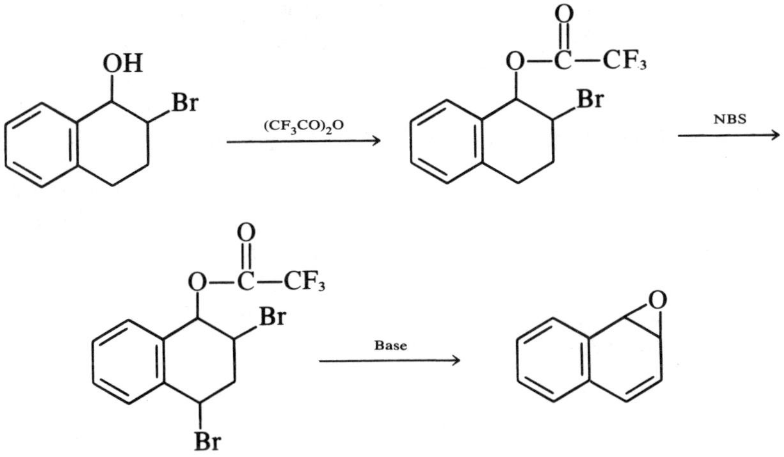

Scheme A

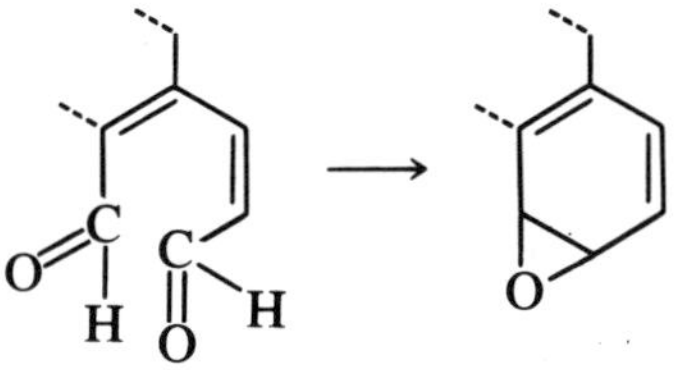

Scheme B

Epoxides can also be prepared by removing water from a *trans* diol either with sulphurane (Martin and Arhart, 1971) or with the dimethylacetal of dimethylformamide (Goh and Harvey, 1973).

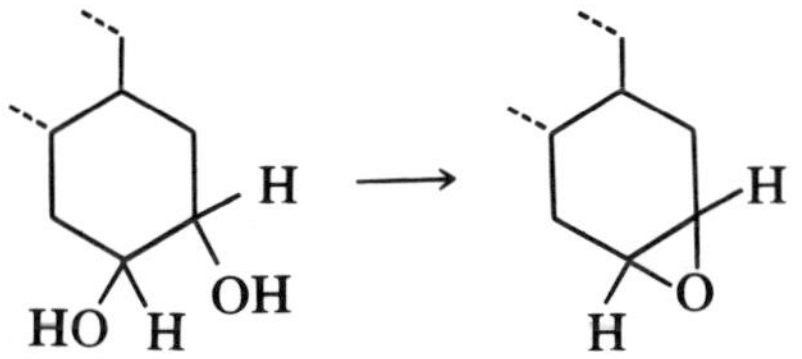

Oxidation

The most widely used method for the preparation of epoxides from olefins is reaction with peracid. The acid of choice appears to be *m*-chloroperbenzoic acid, although it might be necessary to buffer the reaction mixture to prevent further acid attack of the product epoxide. Recently, a two-phase system has been described which is claimed to be suitable for the epoxidation of acid-sensitive compounds (Anderson and Veysoglu, 1973).

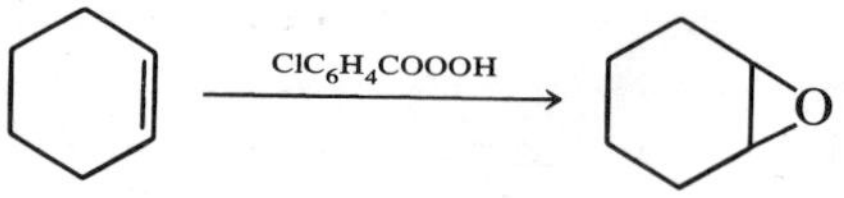

ClC_6H_4COOOH

BIOLOGICAL REACTIONS OF EPOXIDES

Because of the strained ring system, epoxides are reactive. From a biological viewpoint the most important reactions which epoxides undergo are those with nucleophiles, that is, electron-rich compounds. Some epoxides will readily react with water to give *trans* glycols, whereas others have poor spontaneous reactivity but may be hydrated by the microsomal enzyme system, epoxide hydrase (Oesch, 1973).

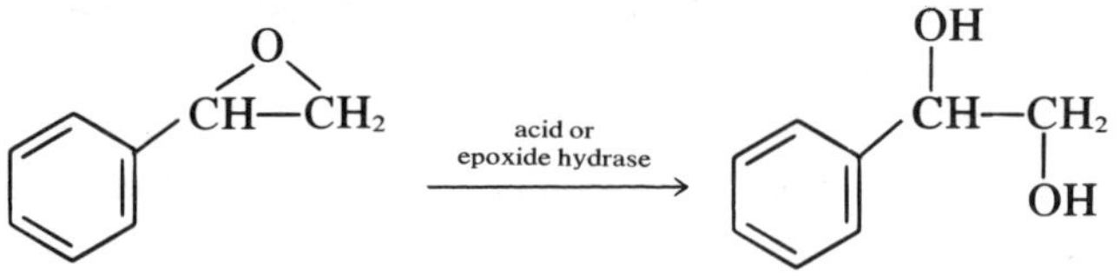

acid or epoxide hydrase

The importance of this enzyme will be discussed later. Sometimes aromatic epoxides are so unstable that under physiological conditions they rapidly rearrange to phenols, as in the conversion of benzo[*a*]pyrene-7,8-oxide to 7-hydroxybenzo[*a*]pyrene (Waterfall and Sims, 1972).

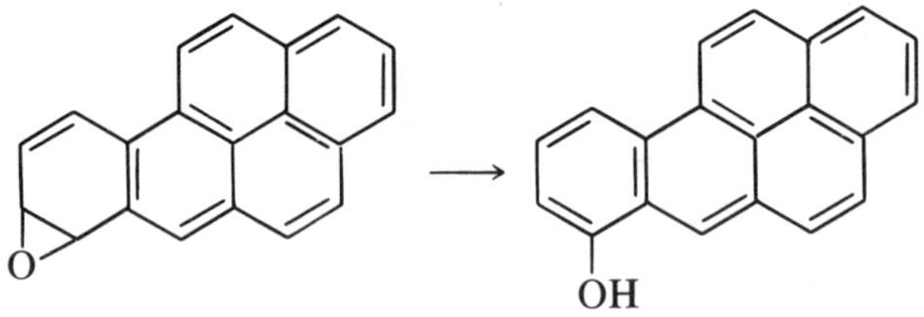

A further common reaction of epoxides in biological systems is with sulphur-containing amino acids, particularly glutathione (GSH). Thus, after administration of aromatic compounds, sulphur-containing conjugates are often excreted in the urine or in the bile. This reaction may be nonenzymic (Boyland and Chasseaud, 1969) or it can be catalysed by glutathione S-transferases, a liver cytoplasmic enzyme system (Boyland and Williams, 1965; Jakoby and Fjellstedt, 1972).

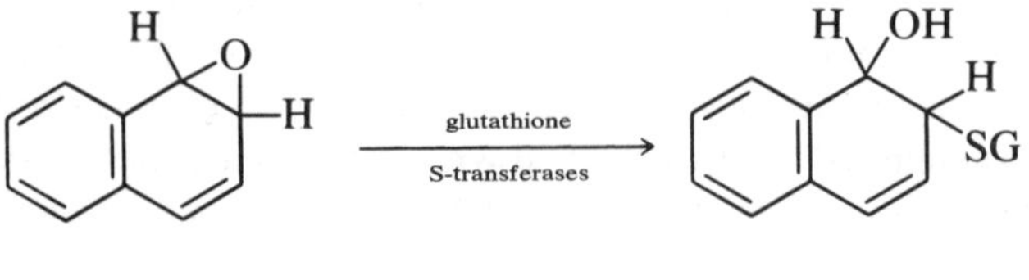

glutathione S-transferases

These glutathione conjugates are further converted in the body to premercapturic acids (hydroxymercapturic acids), and it is these metabolites which appear in the urine (Boyland and Sims, 1964).

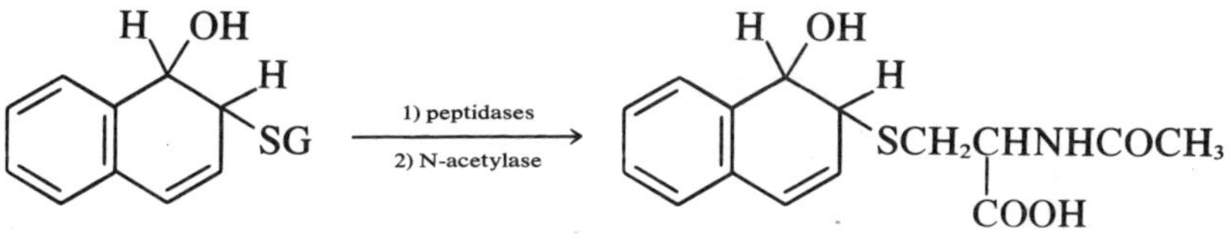

1) peptidases
2) N-acetylase

It is probable that the protein binding of hydrocarbons in mouse skin demonstrated by Heidelberger, may also be to a sulphur-containing amino acid (Abell and Heidelberger, 1962). Epoxides are also capable of reacting with nucleic acids, appearing specifically to attack purine bases (Grover and Sims, 1973).

EVIDENCE FOR THE FORMATION OF EPOXIDES

Epoxides from Olefinic Compounds

As previously mentioned, olefinic compounds can be easily converted chemically to epoxides by reaction with peracids, such as *m*-chloroperbenzoic acid. The evidence that such a conversion can be carried out biologically was first demonstrated for the insecticide heptachlor (Davidow and Radomski, 1953).

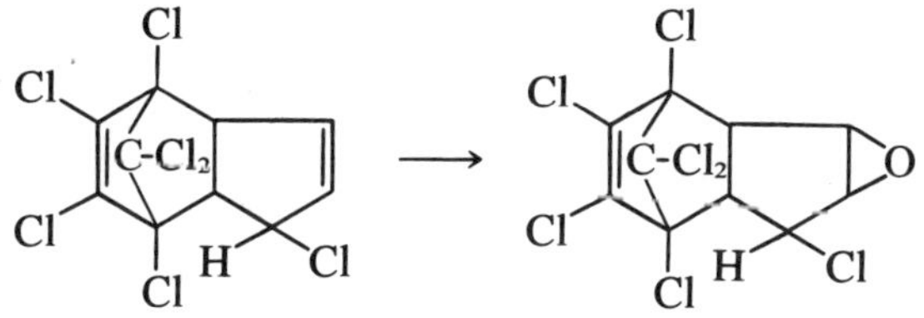

They found that dogs which were fed this insecticide had high levels of the epoxide in their body fat. The epoxides of a number of organochlorine insecticides are stable molecules and are therefore readily isolated. These workers suggested that not only might olefinic bonds be attacked to form epoxides, but that bonds with aromatic character might also be epoxidized. The mechanism of aromatic hydroxylation might therefore proceed through an epoxidative pathway rather than through attack by OH^- or $OH^{\cdot}$, which was a view current at that time. Further studies showed that rats were also able to convert heptachlor to its epoxide, this metabolite accumulating in the body fat. The concentration of the epoxide was highest in the liver, suggesting that epoxide formation occurred in this organ. A sex difference was found in the conversion, female rats producing more than males (Radomski and Davidow, 1953).

Indene has been shown to be metabolized by both the rat and the rabbit to a mixture of *cis*- and *trans*-1,2-dihydroxy-1,2-dihydroindanes, through the intermediate formation of the 1,2 epoxide (Brooks and Young, 1956). Oestratriene-3-ol was reported to be converted by rat liver to an epoxide which then underwent subsequent enzymic hydration to the *trans* dihydrodiol (Breuer and Knuppen, 1961).

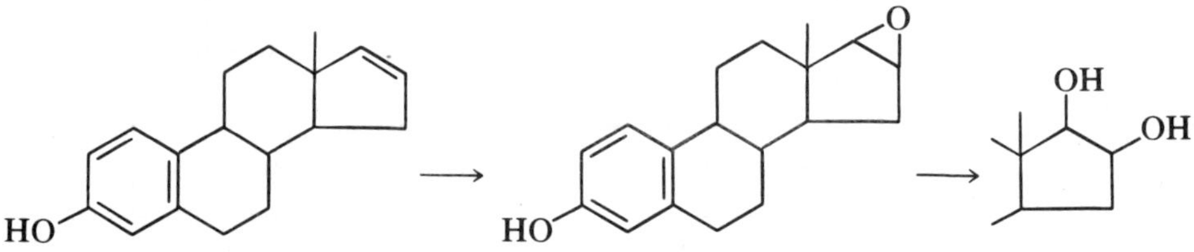

HO → HO O → OH OH

A series of three olefinic hydrocarbons, n-1-octene, n-4-octene and 3-ethyl-2-pentene were converted by rat-liver microsomes to their respective *trans* diols. The reaction required NADPH and oxygen, which are essential for the activity of microsomal mixed-function oxidases. Interestingly, alkyl substitution of one of the vinylic hydrogens as in 3-ethyl-2-pentene is known to increase the chemical rate of epoxide formation by peracid oxidation, but was found to slow the rate of epoxide production enzymically. Probably steric factors, due to the angular methyl group, over-ride the increase in reactivity exerted by the inductive effect. The epoxide hydrase which converted the olefinic epoxides to their *trans* dihydrodiols did not require Mg^{2+} or NADPH and was localized in the microsomal fraction. 1,2-Epoxy-n-octane inhibited the hydrase and was thus used to isolate 4,5-epoxy-n-octane during the metabolism of n-4-octene (Maynert *et al*, 1970).

In a more detailed study on the metabolism of indene by rat- and rabbit-liver microsomes *in vitro*, it was found, contrary to the earlier *in vivo* study (Brooks and Young, 1956), that only the *trans* glycol was formed, and no *cis* isomer. Synthetic *cis* diol could not be converted to the *trans* isomer by the microsomal system. Thus if the 1,2 epoxide of indene was incubated with microsomes, the same product was obtained as was found after incubation of indene, namely the *trans* diol. Previous treatment of animals with phenobarbitone, which increases the activity of liver mixed-function oxidases, enhanced diol production from indene (Leibman and Ortiz, 1968). Styrene and cyclohexene could also be converted by rabbit-liver microsomes in an NADPH-dependent reaction to their respective epoxides (Leibman and Ortiz, 1970). Rabbits and rats metabolize both these compounds to hydroxymercapturic acids (James and White, 1967; James *et al*, 1971), which may arise by conjugation of the intermediate epoxides with glutathione.

These data strongly support the concept that metabolism of olefins proceeds via an initial epoxidation of the double bond; the epoxide often then undergoes further metabolism to a *trans* glycol. Other instances of olefinic epoxidation will be mentioned later.

Epoxides from Aromatic Compounds

One of the first metabolic transformations to be recognized in animals and man was the conversion of benzene to phenol (Schulzen and Naunyn, 1867). It was generally assumed for a long time that the introduction of the hydroxyl group was a substitution reaction mediated by attack of OH^- or $OH^{\cdot}$ on the aromatic ring. A number of reports did not substantiate this mechanism of hydroxylation, particularly the finding by Boyland and Levi (1935) that 1,2-dihydroxy-1,2-dihydroanthracene could be isolated from the urine after administration of anthracene to animals. Since the configuration of the diol was unknown, it was not possible to resolve the mechanism of diol formation. There were suggestions that the reaction proceeded in an analogous manner to oxidation by osmium tetroxide. For instance, oxidation by osmium tetroxide of benz[*a*]anthracene gave 5,6-dihydro-5,6-dihydroxybenz[*a*]anthracene, a known metabolite of benz[*a*]anthracene (Cook and Schoental, 1948).

In 1950, Boyland suggested on the basis of his studies with aromatic hydrocarbons, that epoxides might be intermediates in their metabolism and that such intermediates could be expected to give rise to all the other known products found during hydrocarbon metabolism. It was also discovered that *meta* and *para* hydroxylation occurred during the metabolism of cyanobenzene, whereas the cyano group being *meta* directing, only the *meta* product would have been expected. Smith and Williams (1950) proposed that hydroxylation occurred either via a free-radical mechanism or by the formation of a diol and subsequent rearrangement to either the *meta* or *para* phenol. In the mid-fifties, while studying the enzymic oxidation of 3,4-dimethylphenol to 3,4-dimethylcatechol, Mason and his collaborators discovered that the atom of oxygen incorporated in the product was derived from atmospheric oxygen and not from water. If the metabolism was carried out in an atmosphere of oxygen-18, one atom of heavy oxygen was incorporated into each molecule of product whereas in the presence of $H_2^{18}O$, no heavy atom incorporation was found (Mason, 1957). Thus the concept that aromatic hydroxylation by mono-oxygenases proceeded via attack of either OH^- or $OH^{\cdot}$ had to be abandoned. However, it was another ten years before the mechanism of aromatic hydroxylation was studied in more detail. During this interim period a great deal of work was carried out on what have become known as the mixed-function oxidases, that is, the enzymes responsible for the oxidative metabolism of many foreign compounds. The mechanism of action, localization and properties of these enzymes have been extensively reviewed (Gillette, 1966; Conney, 1967; Gillette *et al*, 1969; Estabrook *et al*, 1973).

During studies to find a rapid assay of liver microsomal mixed-function oxidase activity, Guroff *et al* synthesized 4-tritioacetanilide for use as a substrate.

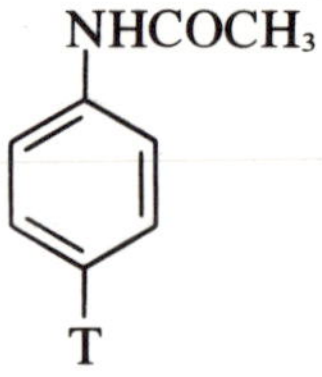

$NHCOCH_3$

T

The intention was that the tritium would be displaced by hydroxylation at the 4 position and the amount displaced could then be measured as tritiated water (Guroff *et al*, 1967). However, only a small amount of tritium was incorporated into water during metabolism, the majority being still associated with acetanilide. The experiment was abandoned in the belief that in the tritium-labelling procedure, positions other than the 4 position were labelled. In other studies, attempts were made to measure tryptophan-5-hydroxylase activity using 5-tritiotryptophan as substrate.

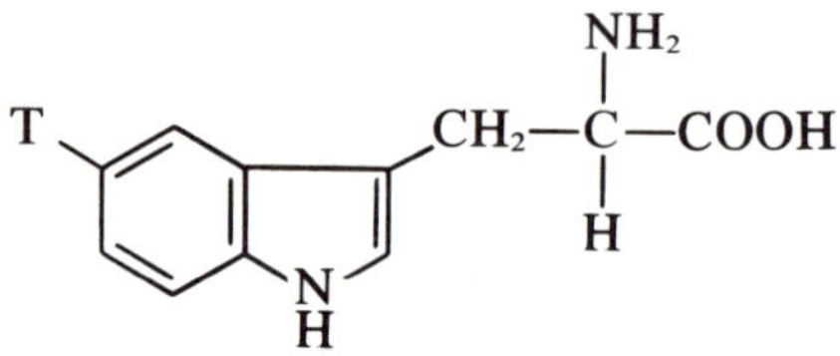

NH_2

T CH_2—C—COOH

H

N
H

Again, little release of tritium was found. Either there was something basically wrong with the labelling procedure and the 5 position was not specifically labelled or the displaced tritium was migrating to another position in the molecule. To clarify this problem 4-deuterophenylalanine was synthesized, the position of deuteration being confirmed by nuclear magnetic-resonance spectroscopy, and used as a substrate for liver or bacterial phenylalanine hydroxylase. Sixty to seventy per cent of the deuterium was retained by the product (Guroff *et al*, 1966a). Further work showed that during metabolism the deuterium had migrated from the 4 position to the 3 position. Chlorine and bromine substituents were also found to undergo migration (Guroff *et al*, 1966b).

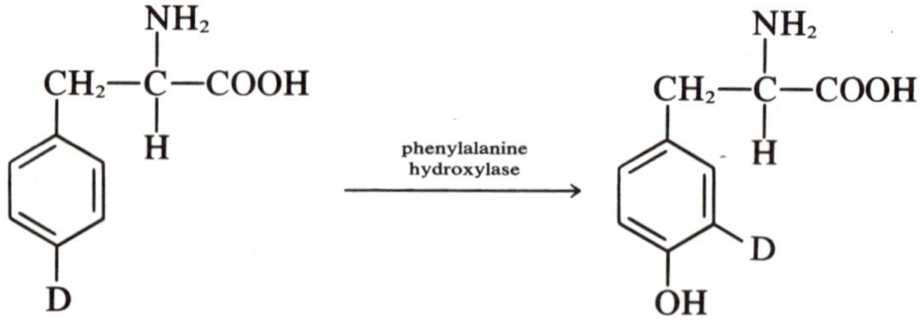

NH_2 NH_2

CH_2—C—COOH CH_2—C—COOH

H phenylalanine hydroxylase → H

D

D OH

As previously mentioned, when 4-tritioacetanilide was metabolized by rabbit-liver mixed-function oxidases, considerable amounts of tritium were retained in the product (4-hydroxyacetanilide) due to migration of the tritium. A similar finding was observed *in vivo* on administration of this compound. In a search for the possible mechanism of migration, in what has become known as the 'NIH shift' (Daly *et al*, 1972), after the institution in which the work was performed, various model systems were sought. Both Fenton's reagent (hydrogen peroxide, EDTA and Fe^{2+}) or Udenfriend's system (ascorbic acid, Fe^{2+} and oxygen) showed no significant retention of label. Clearly these two systems are not suitable models for aromatic hydroxylation (Guroff *et al*, 1967).

Aromatic hydroxylation thus involves formation of a cationic intermediate during the metabolism of the substrate, and figure 1 shows the products and postulated intermediates formed by the action of phenylalanine hydroxylase on 4-chlorophenylalanine (Guroff *et al*, 1966b).

The formation of an epoxide is the initial step in the hydroxylation; the cyclic epoxide ring subsequently opens and a cationic intermediate is formed. The extent of migration will be a function of the stabilization of this intermediate. High migration and retention would be expected with compounds containing either electron-donating (methoxy or methyl) or withdrawing (chloro) groups (Daly *et al*, 1968). If the substrate contains a substituent capable of undergoing ionization to form a neutral intermediate, this will favour release of the label in the hydroxylated position and little retention or migration. In such cases, since the degree of ionization will be pH dependent, retention and migration will be altered under various conditions of pH. Thus, during the 4-hydroxylation of acetanilide by rabbit-liver microsomes, the per-cent migration together with the retention of deuterium in the 4 position decreased from over 40% to 20% in the pH range 6–10. Nonionizable substrates, such as biphenyl, show no pH dependency.

Further evidence that the oxygen atom incorporated during aromatic hydroxylation is derived from air and not water was the incorporation of ^{18}O into naphthalene when incubated with liver microsomes in an atmosphere of oxygen-18. This conclusion was based on mass-spectral examination of the product 1,2-dihydro-1,2-dihydroxynaphthalene containing the heavy oxygen atom (Holtzmann *et al*, 1967) which could have only arisen through intermediate epoxide formation. Definitive evidence that naphthalene was converted to an epoxide during its metabolism was provided by Jerina *et al* (1970). Knowing from the earlier work of Boyland and co-workers (Booth *et al*, 1960) that naphthalene was converted by rat-liver homogenates to 1,2-dihydro-1,2-dihydroxynaphthalene, 1- and 2-naphthol and S-(1,2-dihydro-2-hydroxynaphthyl)glutathione, Jerina *et al*, synthesized the unstable 1,2-naphthalene oxide and studied its metabolism. All the expected metabolites were found when the oxide was incubated with rat liver homogenate, the diol having the same stereochemistry as that formed during

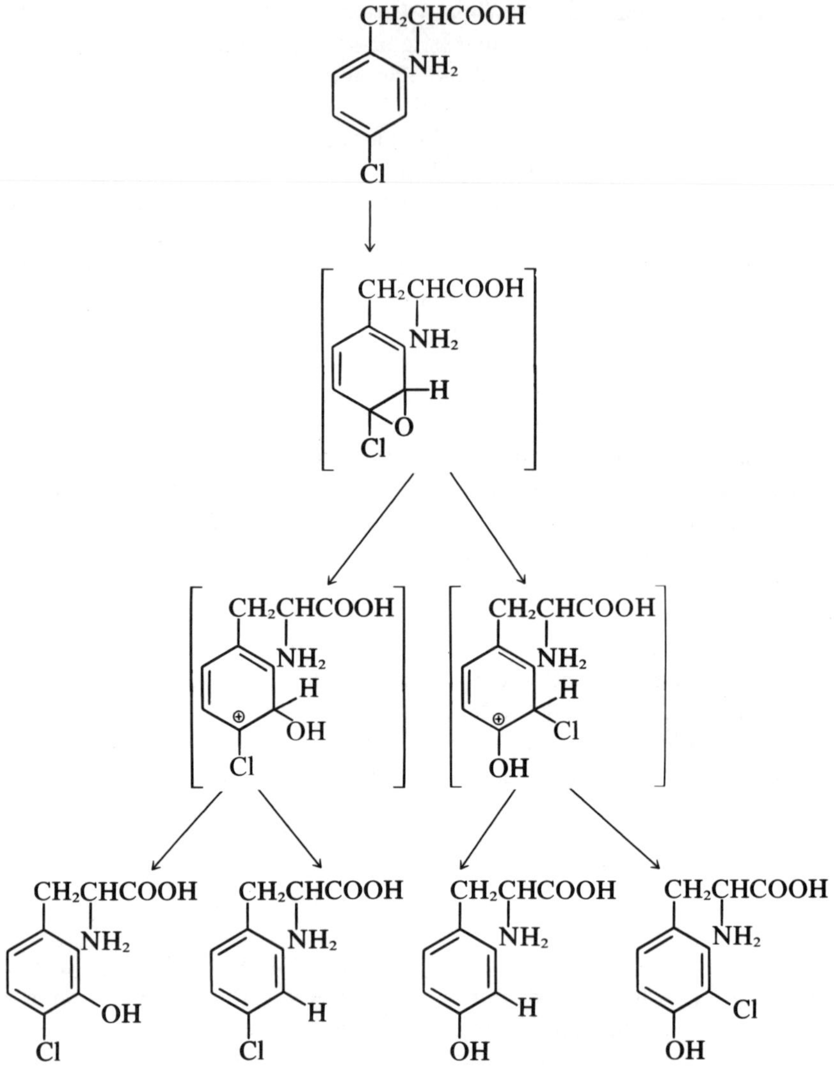

Figure 1. Metabolism of 4-chlorophenylalanine (Guroff *et al*, 1967)

the metabolism of naphthalene. Furthermore, it was possible to isolate the oxide as a metabolite of naphthalene using radiotracer techniques and carrier oxide. These results establish epoxide formation during naphthalene metabolism. It is probable that all *trans* dihydrodiols formed during aromatic hydroxylation result through epoxide formation. It should not, however, be assumed that all diols formed metabolically are in the *trans* configuration. A *Pseudomonas* species converts naphthalene to a 1,2 diol, but the diol was found by n.m.r. spectroscopy to be in the *cis* configuration. This particular diol is probably formed through a cyclic peroxide intermediate and not through an epoxide (Jerina *et al*, 1971).

The formation and metabolism of epoxides (arene oxides) have been reviewed in detail (Daly *et al*, 1972).

With regard to the mechanism of epoxidation and the molecular species involved, Ullrich *et al* (1968) compared the products obtained with 4-halogenoacetanilide, using model systems which operated by (i) a typical free-radical mechanism, (ii) an electrophilic-radical mechanism, and (iii) an electrophilic polar-hydroxylation mechanism. Peracid oxidation with trifluoroperacetic acid was the only good model for the migration of substituents. The most likely mechanism of epoxidation is therefore attack of the double bond by an oxene intermediate (an oxygen atom with 6 electrons), analogous to attack by carbene or nitrene (Daly *et al*, 1972).

EXAMPLES OF METABOLIC EPOXIDATION

Both olefinic and aromatic double bonds can be metabolized to epoxides as already described. It is not surprising therefore, since nearly all foreign compounds and a great number of endogenous compounds contain such bonds, that epoxidation is an extremely important metabolic conversion. It is probably true to say that epoxidation generally results in a potentially more toxic compound than the parent molecule. However, the factors which are important for toxicity are not whether an epoxide is produced, but how much is produced and where, and how rapidly it is converted to a phenol, dihydrodiol or a conjugate. Some compounds are converted to epoxides and are relatively nontoxic, yet others produce severe toxicity.

The main classes of compounds which are known to be epoxidized will be mentioned in this section together with some speculation on other compounds which might be epoxidized but have not as yet been studied in sufficient detail.

Epoxides from Drugs

Hydroxylation of aromatic rings is a general biotransformation process which increases the polarity of the compound and therefore both aids its excretion and provides a focus for conjugation. As already discussed, hydroxylation usually proceeds through formation of an intermediate epoxide which might rearrange at physiological conditions to a phenol, be hydrated to a *trans* dihydrodiol or conjugate with glutathione. Phenols may be further converted to ethereal sulphates, phosphates or glucuronides, while dihydrodiols may be conjugated with glucuronic acid. It is not intended to list the known aromatic hydroxylations found in the metabolism of drugs. These have been discussed and reviewed elsewhere (Williams, 1959; Parke, 1968).

A number of reports have appeared recently on the metabolism of some allyl barbiturates, which indicate that these compounds are converted to epoxides. However, it is thought that the parent compounds are responsible for the sedative and hypnotic effects of this group of compounds and that metabolism is important for excretion. The rate of metabolism will therefore affect their duration of action. Epoxides of diallyl-, 5-allyl-5-phenyl- and 5-allyl-5-(1-methylbutyl)barbituric acid were identified in the urine of rats given the parent compounds (Harvey *et al*, 1972a).

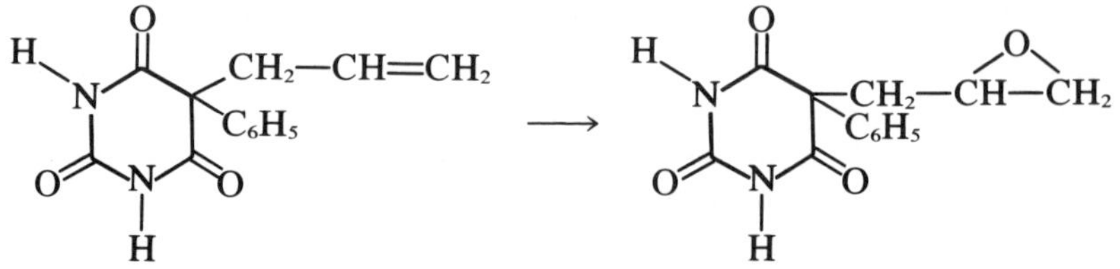

Diols formed by the hydration of the epoxides were detected as major metabolites in all three cases, the hydration being partially enzymic. It was suggested that the epoxide intermediates were the metabolites responsible for the toxicity of these barbiturates, so that the rate of hydration would have an important bearing on the severity of the side effects produced.

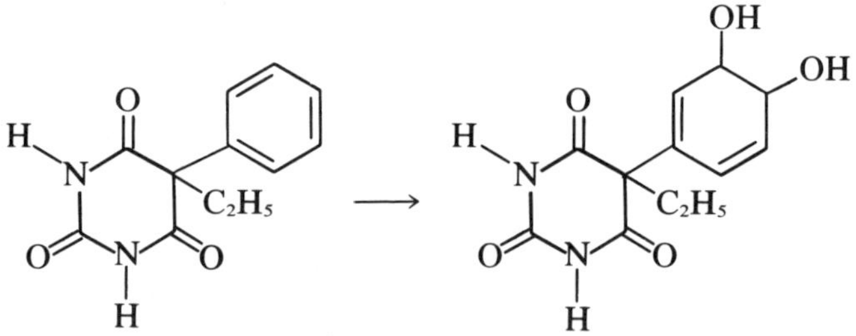

5-(3,4-Dihydroxycyclohexadienyl-1-yl) metabolites were also identified during the metabolism of either phenobarbitone or mephobarbitone in the rat, guinea pig and human (Harvey *et al*, 1972b). There are a number of other olefinic and aromatic barbiturates substituted at the 5 position and it is possible that a number of these might be converted to epoxides during their metabolism (Table 1).

Trichloroethylene, once used as an anaesthetic or dry-cleaning agent, is converted by rat-, rabbit- and dog-liver microsomes in an NADPH-dependent reaction to chloral hydrate. The metabolism is thought to proceed through an intermediate epoxide derivative as set out below (Byington and Leibman, 1965).

In the presence of warfarin, vitamin K is converted to its oxide by rat liver. The oxide still retains vitamin-K activity, and traces of it can be found in the liver and heart of rats fed vitamin K (Matschiner *et al*, 1970).

Table 1 Some barbiturates which may be converted to epoxides

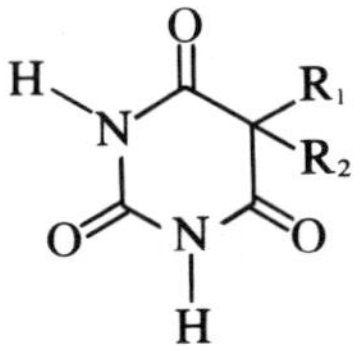

Compound	R_1	R_2
Aprobarbitone	allyl	isopropyl
Cyclobarbitone	ethyl	cyclohexenyl
Heptabarbitone	ethyl	1-cyclohepten-1-yl
Vinbarbitone	ethyl	1-methyl-1-butenyl
Hexobarbitone	methyl	cyclohexenyl

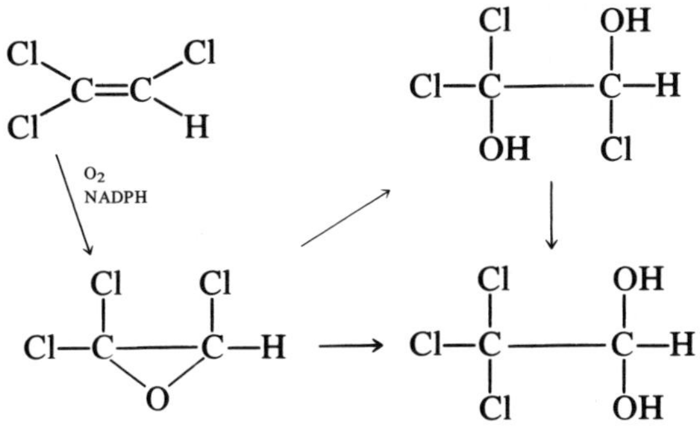

$Cl_2C{=}CHCl \xrightarrow{O_2,\ NADPH}$ Cl—C(Cl)(Cl)—C(Cl)(H) epoxide (O) $\longrightarrow$ CCl_3—CH(OH)(OH); epoxide $\rightarrow$ $CCl_2(OH)$—CH(OH)Cl $\rightarrow$ CCl_3—CH(OH)(OH)

Whether the oxide of vitamin K is important for vitamin-K activity is not known. Interestingly, after vitamin K administration the compound is quickly eliminated, indicating rapid metabolism. Patients with liver disease or injury suffer from hypoprothrombinaemia and this usually parallels the extent of liver injury. Often these patients fail to respond to vitamin-K administration, perhaps because of a failure to convert the compound to its oxide.

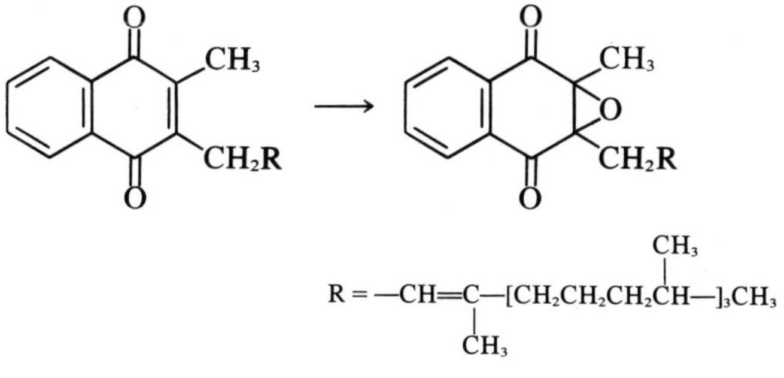

$R = $ —CH=C(CH_3)—[$CH_2CH_2CH_2CH(CH_3)$—]$_3CH_3$

Epoxides from Steroids

There have been only a few reports on the conversion of steroids to epoxides but this may be because not much work has been done in this area rather than because epoxidation is a rare event. Incubation of 16α,17α-oestratriene-3-ol with rat-liver slices converted the compound to its 16α,17α-epoxy derivative. The epoxide could be hydrated enzymically to the trans dihydrodiol (Breuer and Knuppen, 1960).

Using ^{14}C squalene, it has been demonstrated that rat-liver homogenates convert this molecule to its 2,3 oxide and that this epoxidation is a prerequisite for lanosterol formation (Corey *et al*, 1966a).

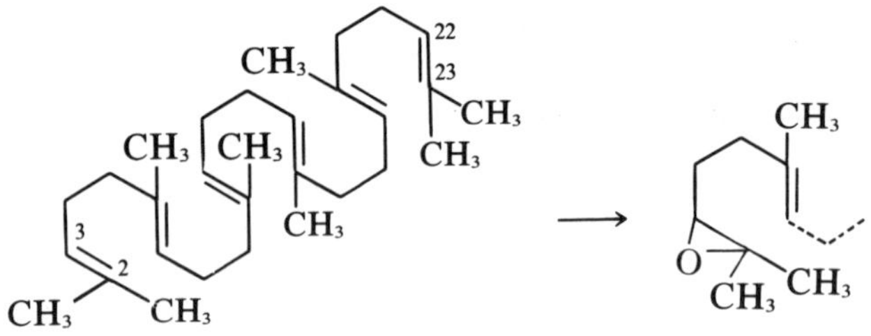

If 10,11-*all trans*-dihydrosqualene was used in place of squalene, no cyclization to lanosterol took place. It could be shown, however, that both the 22,23 as well as the 2,3 double bond had been epoxidized, but the resulting compound was unable to undergo the cyclization reaction to lanosterol (Corey and Russey, 1966). The microsomal enzyme carrying out this epoxidation, squalene epoxidase, requires NADPH and oxygen but does not follow the normal pattern of mixed-function oxidations since a supernatant factor is said to be also required for activity. The enzyme is relatively resistant to inhibition by carbon monoxide and is not affected by either potassium cyanide or sodium azide. Unsaturated fatty acids, such as oleate and linoleate, are potent inhibitors of the enzyme (Yamamoto and Bloch, 1970).

These examples of steroid epoxidation are advantageous to the host animal but not all epoxidations might be so. It is known that there is a close correlation between exposure to strong sunlight and the incidence of human-skin cancer. Most workers would probably ascribe this correspondence to the formation of thymine–thymine dimers in the DNA of the epithelial cells induced by the ultra-violet light. Support for this concept stems from the fact that certain people who have a genetic deficiency in the enzyme required to repair this damaged DNA are much more susceptible to skin cancer than normal individuals (Cleaver and Trosko, 1970). However, there are a group of patients who exhibit all the symptoms of this genetically linked disease known as *xeroderma pigmentosum*, but whose skin cells have normal DNA-repair ability (Robbins and Burk, 1973). Some other mechanism of skin-cancer induction must be postulated to occur in these patients. One such alternative has been proposed by Black and his co-workers. They have suggested that ultra-violet light converts steroids in the skin to carcinogenic molecules: thus cholesterol is converted to cholesterol-α-oxide (Black and Lo, 1971) in human skin. This molecule has been shown to have weak carcinogenic properties in both mouse and rat skin (Bischoff, 1969). In hairless mice the production of the oxide was proportional to the amount of irradiation; the skin concentration of the oxide increased with chronic exposure up to a maximum just prior to the first appearance of tumours (Black and Douglas, 1973). Whether one can regard oxide formation as a tumour-promoting as opposed to an initiating event has not been investigated.

9,11-Dehydrocortexolone is converted by 11β-hydroxylase of adrenal cortex mitochondria in the presence of NADPH and oxygen to 9β,11β-oxidocortexolone (Sih, 1949).

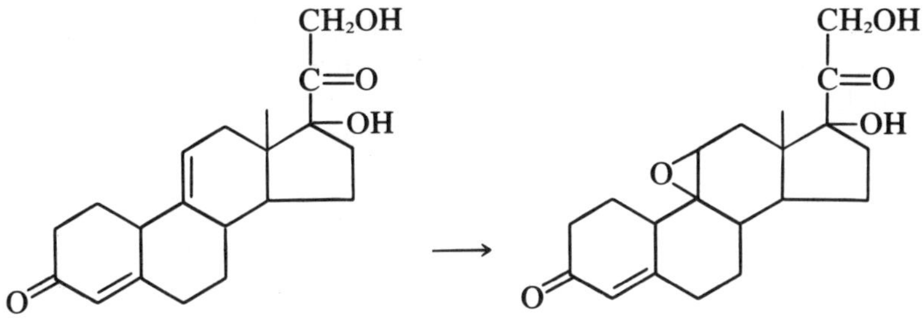

It is probable that a number of other steroids are epoxidized since they have the necessary structural features for such a conversion, e.g. allyl and ethinyloestranol. Also 1,2 and 3,4 epoxides may be produced during the formation of oestrogen–glutathione conjugates (Chasseaud, 1973). After 2-hydroxylation of 17β-oestradiol, the product 2-hydroxy-17β-oestradiol undergoes the complete mercapturic acid biosynthesis *in vitro* (Elce, 1971) and *in vivo* (Elce, 1970; Elce and Harris, 1971).

Epoxides from Pesticides

As mentioned previously, the epoxide of heptachlor was the first biologically produced epoxide to be isolated (Davidow and Radomski, 1953). A number of other insecticide epoxides have been demonstrated during olefinic insecticide metabolism, probably because they are stable molecules and poor substrates for epoxide hydrase (Oesch *et al*, 1971a).

Male and female rat-liver microsomes can convert aldrin, isodrin (the *endo–exo* isomer of aldrin) and heptachlor to their corresponding epoxides (Wong and Terriere, 1965).

In all cases, female rats produced less than males, this perhaps accounting for their greater resistance to the toxic effects of aldrin and heptachlor.

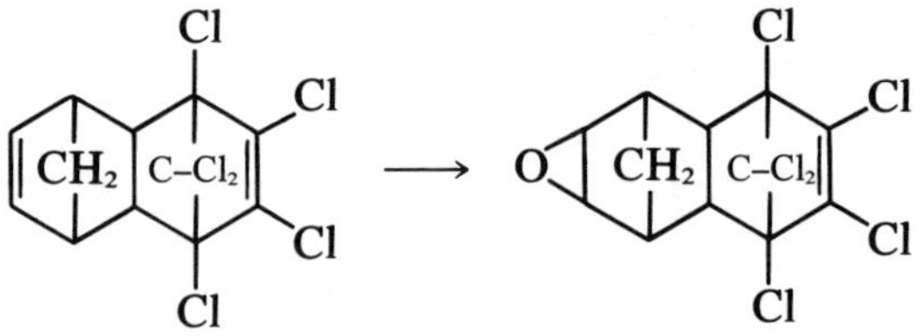

Aldrin → Dieldrin

Interestingly, only the epoxides were identified as metabolites, there being no further conversion to dihydrodiols. It should be pointed out that the insecticidal activity of pesticides, such as aldrin, is probably dependent on conversion to an epoxide; aldrin is converted to dieldrin which is considerably more toxic and persistent (Wilkinson *et al*, 1964).

Rabbit-liver microsomes have been reported to convert aldrin, isodrin and heptachlor, to their respective epoxides in an NADPH-dependent reaction (Nakatsuguwa *et al*, 1965). Epoxidation was inhibited by SKF-525A, piperonyl butoxide, parathion and benzenehexachloride. Epoxidase activity was also detected in insect homogenates. Udenfriend's system was not able to simulate the microsomal epoxidase, a finding in agreement with results discussed earlier.

In a very elegant experiment to demonstrate that aldrin must be converted to dieldrin for insecticidal activity, Brooks and his colleagues showed that flies given aldrin but kept in an atmosphere of nitrogen, showed no ill effects. As soon as the nitrogen was replaced by oxygen, knockdown ensued (Brooks *et al*, 1963). If the insects were administered dieldrin, knockdown took place immediately, even if they were in a nitrogen atmosphere. This demonstrated that epoxidation was essential for insecticidal activity. Besides insects and mammals, freshwater fish can also convert aldrin to dieldrin, clearly showing that fish have the ability to form epoxides (Ludka *et al*, 1972).

There do appear to be certain stereochemical requirements for the toxicity of particular insecticide epoxides. For example, compound **1** has an LD_{50} of 0·01 μg whereas the LD_{50} for compound **2** is 0·12 μg per female housefly (Brooks and Harrison, 1965).

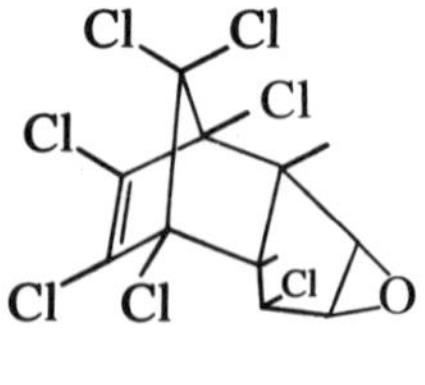

(1) 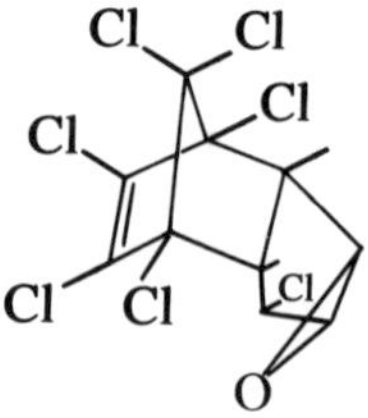 **(2)**

There is also a stereochemical specificity for conversion of insecticidal epoxides to dihydrodiols. Pig-liver microsomes will metabolize only half of a *cis–trans* mixture of chlordane or hexachloronaphthalene to the *trans* diol indicating that epoxide hydrase will attack only one enantiomer of the racemic mixture (Brooks *et al*, 1968).

In this chapter, epoxidation of carbon–carbon double bonds has so far been discussed. In what are probably the only examples demonstrated to date of epoxidation of non-carbon–carbon double bonds, Ptashne and Neal (1972) in studies of the metabolism of parathion and malathion suggested that epoxidation of a phosphorus–sulphur bond occurs. In a model system using peroxytrifluoroacetic acid they found that these two insecticides were converted to products identical to those formed during their biological oxidation.

$$(H_5C_2O)_2—P(\rightarrow S)—O—C_6H_4—NO_2 \longrightarrow [(H_5C_2O)_2—P(—O—S)—O—C_6H_4—NO_2] \longrightarrow (H_5C_2O)_2—P(\rightarrow O)—O—C_6H_4—NO_2$$

Parathion

Paraoxon

Since it has been previously demonstrated that peroxytrifluoroacetic acid is a good model for metabolic transformations through an epoxide mechanism, it is probable that the conversion of these phosphorothionate insecticides proceeds via the same route. Support for this is the observation that one atom of oxygen-18 is incorporated into parathion during its metabolism to the bioactive paraoxon (Ptashne *et al*, 1971).

Epoxides from Polycyclic Hydrocarbons

These compounds are made up of a number of fused benzene rings joined together in a variety of ways. Although at least four such rings are apparently necessary for carcinogenic activity, this section will also consider the metabolism of benzene to show the major biotransformation steps that this group of compounds can undergo. The polycyclic hydrocarbons are intimately associated with certain human cancers and may be the causative agents of a number of others. They are widely distributed in the environment and are associated with pyrolysed organic matter, ranging from cigarette smoke, through well-cooked steak, to car-exhaust fumes. The first well-documented report of polycyclic-hydrocarbon-associated cancer was presented in 1775 when a London surgeon, Percivall Pott, described the high incidence of scrotal cancer in chimney sweeps, and suggested that this was because of gross contact with soot. The historical aspects of hydrocarbon carcinogenesis have been extensively reviewed (Clayson, 1962; Hueper and Conway, 1964). Coal tar induced carcinomas of the skin of rabbits' ears (Yamagiwa and Ichikawa, 1918) were the first experimentally induced animal tumours to be reported, and dibenz[*a*,*h*]anthracene was the first pure chemical to be isolated and shown to induce cancer in animals (Kennaway and Hieger, 1930). Extensive studies have been carried out since this time on structure-activity relationships and their importance for carcinogenesis. Most of these studies have only used two methods of application—skin painting or subcutaneous injection in mice. Neither of these test systems is entirely satisfactory so that much of the old data might have to be re-evaluated. For a critique of what is now known about hydrocarbons, the IARC monograph (1973) should be consulted. It is not proposed to list all the polycyclic hydrocarbons known, their carcinogenic activity or the influence of substituents, but to discuss what is known about hydrocarbon metabolism and what the importance of epoxide formation might be for carcinogenic activity. A more detailed review of this group of compounds is well presented by Sims and Grover (1974).

Typical metabolites found after biotransformation of aromatic compounds. Earlier on in this chapter, the evidence for epoxide formation during aromatic hydroxylation was discussed. Much of what is known about polycyclic-hydrocarbon metabolism stems from the work of Boyland, Sims and Grover.

Levi and Boyland showed, as long ago as 1935, that the rat converted anthracene to 1,2-dihydroxy-1,2-dihydroanthracene which appeared in the urine together with a mercapturic acid derivative. As the configuration of the two alcoholic groups was not known, these workers were not able to suggest a mechanism of diol formation. Cook and Schoental (1948) noted that chrysene, 3-methylcholanthrene and benz[*a*]anthracene were converted by osmium tetroxide to diols which were later shown to resemble those found after the metabolism of these compounds in animals. It was at first thought that diol formation might arise through an osmium-tetroxide type of attack in which a *cis* diol would be produced. Boyland (1950) suggested that all the known metabolites of the hydrocarbons could arise through formation of an intermediate epoxide, but it was not possible to prove this hypothesis for a long time because of difficulties in preparing polycyclic hydrocarbon epoxides. Pullman and Pullman (1955) used a molecular-orbital approach to calculate the activation energy of the phenanthrenoid bond which is the most reactive bond for a number of carcinogenic hydrocarbons and has considerable double-bond character. The bond was called the K-region double bond and was considered to be essential for carcinogenicity.

As discussed earlier, once the hydrocarbon epoxides could be chemically synthesized, it was not long before they were identified during hydrocarbon metabolism. The identification of naphthalene epoxide as a metabolite during the metabolism of naphthalene is an example.

General pattern of metabolites found after aromatic hydroxylation. The metabolism of benzene can be used as a model for hydrocarbon metabolism since most of the products formed typify those found during polycyclic-hydrocarbon metabolism. Metabolites of benzene which have been identified are a mercapturic-acid derivative found in the urine of animals administered benzene (Knight and Young, 1958); a dihydrodiol (Sato *et al*, 1963) and phenol. The phenolic group can be inserted in a number of positions depending on which double bond is epoxidized and also which rearrangement is the more energetically favoured. For example, toluene is hydroxylated at the *ortho* and *para* positions because either the 1,2 or the 3,4 double bond is epoxidized. Rearrangement of benzene epoxide to phenol is probably a nonenzymic reaction despite earlier reports suggesting that it was protein catalysed (Jerina *et al*, 1968). Thus, Sims and co-workers did not find that denatured protein catalysed the rearrangement of polycyclic-hydrocarbon epoxides to phenols (Swaisland *et al*, 1973).

The phenols formed during metabolism may themselves be further conjugated with sulphate or glucuronic acid by enzymes in the liver and the conjugates are then excreted in the urine. Figure 2 shows the various pathways for benzene metabolism and the enzymes responsible.

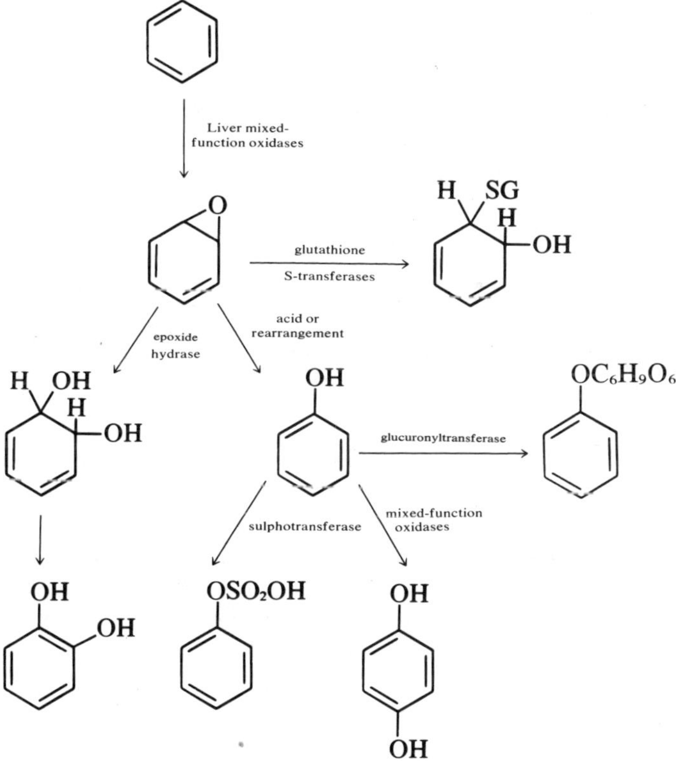

Figure 2 Metabolic pathway of benzene

Levels as low as 400 ppm of benzene are sufficient to induce blood dyscrasias in exposed persons, aplastic anaemia being a common finding. It is likely that benzene epoxide is responsible for those toxic symptoms since administration of phenol, although toxic, does not induce such blood disorders and benzene itself is chemically rather inert. Some patients with aplastic anaemia due to benzene exposure have later developed leukaemia.

Metabolism of well-known polycyclic hydrocarbons and the biological activity of some of the metabolites. Since the polycyclic hydrocarbons are aromatic compounds, they can be hydroxylated at any one of several double-bond positions in the rings. Work has beem mainly concerned with metabolism at the K-region, this being the most reactive position, and epoxides at the K-region seem to be easier to prepare than at other positions.

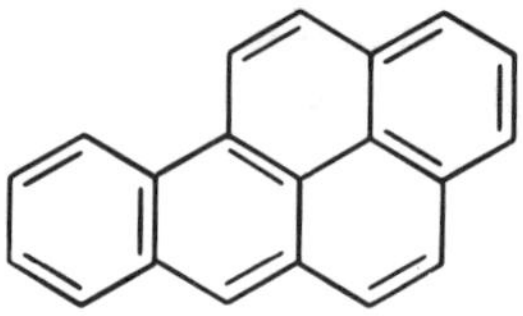

K-region

From the hypothesis of the Pullmans, it might be expected that metabolism at the K-region is essential for carcinogenicity of this group of compounds since molecules without a K-region are apparently noncarcinogenic. Other alternative activation mechanisms to epoxide formation will be discussed later.

In this section, it is not intended to examine in depth the metabolism of each polycyclic hydrocarbon but to discuss the biological activity of some derivatives formed during metabolism. In Table 2 the structures of a number of hydrocarbons are set out together with some of the known metabolites.

Phenanthrene. Under conditions in which the activity of epoxide hydrase was inhibited, production of the 9,10 epoxide has been demonstrated *in vitro* using rat-liver microsomes (Grover *et al*, 1971a). Phenanthrene is a noncarcinogen, and the 9,10 oxide has little biological activity. It is nonmutagenic to *Salmonella typhimurium* (Ames *et al*, 1972) or T_2 *phage* (Cookson *et al*, 1971) although it has some reactivity towards cellular macromolecules of cells in culture. The 9,10 oxide had greater reactivity with DNA, RNA and protein in polyoma virus-transformed and normal baby-hamster kidney cells, than phenanthrene, the 9,10 dihydrodiol or the 9 phenol, although the extent of reaction was less than with benz[*a*]anthracene-5,6-oxide (Grover *et al*, 1971b). The extent of reaction *in vitro* with DNA, RNA and apurinic

Table 2 Polycyclic hydrocarbon metabolites identified *in vivo* or *in vitro* (figures in parenthesis are to references which can be found at the end of the table)

Compound	Position metabolized	Dihydroxydihydro	Phenol	Glutathione conjugate	Epoxide	Others
Toluene 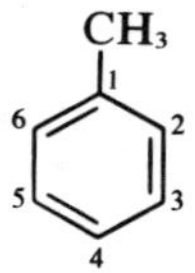	1,2- 3,4-	1,2-[16]	2-[17] 4-[17] 2,4- 2,4,6-	2-[18]		
Naphthalene 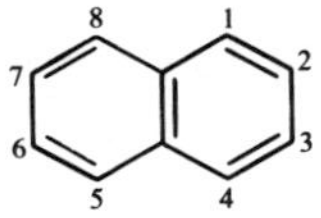	1,2-	1,2-[13,15]	1-[13] 2-[13]	1-[13]	1,2-[12]	
Anthracene 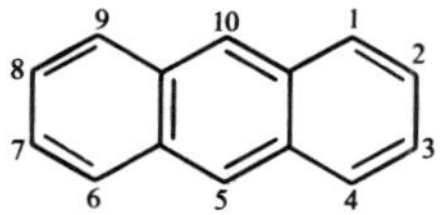	1,2-	1,2-[14]	1- 2-			
Phenanthrene 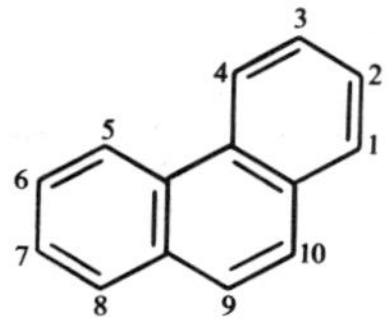	1,2- 3,4- 9,10-	9,10[11,15]	1-[2] 2- 3- 4- 9- 10-	9-[20]	9,10-[9]	

Table 2 *Cont'd*

Compound	Position metabolized	Dihydroxydihydro	Phenol	Glutathione conjugate	Epoxide	Others
Pyrene 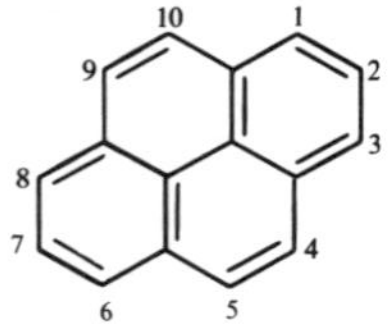	1,2- 4,5-	4,5-[8]	1-[32] 2-[32] 4-[2,8]		4,5-[8]	
3-Methylcholanthrene 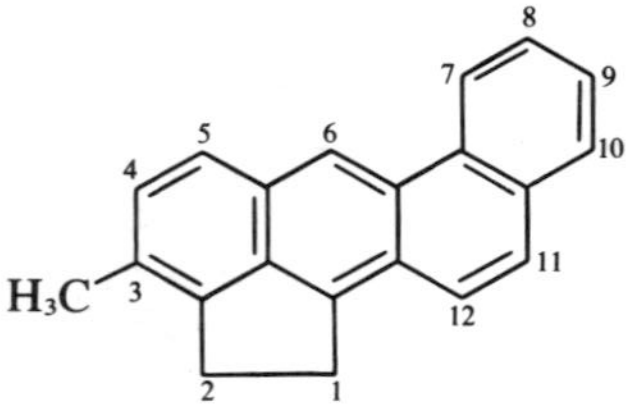	1- 2- 3- 11,12-	11,12-[30]	11-[30]	11-[31]		3-Hydroxymethyl 1-Hydroxy 2-Hydroxy 1,2-Hydroxy 1-Keto 2-Keto 1,2-Diketo
Benzo[*a*]pyrene 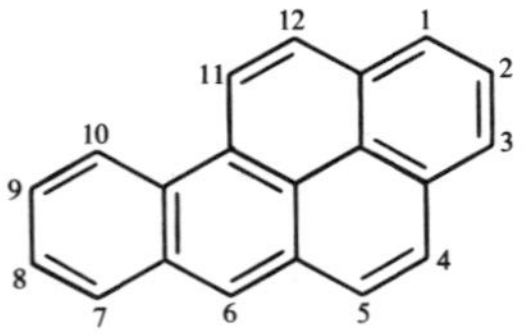	1,2- 2,3- 4,5- 7,8- 9,10-	4,5-[6,8] 7,8-[6,30] 9,10-[6,8,30]	1-[7] 4-[8] 6-[7] 7-[29] 3-[7] 8-[7] 9-[7]		4,5-[8]	1,6-Quinone[6] 3,6-Quinone[6]

Benzo[*e*]pyrene 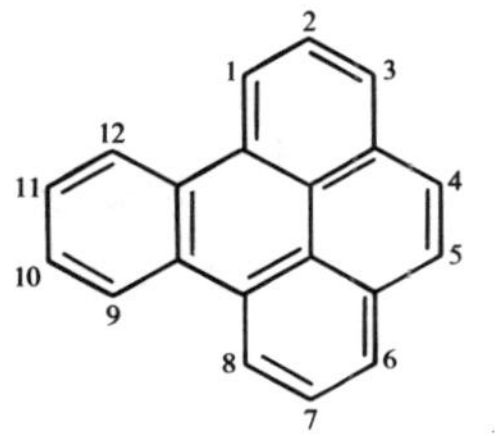	4,5-	4,5-[2]	4- 5-	
Dibenz[*a*,*c*]anthracene 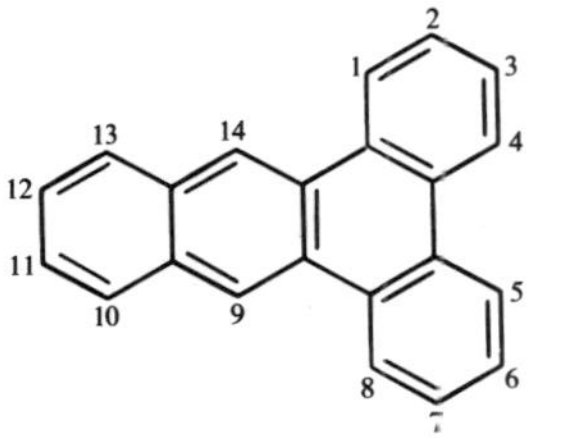	10,11-	10,11-[27]	10-[27]	
Dibenz[*a*,*h*]anthracene 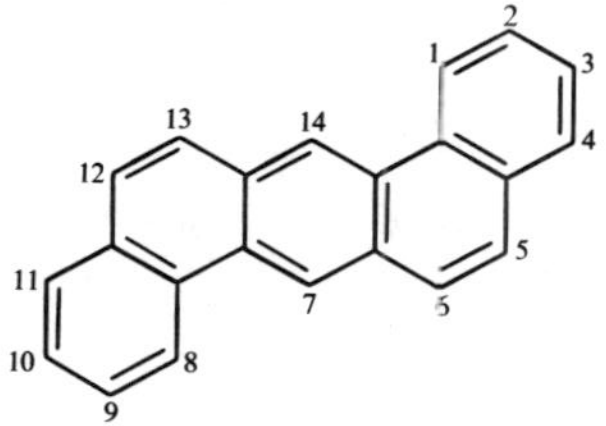	1,2- 3,4- 5,6- 9,10- 7- 14-	3,4- 5,6-	3- 4- 5-[10]	5,6-[9]

Table 2 *Cont'd*

Compound	Position metabolized	Dihydroxydihydro	Phenol	Glutathione conjugate	Epoxide	Others
Benz[*a*]anthracene	1,2-		2-			
	3,4-		4-			
	5,6-	5,6-[10]	5-[21]	5-[10]	5,6-[9,29]	
	8,9-	8,9-[23]	8-[10]			8-[24]
	10,11-		9-[23]			
Chrysene	1,2-	1,2-	1-[2]			
	3,4-	3,4-	2-			
	5,6-		3-			
			4-			
			5-			
			6-			
7-Methylbenz[*a*]anthracene	3,4-		3-		5,6-[20]	7-Hydroxy[28] methyl
	5,6-	5,6-[28]	4-			
	8,9-	8,9-[2,3,4]	5-			
	10,11-	10,11-[3,4,28]				
	7-methyl					

	3,4-	8,9-	3-			methyl
	5,6-		4-			
	8,9-					
	10,11-					
	12-methyl					
7,12-Dimethylbenz[*a*]anthracene	2,3-		2-			
	3,4-		3-			
	5,6-	5,6-[19,25,28]	4-			
	8,9-	8,9-[2,3,4,19]	5-[20]	5-[4,5,20,26,28]	5,6-[5,20]	7-Hydroxy[1,22] methyl or 12-hydroxy[1,22] methyl
	10,11-					
	7-methyl	10,11-[3,4,28]				
	12-methyl					

1. Boyland, E. and Sims, P. (1965), *Biochem. J.*, **95**, 780.
2. Sims, P. (1970), *Biochem. Pharmacol.*, **19**, 795.
3. Sims, P. (1970), *Biochem. Pharmacol.*, **19**, 2261.
4. Booth, J., Keysell, G. R. and Sims, P. (1973), *Biochem. Pharmacol.*, **22**, 1781.
5. Keysell, G. R., Booth, J., Sims, P., Grover, P. L. and Hewer, A. (1972), *Biochem. J.*, **129**, 41.
6. Borgen, A., Darvey, H., Castagnoli, N., Crocker, T. T., Rasmussen, R. E. and Wang, I. Y. (1973), *J. Med. Chem.*, **16**, 502.
7. Sims, P. (1967), *Biochem. Pharmacol.*, **16**, 613.
8. Grover, P. L., Hewer, A. and Sims, P. (1972), *Biochem. Pharmacol.*, **21**, 2713.
9. Grover, P. L., Hewer, A. and Sims, P. (1971), *FEBS Lett.*, **18**, 76.
10. Boyland, E. and Sims, P. (1965), *Biochem. J.*, **97**, 7.
11. Boyland, E. and Sims, P. (1962), *Biochem. J.* **84**, 571.
12. Jerina, D. M., Daly, J. W., Witkop, B., Zaltzmann-Nirenberg, P. and Udenfriend, S. (1970), *Biochemistry*, **9**, 147.
13. Booth, J., Boyland, E., Sato, T. and Sims, P. (1960), *Biochem. J.*, **22**, 182.
14. Boyland, E. and Levi, A. A. (1935), *Biochem. J.*, **29**, 2679.
15. Young, L. (1947), *Biochem. J.*, **41**, 417.
16. Sato, T., Fukuyama, T., Suzuki, T. and Yoshikawa, H. (1963), *J. Biochem.* (Japan), **53**, 23.
17. Jerina, D., Daly, J., Witkop, B., Zaltzmann-Nirenberg, P. and Udenfriend, S. (1968), *Arch. Biochem. Biophys.*, **128**, 176.
18. Knight, R. H. and Young, L. (1958), *Biochem. J.*, **70**, 111.
19. Boyland, E. and Sims, P. (1967), *Biochem. J.*, **104**, 394.
20. Keysell, G. R., Booth, J., Grover, P. L., Hewer, A. and Sims, P. (1973), *Biochem. Pharmacol.*, **22**, 2853.
21. Sims, P., Grover, P. L., Kuroki, T., Huberman, E., Marquardt, H., Selkirk, J. K. and Heidelberger, C. (1973), *Biochem. Pharmacol.*, **22**, 1.
22. Boyland, E. and Sims, P. (1965), *Biochem. J.*, **95**, 780.
23. Boyland, E. and Sims, P. (1964), *Biochem. J.*, **91**, 493.
24. Sims, P., (1971), *Biochem. J.*, **125**, 159.
25. Sims, P. and Grover, P. L., (1968), *Biochem. Pharmacol.*, **17**, 1751.
26. Sims, P. (1973), *Biochem. J.*, **131**, 405.
27. Sims, P. (1972), *Biochem. J.*, **130**, 27.
28. Sims, P. (1967), *Biochem. J.*, **105**, 591.
29. Waterfall, J. F. and Sims, P. (1972), *Biochem. J.*, **128**, 265.
30. Sims, P. (1966), *Biochem. J.*, **98**, 215.
31. Grover, P. L., Hewer, A. and Sims, P. (1973), *FEBS Lett.*, **34**, 63.
32. Boyland, E. and Sims, P. (1964), *Biochem. J.*, **90**, 391.
33. Sims, P. (1967), *Biochem. Pharmacol.*, **16**, 613.

acid, was 0·015, 0·007 and 0·007 mmol/mol phosphorus respectively (Grover and Sims, 1972). 9,10-Epoxyphenanthrene rearranges only slowly to 9-phenanthrenol at neutral pH compared with some of the epoxides of the methyl-substituted hydrocarbons (Swaisland *et al*, 1973).

It is perhaps surprising that an epoxide of a noncarcinogenic hydrocarbon binds to cellular macromolecules if such binding is important in the carcinogenic or mutagenic process. It should be emphasized, however, that it may not be the amount of binding which is important but the rate of removal of the bound form or the fidelity of insertion of the correct base sequences into the gaps remaining after excision of the alkylated bases from nucleic acids.

Chrysene. This hydrocarbon is generally considered a noncarcinogen although it may have weak tumour-initiating activity in mouse skin (van Duuren *et al*, 1966). The compound is metabolized at the 1,2; 3,4 and perhaps at the 5,6 positions (Sims, 1970). Although the 5,6 oxide can be synthesized, it has not been identified as a metabolite although the 5-hydroxy derivative has. Chrysene 5,6 oxide is nonmutagenic to *Salmonella typhimurium* (Ames *et al*, 1972) and to T_2 *phage* (Cookson *et al*, 1971) and does not transform mouse prostate cells in culture (Marquardt *et al*, 1972), but does transform hamster embryo cells (Huberman *et al*, 1972) while the parent hydrocarbon does not.

Benz[a]anthracene. Metabolism has been shown for this compound, which is a weak carcinogen, at the 1,2; 3,4; 5,6; 8,9 and 10,11 double bonds (Sims, 1970, 1971). The 5,6 oxide (K-region) was mutagenic to *Salmonella typhimurium* whereas the 8,9 oxide (non-K-region) was inactive (Ames *et al*, 1972); the 5,6 oxide was nonmutagenic to T_2 *phage* (Cookson *et al*, 1971). The 5,6-oxide transformed mouse prostate cells while the 8,9 oxide had only weak activity (Marquardt *et al*, 1972). The 5,6 dihydrodiol had some transforming activity in these cells but the phenol and the parent hydrocarbon were inactive although the phenol was cytotoxic (Grover *et al*, 1971b). The 5,6 oxide has been definitely established as a metabolite produced by rat-liver microsomes (Grover *et al*, 1971a) and human lung (Grover *et al*, 1973). In hamster embryo cells, the 5,6 oxide bound more to protein than to RNA or DNA and reacted with these more extensively than did the 5 phenol, 5,6 dihydrodiol or benz[*a*]anthracene (Kuroki *et al*, 1971/2). In studies on the metabolism of 5,6 oxide in these cells, the major metabolite identified was the 5,6 dihydrodiol (Sims *et al*, 1973). There was little difference between the rate of rearrangement of the 5,6 oxide and the 8,9 oxide to their respective phenols (Swaisland *et al*, 1973). The 5,6 oxide stimulated unscheduled DNA-repair synthesis in cultured human lymphocytes and fibroblasts whereas the 5,6 dihydrodiol and the parent compound did not (Stich and San, 1973).

Dibenz[a,c]anthracene. This compound does not possess a K-region and is only weakly active as a carcinogen. Metabolism of the compound occurs at the 10,11 double bond; a 10,11-dihydrodiol derivative is formed on metabolism by rat-liver homogenate. Synthetic 10,11 oxide was converted to the dihydrodiol by rat-liver homogenate, a reaction catalysed by epoxide hydrase. Surprisingly, the oxide did not react enzymically or nonenzymically with glutathione but was rapidly converted to the 10, or 11 phenol by acid. Compared to the 5,6 oxide of dibenz[*a,h*]anthracene the 10,11 oxide was much less reactive as an alkylating agent (Sims, 1972a).

Dibenz[a,h]anthracene. This compound is carcinogenic both by skin painting and subcutaneous injection. It is metabolized at positions 1,2; 3,4; 5,6; 9,10; 7 and 14. The 5,6 oxide is only a weak carcinogen compared to the parent hydrocarbon in the mouse-skin initiation test (van Duuren *et al*, 1967), and is nonmutagenic to a *Salmonella typhimurium* strain which appears to be impermeable while the same strain with a permeable cell wall can be mutated (Ames *et al*, 1972). An epoxide has been positively identified as a metabolite of the parent compound in rat-liver microsomal preparations (Grover *et al*, 1971a; Selkirk *et al*, 1971) and the 5,6 oxide has a number of biological activities. It is mutagenic to T_2 *phage* (Cookson *et al*, 1971) and will transform hamster embryo (Huberman *et al*, 1972) and mouse-prostate cells in culture (Marquardt *et al*, 1972). The parent hydrocarbon, the *trans*- or *cis*-5,6 dihydrodiol and the 5 phenol were much less active or inactive. The oxide reacted equally with DNA or RNA and much less with apurinic acid, and the extent of reaction was much greater than with phenanthrene oxide (Grover and Sims, 1972). Hamster embryo cells converted more of the oxide to the phenol than to the dihydrodiol (Sims *et al*, 1973).

7-Methylbenz[a]anthracene. Substitution of the anthracene nucleus with a methyl group in any position increases the carcinogenicity of this compound. 7-Methylbenz[*a*]anthracene is a potent carcinogen in the mouse when applied to the skin or by subcutaneous injection (Heuper and Conway, 1964). Not only can the compound be attacked at the 2,3; 3,4; 5,6; 8,9 or 10,11 double bonds, but the methyl group can be also hydroxylated. The 5,6 oxide of 7-methylbenz[*a*]anthracene is mutagenic to *Salmonella typhimurium* (Ames *et al*, 1972) and T_2 *phage* (Cookson *et al*, 1971), reacts extensively with DNA or RNA *in vitro* (Grover and Sims, 1972) and will transform hamster-embryo cells (Huberman *et al*, 1972). However, the compound was only weakly carcinogenic in the mouse (Miller and Miller, 1967) compared to the parent hydrocarbon. The 5,6 oxide of 7-hydroxymethylbenz[*a*]anthracene was less reactive with 4-(*p*-nitrobenzyl) pyridine than the 5,6 oxide of 7-methylbenz[*a*]anthracene (Sims, 1972b).

7,12-Dimethylbenz[a]anthracene. This compound, which has been extensively studied, is a very strong carcinogen for mouse skin although it induces a lower tumour incidence than 3-methylcholanthrene or benzo[*a*]pyrene; however, it has a latent period only half as long as these two chemicals. It is metabolized at the 2,3; 3,4; 5,6; 8,9 and 10,11 positions besides being hydroxylated on the 7- or 12-methyl groups (Sims, 1970). The 5,6 oxide has been identified as a metabolite in rat-liver microsomes in which the activity of epoxide hydrase was inhibited (Keysell *et al*, 1972; Keysell *et al*, 1973). The 5,6 oxide transformed mouse-prostate cells but was not as active as the parent compound. 7-Bromomethylbenz[*a*]anthracene and 7-bromomethyl-12-methylbenz[*a*]anthracene, two compounds which have been synthesized as models of the ultimate electrophilic species of the two parent hydrocarbons (Dipple and Slade, 1972) were not as active as the parent compounds in transforming mouse-prostrate (Marquardt *et al*, 1972) or hamster-embryo cells (Huberman *et al*, 1972). It has been proposed that the formation of the 7-hydroxymethyl derivatives may be the first step in tumour initiation by 7,12-dimethylbenz[*a*]anthracene (Flesher and Sydnor, 1971), but this may not be the case as the hydroxymethyl derivative can be further metabolized to a 5,6 oxide (Keysell *et al*, 1973). The 5,6 oxides of 7-hydroxymethyl-12-methylbenz[*a*]anthracene and 7,12-dimethylbenz[*a*]anthracene-5,6-oxide were more active than the 5,6 oxides of 7-methylbenz[*a*]anthracene and benz[*a*]anthracene in alkylating 4-(*p*-nitrobenzyl)pyridine (Sims, 1973).

Benzo[*a*]*pyrene*. This compound has been extensively investigated because of its wide distribution in the human environment and also because it is a potent animal carcinogen. The compound is metabolized at the 1,2; 2,3; 4,5; 7,8 and 9,10 double bonds. The epoxide at the 4,5 position has been definitely identified as a metabolite formed during metabolism by rat-liver microsomes (Grover *et al*, 1972) and an epoxide has been shown to react with DNA (Wang *et al*, 1972) after isolation from a hamster-liver microsomal system. The non-K-region epoxides at the 7,8 and 9,10 positions have been synthesized. They easily rearrange to the respective phenols and are converted by rat-liver homogenates to the *trans* dihydrodiols. There was little evidence for formation of glutathione conjugates during the *in vitro* metabolism (Waterfall and Sims, 1972). Production of an active metabolite of benzo[*a*]pyrene by liver microsomes, which could bind to DNA, was one of the first reports to indicate that a metabolite of a hydrocarbon probably had chemical reactivity (Grover and Sims, 1968; Gelboin, 1969) although Brookes and Lawley (1964) had shown earlier that benzo[*a*]pyrene would bind to mouse-skin DNA. Interestingly, 7,8-dihydrobenzo[*a*]pyrene proved to be a powerful subcutaneous carcinogen in the mouse, indicating that the 7,8 double bond is not important for biological activity (P. Sims, unpublished results). If 7,8-dihydro-7,8-dihydroxybenzo[*a*]pyrene is used in a microsomal activation assay with DNA, ten times as much metabolite is bound to the DNA than if benzo[*a*]pyrene is used (Borgen *et al*, 1973).

3-Methylcholanthrene. This compound is a potent carcinogen (Hueper and

Conway, 1964) and is metabolized by rat-liver homogenate at the 1, 2, 3-methyl and 11,12 positions (Sims, 1966). The 1,2-methylene bridge appears to be equivalent to methyl groups at the 1 and 2 positions in terms of carcinogenic potency. The 11,12 oxide is nonmutagenic to *Salmonella typhimurium* (Ames *et al*, 1972) but will mutate T_2 *phage* (Cookson *et al*, 1972). It will transform hamster-embryo (Huberman *et al*, 1972) and mouse-prostate cells (Marquardt *et al*, 1972) and is more potent than the parent hydrocarbon.

Cyclopenta[*a*]*phenanthrenes.* This group of compounds has the same ring system as naturally occurring steroids. Some of them are potent carcinogens, particularly compounds which are substituted at the 11 or 17 position (Coombs *et al*, 1973). They are of interest because they might be formed by abnormal steroid metabolism to produce endogenous carcinogens (Hill *et al*, 1971). One of the metabolites of 11-methyl-17-ketocyclopenta[*a*]phenanthrene found in the urine has been recently shown to have the rather unusual oxepine structure indicated below (Coombs, personal communication).

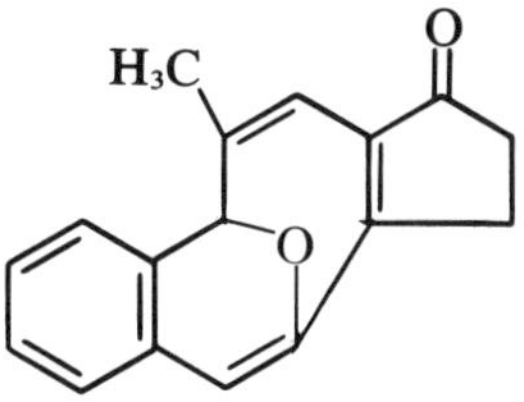

Other possible activation mechanisms. Although the K-region epoxides of a number of hydrocarbons are much more active than the parent compound in mutagenicity assays with bacteria or mammalian cell transformation, the pattern of products seen after reaction of these compounds with macromolecules might not be the same as that found after metabolism of the parent molecule (Baird and Brookes, 1973; Baird *et al*, 1973). When tested for carcinogenicity, a number of K-region epoxides have been found to be considerably less active than the parent compound although this may be because of reaction with noncritical targets within the cell such as glutathione. Consequently, too low a concentration of hydrocarbon epoxides may reach and react with critical cell components. It has been known for some time that irradiation of compounds, such as benzo[*a*]pyrene, in the presence of DNA leads to covalently bound molecules (T'so and Lu, 1964). Using γ-irradiation as much as one molecule of benzo[*a*]pyrene can be bound per 100 nucleotides and not surprisingly, template function of the DNA is impaired (Chan and Ball, 1971; Maher *et al*, 1971). Covalent binding of benzo[*a*]pyrene can also be induced by iodine [Hoffman *et al*, 1970], ferrous iron (Lesko *et al*, 1969) and X-irradiation (Rapaport and T'so, 1966). All these reactions are thought to occur through radical-cation formation. Recently there has been a report that a phenoxide radical of benzo[*a*]pyrene is important for carcinogenicity of this compound (Nagata *et al*, 1973). Injection of Fenton's reagent together with hydrogen peroxide and benzo[*a*]pyrene gave a statistically higher tumour incidence than injection of any of the components alone. Since Fenton's reagent produces the 5-phenoxide radical of benzo[*a*]pyrene, it was proposed that this molecule is the active intermediate.

Although free-radical formation cannot be discounted, so far there is very little biological evidence that such radicals are formed during metabolism of benzo[*a*]pyrene. Experiments must be performed to demonstrate for example an e.s.r. signal during metabolism of the compound. Do these compounds stimulate lipid peroxidation, a common property of free radicals? Until such experiments are done it will not be possible to decide which of the mechanisms are responsible for generation of activated polycyclic-hydrocarbon metabolites.

In summary, the relationship between carcinogenicity and polycyclic-hydrocarbon metabolism is extremely confused. If it is really desired to determine the mechanism of activation then the chemical nature of the macromolecular-bound metabolites must be identified, a tedious but probably fruitful line of research. At the present time the body of evidence still supports the view that hydrocarbons are active through epoxide intermediates, although it may be that these will turn out to be non-K-region epoxides.

Epoxides from Aflatoxins and Related Mycotoxins

These compounds are produced by various species of *Aspergillus*, particularly *Aspergillus flavus*. These are four naturally occurring aflatoxins—B_1, B_2, G_1 and G_2, the structures of which are given below:

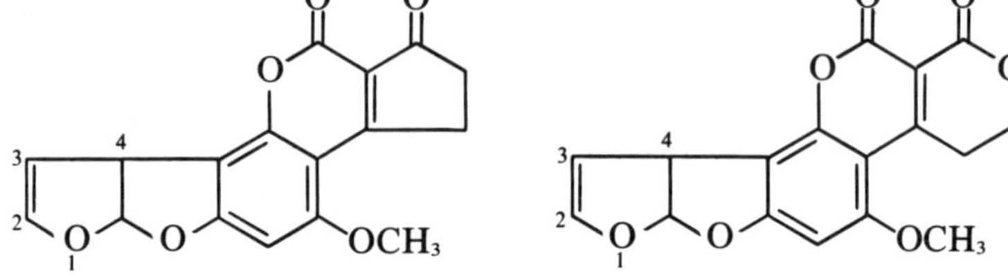

Aflatoxin B_1
Aflatoxin B_2 = 2,3-dihydroaflatoxin B_1

Aflatoxin G_1
Aflatoxin G_2 = 2,3-dihydroaflatoxin G_1

There have been a number of comprehensive reviews on all aspects of the aflatoxins, which should be consulted for a more detailed account (Goldblatt, 1969; Detroy *et al*, 1971).

Aflatoxin B_1, the chief aflatoxin produced by *Aspergillus flavus*, is the most potent liver carcinogen known for the rat. A total dose of less than 100 μg per rat is sufficient to induce a 100% tumour incidence (Wogan and

Newberne, 1967), when given over a 68-week period. If this amount was given as a single injection, no tumours resulted. For development of liver cancer by aflatoxin, continuous exposure to low amounts is essential for tumour induction. Liver tumours have been induced by a single administration of aflatoxin B_1, but a dose of 7 mg/kg, equivalent to an LD_{50} dose, was used (Carnaghan, 1967).

The economic importance of the aflatoxins lies in their widespread distribution in certain areas of the world. A recent report has provided strong evidence that aflatoxin contamination of foods is associated with an increased human-liver cancer incidence (Peers and Linsell, 1973). It is important therefore to know the factors which might affect aflatoxin B_1 carcinogenicity in order to determine what protective measures might be feasible. It should be emphasized that aflatoxin contamination of foods is not only a problem in warm humid climates, but also in the western world which imports large quantities of food from these areas. The human-liver cancer incidence is low in the United Kingdom, for example, but one should at the same time remember that tumours can be induced at sites other than the liver by aflatoxin. A surprising finding is that vitamin-A deficient rats can develop colon carcinomas when given low amounts of aflatoxin B_1 (Newberne and Rogers, 1973). A low incidence of kidney tumours can be induced by aflatoxim B_1 in rats and a number of tumours at other sites have been seen (Butler *et al*, 1969).

Little is known about the mechanism of tumour induction by the aflatoxins, although there have been a large number of reports on the biochemical and pathological changes seen after aflatoxin administration in a wide variety of species. Knowledge of the early events occurring after aflatoxin administration, in particular, the metabolism of the compound is necessary. It is now thought that the first important event after administration of any chemical carcinogen is the conversion of the compound to an electrophilic species, which can occur in one or more steps. The final form has been called by Miller (1970) 'the ultimate carcinogen' and is characterized by its reactivity with nucleophiles. Since within the cell there are a large number of nucleophilic centres, ultimate carcinogens can react with these to give covalently bound conjugates. One or more of these interactions, which can be with DNA, RNA or protein, is thought to initiate the cancer process. It should be emphasized that cancer induction is not solely dependent on these interactions since the latter have been found in noncarcinogenic situations, but will also be governed by other factors such as hormonal and immunological status, cellular replication and repair, etc. For some carcinogens, e.g. nitrosamines (Magee and Barnes, 1967) and aromatic amines (Weisburger and Weisburger, 1973), these initial events are reasonably well understood, whereas for the aflatoxins they are not. If electrophilic attack is a unifying concept of chemical carcinogenesis then it is important to know if the hypothesis fits the most potent chemical carcinogen. However, exactly what hazard aflatoxin exposure is likely to be for man is at present unknown.

Evidence that metabolism of aflatoxin B_1 is important for biological and carcinogenic sensitivity. As already mentioned, aflatoxin B_1 is the most potent of the four naturally occurring aflatoxins and the most studied. It is toxic and/or carcinogenic for a wide species range including fish (Ayres *et al*, 1971), birds, (Carnaghan, 1965), laboratory rodents (Newberne and Butler, 1969) and primates (Adamson *et al*, 1973). This has suggested to some people that metabolic activation may not be a prerequisite for tumour induction, the compound being active *per se*. However, there are a number of facts which do not substantiate this view. Despite the wide species range, there are resistant species to the liver carcinogenic effect, such as adult mice (Wogan, 1969), although new-born mice are sensitive (Vesselinovitch *et al*, 1972). This age difference in sensitivity might be the result of an altered metabolism, but is more likely due to a greater number of liver cells undergoing active DNA replication in the young animals at the time of exposure to the carcinogen. It is known that increased DNA replication increases the tumour incidence for a number of other carcinogens (Warwick, 1971). Other species which are resistant to the carcinogenic effects are the hamster (Herrold, 1969) and possibly the guinea pig (Butler and Barnes, 1963). Such variation is unlikely to occur if the compound did not require metabolic conversion to some other form. There is considerable organ specificity for aflatoxin B_1 tumour induction, the liver being the prime target organ. Tumours have been obtained at other sites as diverse as the submandibular stomach and the Harderian gland (Butler *et al*, 1969). The particular sensitivity of the liver to tumour induction might reside in its capacity to actively convert aflatoxin B_1 to a reactive molecule.

Administration of ^{3}H-labelled aflatoxin B_1 to rats results in covalent binding of radioactivity to cellular macromolecules in the liver (Lijinsky *et al*, 1970). The parent compound is itself unreactive; only weak associations have been found *in vitro* with DNA (Sporn *et al*, 1966; Clifford and Rees, 1967), which is again suggestive of an activated species being formed *in vivo* which binds to macromolecules.

Evidence that aflatoxin B_1 does not resemble actinomycin D in its mode of action. It has been suggested that because of the potent inhibitory action of aflatoxin B_1 on RNA and protein synthesis *in vivo*, its mechanism of action is similar to actinomycin D (Detroy *et al*, 1971). Although the compounds are similar in these two respects, there are many more differences, so that it is probably unhelpful to think of the two together. Actinomycin D co-crystallizes with deoxyguanosine and will intercalate to form a strong complex with DNA between adjacent deoxyguanosine–deoxycytosine residues (Sobell *et al*, 1971), whereas aflatoxin B_1 has only a weak association as mentioned above. Using equilibrium dialysis, a weak association of aflatoxin B_1 with DNA can be demonstrated (Sporn *et al*, 1966), but any complex formed is easily dissociated by *Sephadex* chromatography (Clifford and Rees, 1967).

Probably the strongest argument against the actinomycin D hypothesis is the lack of biological activity of aflatoxin B_1 in those situations in which it cannot be metabolized. For example, RNA synthesis is not inhibited in a cell-free system (Edwards and Wogan, 1970), while chromatin template activity is impaired from liver nuclei of rats pretreated with aflatoxin B_1, but not when aflatoxin B_1 is added directly to the *in vitro* polymerase assay. If, however, DNA is used which has been previously incubated with aflatoxin B_1 and a microsomal enzyme-activation system in the polymerase assay, template activity is impaired [Neal, 1973]. Other instances in which aflatoxin B_1 has biological activity and where metabolism probably occurs are in the induction of mutations in *Neurospora crassa* (Ong and de Serres, 1972) and *Drosophila melanogaster* (Lamb and Lilly, 1971).

Biological activity of identified metabolites of aflatoxin B_1. Since the discovery of aflatoxin B_1 as a potent liver carcinogen in the rat, there has been a considerable amount of work done on its metabolism in a variety of species, particularly laboratory rodents. However, probably more effort has been concentrated on the biological effects of the compound—thus leading to considerable confusion because of the failure to recognize that metabolism is important in biological activity. In figure 3 the structures of the known metabolites of aflatoxin B_1 are set out together with the types of enzyme responsible for their production. The formation of each of these metabolites will be discussed separately and the reasons given why they are probably not the ultimate carcinogenic form of aflatoxin B_1.

Aflatoxin M_1 (milk toxin, 4-hydroxyaflatoxin B_1). This compound was the first metabolite of aflatoxin B_1 to be detected, it being excreted in the milk of lactating cows after aflatoxin B_1 administration (Allcroft and Carnaghan, 1963). The chemical structure of the compound was subsequently determined (Holzapfel *et al*, 1966). It has also been found as a metabolite in the milk of lactating rats (de Iongh *et al*, 1964) and in the urine of sheep (Masri *et al*, 1967) and rats (Steyn *et al*, 1971). Approximately 50% of all aflatoxin M_1 produced is excreted through the bile duct in male rats (R. C. Garner, unpublished results). Aflatoxin M_1 has also been identified as a metabolite of aflatoxin B_1 in human urine, this being the first demonstration of human metabolism of aflatoxin B_1 (Campbell *et al*, 1970).

Aflatoxin M_1 still has considerable biological activity. For example, its toxicity to ducklings is comparable to that of aflatoxin B_1 (Purchase, 1967) and the liver lesions induced are identical to those produced by aflatoxin B_1. Aflatoxin M_1 is also carcinogenic to rainbow trout but is less effective than aflatoxin B_1 (Sinnhuber *et al*, 1970). Synthetic racemic aflatoxin M_1 is as potent as aflatoxin B_1 in suppressing rat-liver nuclear-RNA synthesis and the fine structural changes induced by both compounds were indistinguishable (Pong and Wogan, 1971). Aflatoxin M_1 is nonlethal to *Salmonella typhimurium* but can be converted by liver mixed-function oxidases to a

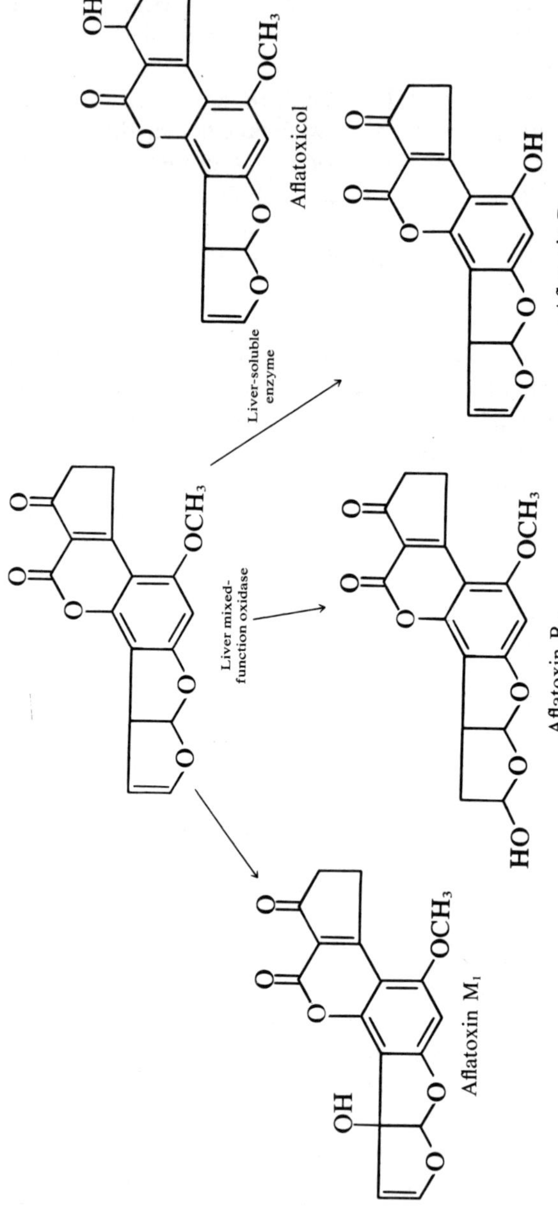

Figure 3 Metabolites of aflatoxin B$_1$

toxic compound (Garner *et al*, 1972).Aflatoxin M_1 fails to inhibit protein synthesis in an *in vitro* system (Sarasin and Moulé, 1973). In long term carcinogenicity studies in the rat, aflatoxin M_1 has been found to be only a weak carcinogen (G. N. Wogan, personal communication), nor is there apparently any correlation between aflatoxin M_1 production and carcinogenic sensitivity since *in vitro* the hamster, a relatively resistant species, produces more aflatoxin M_1 than the rat, a sensitive species (R. C. Garner, unpublished results).

The activity of aflatoxin M_1 in situations where it can be metabolized probably resides in the fact that the compound still has an isolated 2,3 double bond so that further metabolism to an epoxide derivative might still occur. This will be discussed later. However, aflatoxin M_1 is probably a detoxication product of aflatoxin B_1, and because of its greater polarity, is more rapidly excreted once formed.

Aflatoxin B_{2a} (2-hydroxy-2,3-dihydroaflatoxin B_1, aflatoxin B_1 hemiacetal). Treatment of aflatoxin B_1 with mild acid results in the hydration of the 2,3 double bond (Pohland *et al*, 1968), a process which also occurs enzymically in the liver (Patterson and Roberts, 1970). The compound forms a number of tautomers in alkali (figure 4) due to opening up of the furan rings. It has been

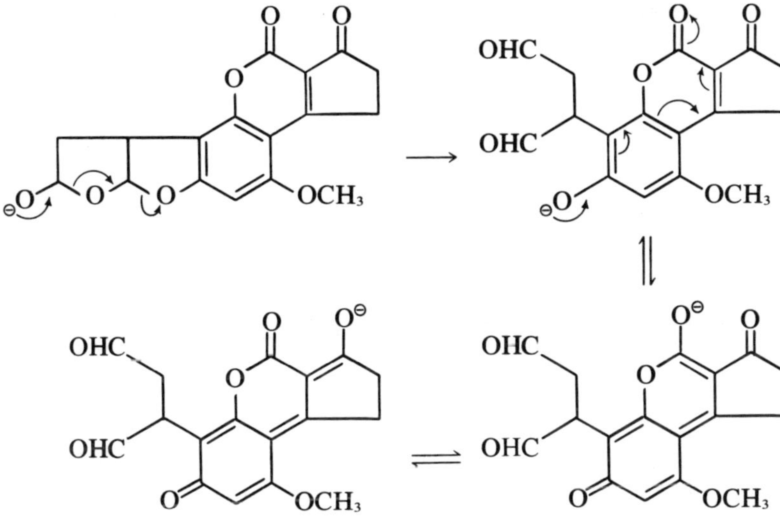

Figure 4 Resonance forms of aflatoxin B_{2a} (Pohland *et al*, 1968)

suggested that aflatoxin B_{2a} will react with amino acids to form a Schiff base (figure 5) and that this might account for some of the biological effects of aflatoxin B_1 (Patterson and Roberts, 1972). Aflatoxin B_{2a} has little or no biological activity, being only weakly toxic to ducklings (Ciegler and Peterson, 1968) and nontoxic to *Salmonella typhimurium* in the presence or

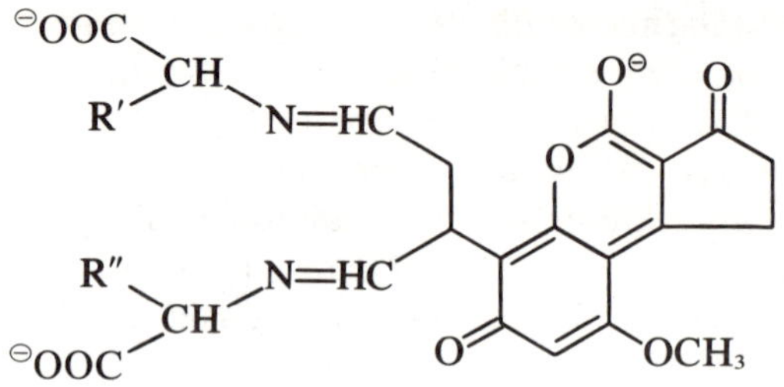

Figure 5 Hypothetical Schiff base formed by reaction of aflatoxin B_{2a} with amino acids (Patterson and Roberts, 1972)

absence of a liver mixed-function oxidase system (Garner *et al*, 1972). It has been proposed that aflatoxin B_{2a} is derived by reduction of an intermediate epoxide formed during metabolism (Patterson and Roberts, 1970) but this is unlikely, since, as will be discussed later, the 2,3 epoxide of aflatoxin B_1 is probably converted to the 2,3-dihydroxy compound which is itself unstable.

Aflatoxin P_1 (desmethylaflatoxin B_1). Monkeys are able to demethylate aflatoxin B_1 to aflatoxin P_1, excreting as much as 60% of a dose of aflatoxin B_1 as this compound conjugated with glucuronic acid (Dalezios and Wogan, 1972). Aflatoxin P_1 has no effect on fertile chicken eggs (Stoloff *et al*, 1972) and is nonlethal to *Salmonella typhimurium* either in the presence or absence of liver mixed-function oxidases (Garner *et al*, 1972). This latter finding is surprising since the compound has a 2,3 isolated double bond which could be epoxidized.

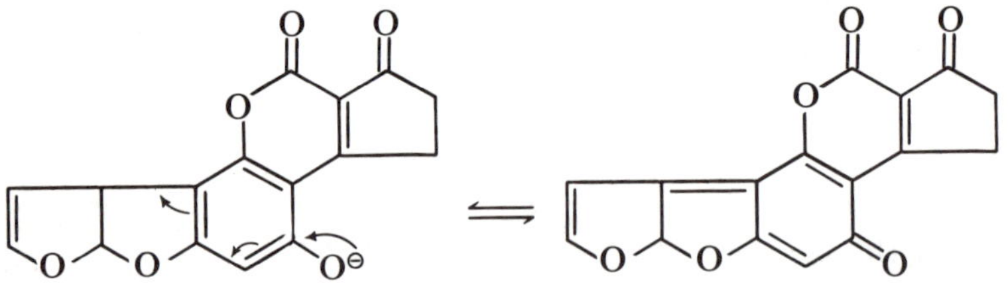

The compound, however, may keto-enolize as above so that the double bond becomes part of a conjugated system and thus less susceptible to epoxidation. This perhaps accounts for the intense yellow colour of the compound in alkaline solution.

Aflatoxicol (aflatoxin F_1). This metabolite of aflatoxin B_1, in which the carbonyl group in the cyclopentenone ring is reduced to an alcohol, is formed by enzymes in the cytoplasmic fractions of avian livers (Patterson and Roberts, 1971) and possibly rat liver (Friedman *et al*, 1972). The compound is as active as aflatoxin B_1 in the fertile chicken-egg test but is relatively nontoxic in the duckling bile-duct hyperplasia test (Detroy and Hesseltine,

1968). Aflatoxicol is also nontoxic to *Salmonella typhimurium* but can be metabolized by rat-liver mixed-function oxidases to a toxic derivative (Garner *et al*, 1972).

Summary of the biological activities of the known metabolites of aflatoxin B_1. All the metabolites so far discussed are not as potent as the parent compound in any of their biological activities. They are all stable, unreactive molecules and do not satisfy the theoretical requirements of an 'ultimate carcinogen', namely electrophilicity, reactivity with nucleophiles and instability. One must therefore postulate a new metabolite which is reactive and able to combine with nucleophiles, since such reaction has already been demonstrated *in vivo* after administration of aflatoxin B_1 (Lijinsky *et al*, 1970).

Evidence that aflatoxin B_1 can be converted to an epoxide and that this metabolite is responsible for biological activity. It is surprising that in view of what has been known for some time about the structure-activity relationships in the aflatoxin group, so little attention has been paid to the isolated 2,3 double bond. It has been known since 1969 (Butler *et al*, 1969) that aflatoxin B_2, the 2,3-dihydro derivative of aflatoxin B_1 is a much less potent carcinogen than aflatoxin B_1. This should have suggested that this bond is important for biological activity since all the other positions are identical in the two compounds. Schoental (1970) in a speculative note without supporting experimental evidence, suggested that generation of 2,3-epoxyaflatoxin B_1 might be important for carcinogenic activity. Other workers have also suggested that aflatoxin B_1 might be converted to a reactive species (Goodall and Butler, 1969; Edwards and Wogan, 1970).

In the past few years, a number of new techniques have been introduced which make it possible to rapidly test compounds that are metabolized to electrophilic species. One such test utilizes induction of mutations and inactivation of bacteria as an indicator of attack on the bacterial DNA by the activated species (Gabridge and Legator, 1969). Using a modification of this technique, it has been possible to demonstrate the formation of a toxic and mutagenic metabolite of aflatoxin B_1 produced by liver mixed-function oxidases *in vitro* (Garner *et al*, 1971; Garner and Wright, 1973) in DNA repair-deficient strains of bacteria. None of the known metabolites of aflatoxin B_1 were toxic to bacteria and only those with an isolated double bond at the 2,3 position could be activated by mixed-function oxidases (Garner *et al*, 1972). The livers of all species tested, including man, could produce this metabolite which not only induced mutations in bacteria but also reacted with cellular macromolecules (Garner, 1973a). On the basis of these results it was suggested that the mutagenic metabolite and that which reacted with macromolecules was one and the same compound, namely 2,3-epoxy-2,3-dihydroaflatoxin B_1. Strong support for the formation of this metabolite has been recently found by chemical methods. Acid hydrolysis of an aflatoxin B_1–RNA conjugate, formed by reaction of the activated aflatoxin B_1 metabolite with RNA, cleaves the aflatoxin B_1 moiety to 2,3-dihydro-2,3-dihydroxyaflatoxin B_1, indicating that an epoxide has reacted with RNA bases (Swenson *et al*, 1973). Similarly one would expect an extremely reactive molecule, such as an epoxide, to react with the most abundant nucleophile in the microsomal incubation medium, namely water, to give a dihydrodihydroxy derivative. This compound is, however, unstable in neutral buffer and breaks down to give water-soluble metabolites. Such metabolites have been found after incubation of aflatoxin B_1 with hamster-liver mixed-function oxidases (Garner, 1973b). These latter two findings demonstrate that aflatoxin B_1 is converted to an epoxide and that this compound reacts with macromolecules. It has not been possible to isolate the compound directly since it is extremely unstable. Chemical methods using peracid oxidation have demonstrated that the 2,3 double bond is extremely sensitive to epoxidation, but that the epoxide formed reacts further with the acid to give a hydroxy ester (figure 6) (Garner, 1973b).

If aflatoxin B_1, peracid and nucleic acid are reacted in a two-phase system and the nucleic acid subsequently reisolated, binding of aflatoxin to the nucleic acid is found. Presumably the epoxide is sufficiently stable to react with other nucleophiles which are present. Enzymic hydrolysis of the carcinogen–DNA complex and molecular-sieve chromatography shows an identical elution pattern to that of DNA isolated from rats given ^{14}C-aflatoxin B_1, there being three major peaks of radioactivity well separated from the four bases. Further work will characterize these fractions (R. C. Garner, unpublished results) which are probably reaction products of the aflatoxin-B epoxide with the bases (possibly guanine and adenine).

Other compounds related to aflatoxin B_1 which are probably epoxidized by liver mixed-function oxidases. Table 3 shows the toxicity to bacteria of a number of mycotoxins related to aflatoxin B_1 when these are incubated with liver mixed-function oxidases and the bacteria. Only those compounds which have an isolated 2,3 double bond are active, aflatoxin G_1 and sterigmatocystin being almost as potent as aflatoxin B_1 itself (Garner *et al*, 1972; Garner and Wright, 1973). A number of other metabolites of aflatoxin B_1 have been tested; only those with an isolated 2,3 double bond are active. As can be seen, a number of compounds active in the microsomal mixed-function oxidase activation assay have not been tested for carcinogenicity although they are contaminants of human foods (Detroy *et al*, 1971). None of the compounds are active alone, and bactericidal activity is lost by heat-inactivating the liver preparation.

It is probably true to say that all these bisfuran compounds are active in the bacterial assay through epoxidation of the 2,3 double bond during metabolism; however, they may have different activities not only because of differences in the rate of epoxidation, but also due to differences in molecular size and shape of the various compounds. Possibly for any

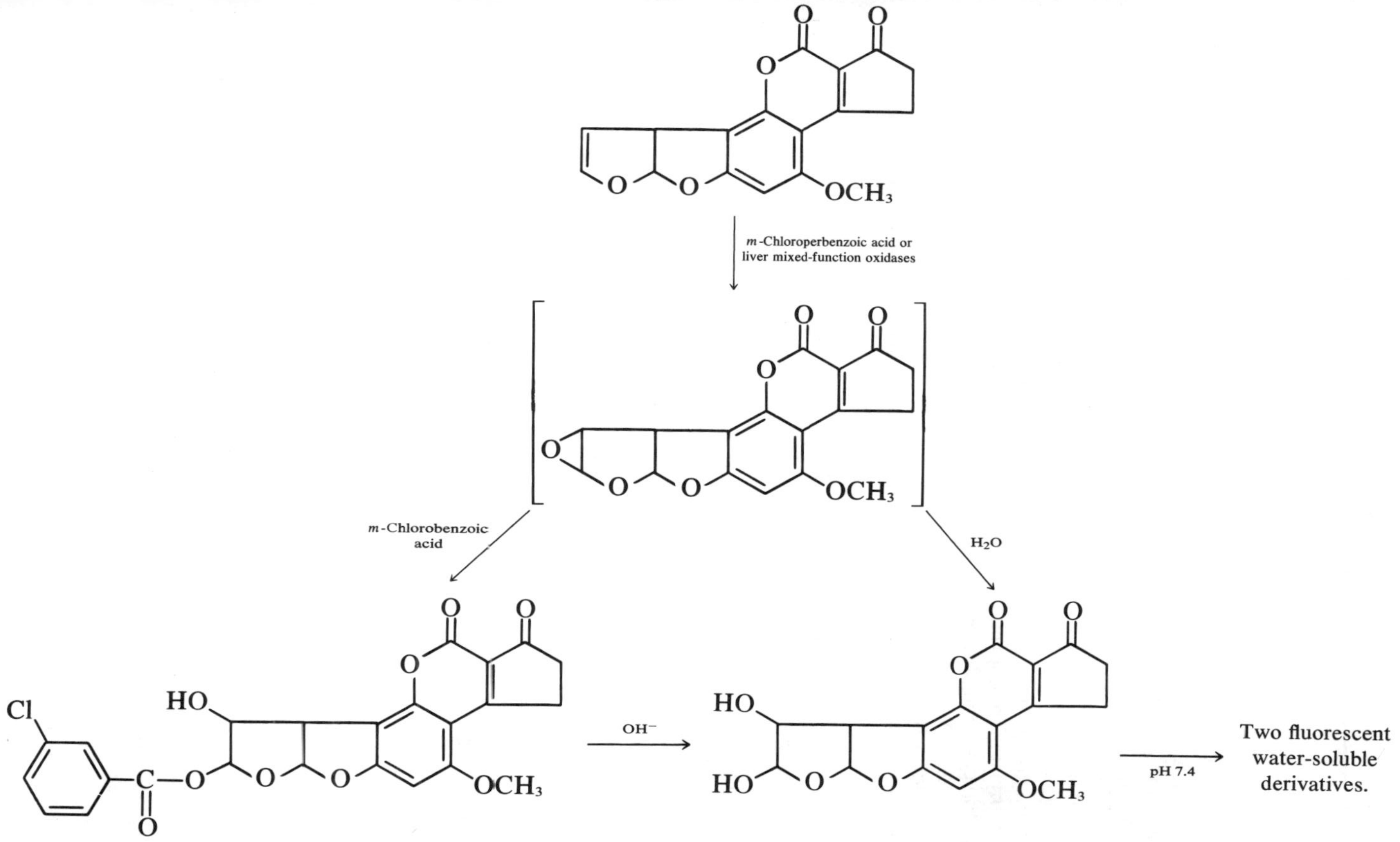

OCH₃
m-Chloroperbenzoic acid or liver mixed-function oxidases
m-Chlorobenzoic acid
H₂O
Cl
HO
OH⁻
pH 7.4
Two fluorescent water-soluble derivatives.

Figure 6 Reaction sequence for chemical or enzymic methods of obtaining the water-soluble derivatives of aflatoxin B_1 (Garner, 1973b)

Table 3 Comparison of carcinogenicity for rat liver with lethality in the microsomal activation assay

	Microsomal activation*	Carcinogenicity*
Aflatoxin B_1	++++	++++
Aflatoxin G_1	+++	+++
Aflatoxin M_1	+	+
Aflatoxin B_2	+	+
Aflatoxin G_2	−	−
Aflatoxin B_{2a}	−	?
Aflatoxin P_1	−	?
Parasiticol	+++	?
Aflatoxicol	++	?
Sterigmatocystin	+++	++
O-Methylsterigmatocystin	++	?
5-Methoxysterigmatocystin	++	?
Versicolorin A	+	?
Versicolorin B	−	?

*+ active, − inactive, ? not tested.

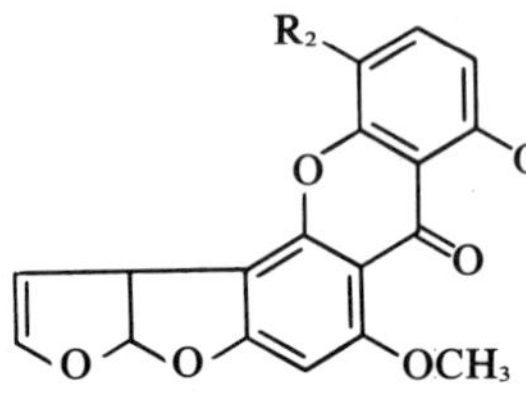

	R_1	R_2
Sterigmatocystin	H	H
O-Methylsterigmatocystin	CH_3	H
5-Methoxysterigmatocystin	H	OCH_3

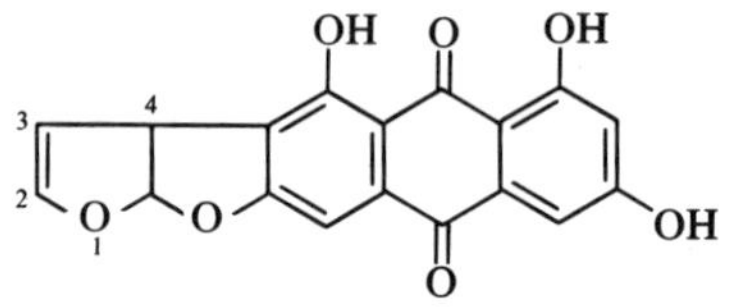

Versicolorin A
Versicolorin B = 2,3-dihydro versicolorin A

bisfuran mycotoxin, the compound is first epoxidized, the ensuing epoxide is then intercalated in the bacterial DNA because of its planar shape, and finally the epoxide ring can react with a nucleic-acid base, probably guanine (Garner, 1973a), to fix the molecule into position. Subsequent replication of the DNA might result in mutation (Garner and Wright, 1973).

Factors that might affect sensitivity to aflatoxin-B_1 carcinogenesis. It has already been mentioned that the livers of all species tested appear to be capable of converting aflatoxin B_1 to its epoxide, and yet differences are found in carcinogenic sensitivity. If the epoxide is the ultimate form of aflatoxin B_1, then quite clearly factors other than simply production of the metabolite are important. Results have been obtained using an *in vitro* system which is artificial in the sense that there is no longer any intracellular compartmentation. Such compartmentation might prevent the reactive metabolite attacking critical cell components, particularly within the nucleus. The amounts of aflatoxin B_1 used are probably in excess in the *in vitro* system whereas they are limiting *in vivo*. Thus, competitive metabolic pathways between activation and deactivation might be much more important in determining the outcome in the *in vivo* situation. No attempt has been made in these assays to add co-factors necessary for conjugation which could lead to detoxication.

Not only might competition between the various metabolic pathways be important for carcinogenicity, but also the rate of removal of base aflatoxin-B_1 conjugates in nucleic acids by repair mechanisms may be of significance. In bacteria there are differences between strains which have their full complement of repair enzymes and those that are deficient. Strains which are sensitive to the toxic and mutagenic actions of ultra-violet light are much more susceptible than wild-type strains to the aflatoxin-B_1 metabolite (Garner and Wright, 1973). Similar differences might be found between animal species in removing the aflatoxin B_1 bound to DNA which could account for differences in carcinogenic sensitivity if such binding is important (see note added in proof).

The results, therefore, using bacteria and a microsomal activation system together with those obtained using chemical techniques, point to 2,3 epoxides of these bisfuran mycotoxins being the ultimate carcinogenic forms. No other metabolites so far identified are as biologically active as aflatoxin B_1. The epoxide satisfies the criteria of an ultimate carcinogen in that it is unstable, electrophilic and reactive. Although other activation mechanisms at the 2,3 double bond, such as free-radical formation, are possible, no evidence has been obtained to support this view. Indeed, when aflatoxin B_1 was incubated in Udenfriend's system, no oxidative attack was found (R. C. Garner, unpublished results).

Epoxides from Other Compounds

The pyrrolizidine alkaloids, obtained from plants of the *Senecio* species, are potent hepatotoxins in the rat and may also be carcinogenic. Although Mattocks (1971) has proposed that these compounds are active through the formation of pyrrolic esters during their metabolism, Schoental (1970) has suggested that epoxidation of the double bond is important for toxic activity.

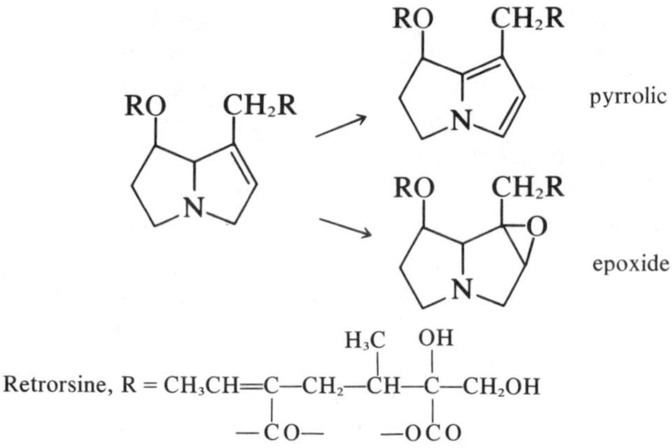

RO CH$_2$R → RO CH$_2$R (pyrrolic)
→ RO CH$_2$R (epoxide)

Retrorsine, R = $CH_3CH{=}C{-}CH_2{-}CH{-}C{-}CH_2OH$ (with H_3C on CH, OH on C; —CO— and —OCO below)

Epoxides of monocrotaline have been synthesized but have shown no carcinogenic activity (Culvenor *et al*, 1971). This may be because the epoxides were so reactive that they reacted with noncritical targets in the cell or that they are not the biologically active metabolites of these compounds.

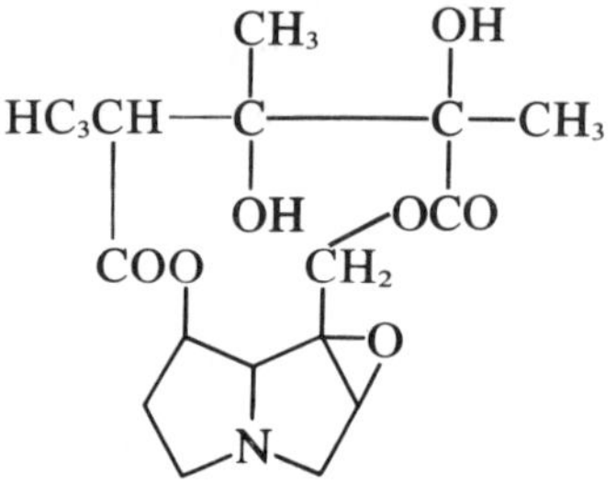

1,2-Epoxymonocrotaline

A simple way to test which mechanism was correct would be to identify the bound forms of these compounds to macromolecules and the macromolecules concerned.

In another speculative paper, Schoental and Gibbard (1972) suggested that the carcinogenic activity of 3,4,5-trimethoxycinnamaldehyde in rats was through the generation of an epoxide at the olefinic double bond. This compound, a normal volatile constituent of wood, induced nasal tumours in rats and might be responsible for the increased incidence of nasal tumours in workers in the furniture industry. However, 3,4,5-trimethoxycinnamaldehyde is probably an electrophile *per se*.

Other compounds which contain olefinic double bonds and are carcinogenic are safrole, diethylstilboestrol and acetylaminostilbene. Whether any of these are metabolized at the double-bond position to an epoxide is a matter for speculation although there is some evidence that the latter compound can be metabolized to a glycol on the bridge carbon–carbon double bond (Neumann *et al*, 1973). Alternatively, acetylaminostilbene could be rendered carcinogenic by N-hydroxylation.

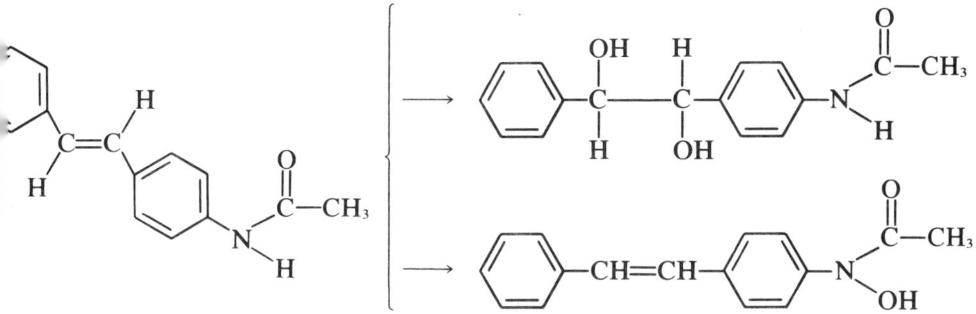

Safrole can be converted to 1′-hydroxysafrole by liver microsomes, and it has been suggested that this compound is a proximate carcinogen (Borchert *et al*, 1973). Metabolites of the carbon–carbon double bond have recently been identified (Horning *et al*, 1974).

OTHER CARCINOGENIC EPOXIDES

Besides those compounds which are converted to epoxides by metabolism, there are a number of synthetic epoxides which have carcinogenic activity. van Duuren and his co-workers have tested several and have found diepoxybutane, 1,2,4,5,-diepoxypentane, 1,2,5,6,-diepoxyhexane, 1,2,6,7-diepoxyheptane and glycidaldehyde to be weak skin carcinogens in the mouse whereas 3,4-epoxycyclohexane, ethyleneoxycyclohexane, limonenemonoxide and epoxycyclooctane were all inactive. It is possible that the long-chain oxides are carcinogenic because unlike the cyclic epoxides, they are able to crosslink DNA (van Duuren *et al*, 1965). The mutagenic activity of these compounds in *Neurospora crassa* parallels their carcinogenic activity. Thus the cyclic epoxide 1,2,3,4-diepoxycyclohexane is inactive as a mutagen whereas 1,2,4,5-diepoxypentane and 1,2,7,8-diepoxyoctane are active (Ong and de Serres, 1972).

FACTORS AFFECTING THE RATE OF EPOXIDE FORMATION AND BREAKDOWN

Clearly the amount of epoxide produced during the metabolism of any of the substances mentioned in this chapter will initially be dependent on the concentration of the parent compound reaching the epoxidase enzymes. These enzymes are localized in the endoplasmic reticulum, probably in a number of tissues, and are in the microsomal electron-transport chain. They have all the characteristics of mixed-function oxidase enzymes, i.e. they require NADPH and atmospheric oxygen, can be inhibited by carbon monoxide, other substrates and compounds such as SKF-525A. The activity of epoxidases can be increased by pretreating animals with many of the substrates which are metabolized by them. For example, pretreatment with many polycyclic hydrocarbons increases the rate of metabolism of other polycyclic hydrocarbons (Gelboin, 1967). Sims (1970) has shown that methylcholanthrene pretreatment can increase the metabolism of the majority of hydrocarbons he has examined. Such increased metabolism need not enhance the toxicity or carcinogenicity of a particular compound, indeed it may sometimes decrease it. However, there is a positive correlation between the inducibility of polycyclic-hydrocarbon metabolism and the susceptibility to hydrocarbon carcinogenesis in animals (Kouri *et al*, 1973) and possibly in humans (Kellerman *et al*, 1973). Induction of the mixed-function oxidase enzymes does not increase the metabolism of all compounds which are epoxidized. For example, steroid hydroxylation in the liver, a mixed-function oxidation, is not increased by prior polycyclic-hydrocarbon pretreatment (Conney, 1967). A similar observation was made during studies on the metabolism of aflatoxin B_1 (Garner and Wright, 1973). On the other hand, steroid hydroxylation and aflatoxin-B_1 epoxidation are increased by pretreatment with phenobarbitone. Epoxidation follows therefore the normal pattern of enzyme induction, inducing agents falling into two classes—those typified by polycyclic hydrocarbons and those typified by phenobarbitone. There are a large number of other potential factors which might alter epoxidase enzyme levels (Conney and Burns, 1972).

Not only will the tissue levels of epoxide be dependent on the amount produced, but also on its stability and rate of conversion to other compounds. The stability of some of the hydrocarbon epoxides has already been discussed. Some of these are stable compounds whereas others rapidly rearrange to their corresponding phenols. It is perhaps surprising that K-region epoxides are at the present time the chief candidates for the ultimate carcinogenic form of these compounds since they do appear to be the most stable epoxides of the hydrocarbon epoxides. In no other class of chemical carcinogens have the ultimate forms been isolated (Miller and Miller, 1971). An ultimate carcinogen would be expected to be a highly reactive molecule, not amenable to isolation from a metabolizing system and difficult to synthesize except at low temperatures.

For example, the N-sulphate of acetylaminofluorene is thought to be one of the ultimate carcinogenic forms of acetylaminofluorene and yet it has not been possible to isolate it (de Baun *et al*, 1970) from a metabolizing system. Perhaps epoxidation at non-K-region positions is important for the carcinogenicity of the polycyclic hydrocarbons. The rate of rearrangement to a phenol will undoubtedly influence the reactivity of any aromatic epoxide with macromolecules.

Besides rearrangement, epoxides can undergo a number of enzymic reactions. Epoxide hydrase is a microsomal enzyme system which hydrates epoxides to give *trans* diols (Oesch and Daly, 1971). The enzyme requires no co-factors and is found in a number of tissues including liver, kidney, lung and intestine (Oesch *et al*, 1973). The activity of the enzyme is increased by prior treatment of rats with 3-methylcholanthrene or phenobarbitone (Oesch *et al*, 1971b) and can be inhibited by a number of synthetic epoxides such as cyclohexene oxide (Oesch *et al*, 1971a). Interestingly, inhibiting epoxide hydrase *in vivo* with cyclohexene oxide did not potentiate the toxic effect of bromobenzene, the epoxide of which is thought to induce liver necrosis. On the contrary, the toxicity was inhibited (Oesch *et al*, 1973). Obviously the toxic effect of bromobenzene cannot be related only to the amount of epoxide produced.

A further enzyme system which can affect the tissue concentration of epoxides formed during metabolism is the glutathione S-transferases (Boyland and Williams, 1965; Chasseaud, 1973). This is a cytoplasmic enzyme system present in the liver and kidneys which can conjugate some epoxides with glutathione (Booth *et al*, 1973). Many of the aromatic hydrocarbon epoxides are substrates for this enzyme system, although some epoxides can react directly with glutathione without an enzyme mediator, albeit more slowly.

Some epoxides will react with macromolecules within the cell and this might be a method of limiting the amount reaching the critical targets for tumour initiation. In studies on the binding of hydrocarbons to cellular macromolecules, it is pertinent to point out that almost invariably the greatest amount of binding is with cellular protein. Whether this binding is involved in tumour initiation or whether it is a detoxication step is a matter of debate at the present time (Miller, 1970; Pitot and Heidelberger, 1963).

For any particular epoxide, its toxicity, carcinogenicity or pharmacological activity will depend on a balance between the various pathways just described. It is reasonable to say that epoxides are always biologically more active than the parent compound; how toxic they are will depend on the rate and extent of their deactivation.

CONCLUSIONS

This chapter has briefly reviewed the evidence for epoxide formation during the metabolism of a number of classes of compound. The published data on this biotransformation process suffers in that only a few classes have been studied in any sort of depth. This is surprising in view of the potent biological properties of many epoxide intermediates. Many drugs have adverse side-effects which could well be due to the formation of an epoxide intermediate during metabolism. In other cases, the epoxide might be the biologically active form of the compound, e.g. vitamin K, some insecticides and perhaps some steroids. We are only at the threshold of discovering the true role of epoxides in bioactivation.

Future examples of epoxidation are likely to be found not only of carbon–carbon double bonds but possibly of carbon–nitrogen bonds and carbon–sulphur bonds. Not only may simple olefinic and aromatic double bonds be epoxidized, but also the double bonds of vinyl and allyl derivatives and of α,β-unsaturated compounds.

The epoxidases are widely distributed throughout the body although certain organs such as the liver have high levels of these enzymes. They are intimately associated with the mixed-function oxidases and are induced by agents which induce the latter enzymes. Since the mixed-function oxidases are subject to nutritional and genetic control, so the amounts of epoxide produced will vary from individual to individual. This might account for the individual variations to the toxic side effects of some drugs, and perhaps the carcinogenic effect of compounds such as the polycyclic hydrocarbons, all compounds having epoxide intermediates. The final effects of epoxides will also be greatly influenced by the epoxide deactivating enzyme systems such as epoxide hydrase and glutathione S-transferases. The levels of the former enzyme are also altered by dietary influences whereas the latter enzyme levels are not known to be, although concentrations of glutathione are.

With regard to 2,3-epoxyaflatoxin B_1, there is now very strong evidence that this metabolite is the 'ultimate' carcinogenic form of the parent compound. This metabolite is formed by an epoxidase enzyme which is inducible by phenobarbitone and not by the polycyclic hydrocarbons. It is extremely unstable and is probably hydrated non-enzymically as judged by the failure of cyclohexene oxide to inhibit conversion to the dihydrodiol. However, the carcinogenic action of aflatoxin B_1 is not solely dependent on the amount of epoxide produced since *in vitro* experiments show the hamster for example to be very active in producing the epoxide but relatively resistant to the carcinogenic activity of aflatoxin B_1. The hamster is also very active in converting aflatoxin to its nontoxic metabolites as well so that the major amount of the compound may be excreted as these derivatives and very little converted to the epoxide.

Other factors which may be of importance in determining carcinogenic sensitivity to aflatoxin may include the extent and faithfulness of repair of the DNA–aflatoxin epoxide conjugate and the immunosuppressant activity of the compound. Reaction of the epoxide with noncritical macromolecules may also affect sensitivity.

A number of other carcinogens containing olefinic aromatic double bonds whose activation steps are not fully understood may have epoxide intermediates. It has been suggested, as already discussed, that safrole may be activated through allylic esterification and that 1′-hydroxysafrole is the proximal carcinogenic form of this compound. An alternative mechanism could involve epoxidation of the olefinic double bond, such metabolites having been identified in recent studies.

The list of likely candidates for epoxidation is endless and it would be possible to speculate at length about other compounds. Are the methyl-substituted polycyclic hydrocarbons generally more active because this group increases the reactivity of double bonds? What other drugs are epoxidized besides the barbiturates? Probably all hydroxy groups introduced into aromatic compounds by mixed-function oxidases arise via an epoxide intermediate as does the formation of a dihydrodiol from an olefinic double bond.

In the final analysis, most knowledge of epoxide formation during metabolism stems from investigations of chemical carcinogens. The data for other classes of compound is very meagre because no great effort has been made in studying these classes. Since epoxides are often biologically active, more research must be concentrated on these other classes of compound if there is to be a better understanding of what the importance of epoxide formation is, other than in carcinogenesis or indeed, whether all epoxides are potential carcinogens.

ACKNOWLEDGEMENTS

I would like to thank the Yorkshire Council of the Cancer Research Campaign for financial support while writing this chapter. I would also like to thank Mrs. M. Davis for typing the manuscript.

REFERENCES

Abell, C. W. and Heidelberger, C. (1962), *Cancer Res.*, **22**, 931.
Adamson, R. H., Correa, P. and Dalgard, D. W. (1973), *J. Nat. Cancer Inst.*, **50**, 549.
Allcroft, R. and Carnaghan, R. B. A. (1963), *Vet. Rec.*, **75**, 259.
Ames, B. N., Sims, P. and Grover, P. L. (1972), *Science*, **176**, 47.
Anderson, W. K. and Veysoglu, T. (1973), *J. Org. Chem.*, **38**, 2267.
Ayres, J. L., Lee, D. J., Wales, J. H. and Sinnhuber, R. O. (1971), *J. Nat. Cancer Inst.*, **46**, 561.
Baird, W. M., Dipple, A., Grover, P. L., Sims, P. and Brookes, P. (1973), *Cancer Res.*, **22**, 2386.
Baird, W. M. and Brookes, P. (1973), *Cancer Res.*, **33**, 2378.
de Baun, J. R., Miller, E. C. and Miller, J. A. (1970), *Cancer Res.* **30**, 577.
Bischoff, F. (1969), *Adv. Lipid Res.*, **7**, 165.
Black, H. S. and Douglas, D. R. (1973), *Cancer Res.*, **33**, 2094.
Black, H. S. and Lo, W. B. (1971), *Nature (Lond.)*, **234**, 306.
Booth, J., Boyland, E., Sato, T. and Sims, P. (1960), *Biochem. J.*, **22**, 182.
Booth, J., Keysell, G. R. and Sims, P. (1973), *Biochem. Pharmacol.*, **22**, 1781.
Borchert, P., Miller, J. A., Miller, E. C. and Shires, T. K. (1973), *Cancer Res.*, **33**, 590.
Borgen, A., Darvey, H., Castagnoli, N., Crocker, T. T., Rasmussen, R. E. and Wang, I. Y. (1973), *J. Med. Chem.*, **16**, 502.
Boyland, E. (1950), *Biochem. Soc. Symp.*, **5**, 40.
Boyland, E. and Chasseaud, L. F. (1969), *Adv. Enzymol.*, **32**, 173.
Boyland, E. and Levi, A. A. (1935), *Biochem. J.*, **29**, 2679.
Boyland, E. and Williams, K. (1965), *Biochem. J.*, **94**, 190.
Breuer, H. and Knuppen, R. (1961), *Biochim. Biophys. Acta*, **49**, 620.
Brookes, C. J. W. and Young, L. (1956), *Biochem. J.*, **63**, 264.
Brookes, P. and Lawley, P. D. (1964), *Nature*, **202**, 781.
Brooks, G. T. and Harrison, A. (1965), *Nature*, **205**, 1031.
Brooks, G. T., Harrison, A. and Cox, J. T. (1963), *Nature*, **197**, 311.
Brooks, G. T., Lewis, S. E. and Harrison, A. (1968), *Nature*, **220**, 1034.
Butler, W. H., Greenblatt, M. and Lijinsky, W. (1969), *Cancer Res.*, **29**, 2206.

Butler, W. H. and Barnes, J. M. (1963), *Brit. J. Cancer*, **17**, 699.
Byington, K. H. and Leibman, K. C. (1965), *Mol. Pharmacol.*, **1**, 247.
Campbell, T. C., Caedo, J. P., Bulatao-Jayme, J., Salamat, L. and Engel, B. W. (1970), *Nature*, **227**, 403.
Carnaghan, R. B. A. (1965), *Nature*, **208**, 308.
Carnaghan, R. B. A. (1967), *Brit. J. Cancer*, **21**, 811.
Chan, E. W. and Ball, J. K. (1971), *Biochim. Biophys. Acta*, **238**, 46.
Chasseaud, L. F. (1973), *Drug Metab. Rev.* **2**, 185.
Ciegler, A. and Peterson, R. E. (1968), *Appl. Microbiol.*, **16**, 665.
Clayson, D. B. (1962), *Chemical carcinogenesis*, Churchill, London.
Cleaver, J. E. and Trosko, J. E. (1970), *Photochem. Photobiol.*, **11**, 547.
Clifford, J. I. and Rees, K. R. (1967), *Biochem. J.*, **103**, 467.
Conney, A. H. (1967), *Pharmacol. Rev.*, **19**, 317.
Conney, A. H. and Burns, J. J. (1972), *Science*, **178**, 576.
Cook, J. W. and Schoental, R. (1948), *J. Chem. Soc.* 170.
Cookson, M. J., Sims, P. and Grover, P. L. (1971), *Nature New Biol.*, **234**, 186.
Coombs, M. M., Bhatt T. S. and Croft, C. J. (1973), *Cancer Res.* **33**, 832.
Corey, E. J. and Russey, W. E. (1966), *J. Amer. Chem. Soc.*, **88**, 4751.
Corey, E. J., Russey, W. E. and Ortiz de Montellano, P. R. (1966), *J. Amer. Chem. Soc.* **88**, 4750.
Culvenor, C. C. J., Edgar, J. A., Smith, L. W., Jacq, M. V. and Peterson, J. E. (1971), *Nature New Biol.*, **229**, 255.
Dalezios, J. I. and Wogan, G. N. (1972), *Cancer Res.*, **32**, 2297.
Daly, J. W., Jerina, D. M. and Witkop, B. (1968), *Arch. Biochem. Biophys.*, **128**, 517.
Daly, J. W., Jerina, D. M. and Witkop, B. (1972), *Experientia*, **28**, 1129.
Davidow, B. and Radomski, J. L. (1953), *J. Pharmacol. Exp. Ther.*, **107**, 259.
Detroy, R. W. and Hesseltine, C. W. (1968), *Nature*, **219**, 967.
Detroy, R. W., Lillehoj, E. B. and Ciegler, A. (1971), *Microbial Toxins*, vol. 6, chapter 1, Academic Press, New York.
Dipple, A. and Slade, T. A. (1970), *Eur. J. Cancer*, **6**, 477.
van Duuren, B. L., Langseth, L., Goldschmidt, B. M. and Orris, L. (1967), *J. Nat. Cancer Inst.*, **39**, 1217.
van Duuren, B. L., Orris, L. and Nelson, A. (1965), *J. Nat. Cancer Inst.*, **35**, 707.
van Duuren, B. L., Sivak, A., Segal, A., Orris, L. and Langseth, L. (1966), *J. Nat. Cancer Inst.*, **37**, 519.
Edwards, G. S. and Wogan, G. N. (1970), *Biochim. Biophys. Acta*, **224**, 597.
Elce, J. S. *Biochem. J.* (1970), **116**, 913.
Elce, J. S. *Biochem. J.* (1972), **126**, 1067.
Elce, J. S. and Harris, J. (1971), *Steroids*, **18**, 583.
Estabrook, R. W., Gillette, J. R. and Leibman, K. C. (ed.) (1972), *Microsomes and drug oxidations*, (*Drug Metab. Disposition*, **1**), Williams and Wilkins, Baltimore.
Flesher, J. W. and Sydnor, K. L. (1971), *Cancer Res.*, **31**, 1951.
Friedman, L., Yin, L. and Verrett, M. J. (1972), *Toxicol. Appl. Pharmacol.*, **23**, 385.
Gabridge, M. G., Legator, M. S. (1969), *Proc. Soc. Exp. Biol. Med.*, **130**, 831.
Garner, R. C. *Chem. Biol. Inter.* (1973a), **6**, 125.
Garner, R. C. (1973b), *FEBS Lett.*, **36**, 261.
Garner, R. C., Miller, E. C., Miller, J. A., Garner, J. V. and Hanson, R. S. (1971), *Biochem. Biophys. Res. Commun.*, **45**, 774.
Garner, R. C., Miller, E. C. and Miller, J. A. (1972), *Cancer Res.*, **32**, 2058.
Garner, R. C. and Wright, C. M. (1973), *Brit. J. Cancer*, **28**, 504.
Gelboin, H. V. (1967), *Adv. Cancer Res.*, **10**, 1.
Gelboin, H. V. (1969), *Cancer Res.*, **29**, 1272.

Gillette, J. R. (1966), *Adv. Pharmacol.*, **4**, 219.
Gillette, J. R., Conney, A. H., Cosmides, G. J., Estabrook, R. W., Fouts, J. R. and Mannering, G. J. (ed.) (1969), *Microsomes and drug oxidations*, Academic Press, New York.
Goh, S. H. and Harvey, R. G. (1973), *J. Amer. Chem. Soc.*, **95**, 242.
Goldblatt, L. (ed.) (1969), *Aflatoxin*, Academic Press, New York.
Goodall, C. M. and Butler, W. H. (1969), *Int. J. Cancer*, **4**, 422.
Grover, P. L., Forrester, J. A. and Sims, P. (1971b), *Biochem. Pharmacol.*, **20**, 1297.
Grover, P. L., Hewer, A. and Sims, P. (1971a), *FEBS Lett.*, **18**, 76.
Grover, P. L. Hewer, A. and Sims, P. (1973), *FEBS Lett.*, **34**, 63.
Grover, P. L. and Sims, P. (1968), *Biochem. J.*, **110**, 159.
Grover, P. L. and Sims, P. (1972), *Biochem. J.*, **129**, 41P.
Grover, P. L. and Sims, P. (1973), *Biochem. Pharmacol.*, **22**, 661.
Guroff, G., Reifsnyder, C. A. and Daly, J. W. (1966a) *Biochem. Biophys. Res. Commun.*, **24**, 720.
Guroff, G., Kondo, K. and Daly, J. W. (1966b), *Biochem. Biophys. Res. Commun.*, **25**, 622.
Guroff, G., Daly, J. W., Jerina, D. M., Renson, J., Witkop, B. and Udenfriend, S. (1967), *Science*, **157**, 1524.
Harvey, D. J., Glazener, L., Stratton, C., Johnson, D. B., Hill, R. M., Horning, E. C. and Horning, M. G. (1972a), *Res. Commun. Chem. Pathol. Pharmacol.*, **4**, 247.
Harvey, D. J., Glazener, L., Stratton C., Nowlin, J., Hill, R. M. and Horning, M. G. (1972b), *Res. Commun. Chem. Pathol. Pharmacol.*, **3**, 557.
Herrold, K. (1969), *Brit. J. Cancer*, **23**, 655.
Hill, M. J., Crowther, J. S., Drasar, B. S., Hawksworth, G., Avies, V. and Williams, R. E. O. (1971), *Lancet*, 95.
Hoffman, H. D., Lesko, Jr. S. A. and Ts'O, P. O. P. (1970), *Biochemistry*, **9**, 2594.
Holtzmann, J. L., Gillette, J. R. and Milne, G. W. A. (1967), *J. Biol. Chem.* **242**, 4386.
Holtzapfel, C. W., Steyn, P. S. and Purchase, I. F. H. (1966), *Tetrahedron Lett.*, 2799.
Horning, M. G., Bell, L., Corman, M. J. and Stilwell, W. G. (1974), *Proc. Amer. Soc. Toxicol.*, **29**.
Huberman, E., Kuroki, T., Marquardt, H., Selkirk, J. K., Heidelberger, C., Grover, P. L. and Sims, P. (1972), *Cancer Res.*, **32**, 1391.
Hueper, W. C. and Conway, W. D. (1964), *Chemical carcinogenesis and cancers*, Charles C. Thomas, Springfield.
IARC Monograph (1973), *Evaluation of carcinogenic risk*, vol. 3, IARC, Lyon.
de Iongh, H., Vles, R. O. and van Pelt, J. G. (1964), *Nature*, **202**, 466.
Jakoby, W. B. and Fjellstedt, T. A. (1972), in *The Enzymes*, 3rd ed., vol. 7, Boyer, P. D. (ed.), p. 199, Academic Press, New York.
James, S. P. and White, D. A. (1967) *Biochem. J.*, **104**, 914.
James, S. P., Jeffery, D. J., Waring, R. H. and White, D. A. (1971), *Biochem. Pharmacol.*, **20**, 897.
Jerina, D. M., Daly, J. W., Witkop, B., Zaltzmann-Nirenberg, P. and Udenfriend, S. (1968), *Arch. Biochem. Biophys.*, **128**, 176.
Jerina, D. M., Daly, J. W., Witkop, B., Zaltzman-Nirenberg, P. and Udenfriend, S. (1970), *Biochemistry*, **9**, 147.
Jerina, D. M., Daly, J. W., Jeffrey, A. M. and Gibson, D. T. (1971), *Arch. Biochem., Biophys.*, **142**, 394.
Kellerman, G., Shaw, C. R. and Luyten-Kellerman, M. (1973), *New Engl. J. Med.*, **289**, 934.
Kennaway, E. L. and Hieger, I. (1930), *Brit. Med. J.*, **1**, 1044.
Keysell, G. R., Booth, J., Sims, P., Grover, P. L. and Hewer, A. (1972), *Biochem. J.* **129**, 41P.

Keysell, G. R., Booth, J., Grover, P. L., Hewer, A. and Sims, P. (1973), *Biochem. Pharmacol.*, **22**, 2853.
Knight, R. H. and Young, L. (1958), *Biochem. J.*, **70**, 111.
Kouri, R. E., Salerno, R. A., and Whitmire, C. E. (1973), *J. Nat. Cancer Inst.*, **50**, 363.
Kuroki, T., Huberman, E., Marquardt H., Selkirk, J. K., Heidelberger, C., Grover, P. L. and Sims, P. (1971/2), *Chem. Biol. Inter.* **4**, 389.
Lamb, M. J. and Lilly, L. J. (1971), *Mutation Res.*, **11**, 430.
Leibman, K. C. and Ortiz, E. (1968), *Mol. Pharmacol.*, **4**, 201.
Leibman, K. C. and Ortiz, E. (1970), *J. Pharmacol. Exp. Ther.*, **173**, 242.
Lesko, jr. S. A., Ts'O, P. O. P. and Umans, R. S. (1969), *Biochemistry*, **8**, 2291.
Lijinsky, W., Lee, K. Y., and Gallagher, C. H. (1970), *Cancer Res.*, **30**, 2280.
Ludka, J. L., Gibson, J. R. and Lusk, C. I. (1972), *Toxicol. Appl. Pharmacol.*, **21**, 89.
Magee, P. N. and Barnes, J. M. (1967), *Adv. Cancer Res.*, **10**, 163.
Maher, V. M., Lesko, S. A., Straat, P. A. and Ts'O, P. O. P. (1971), *J. Bacteriol*, **108**, 202.
Marquardt, H., Kuroki, T., Huberman, E., Selkirk, J. K., Heidelberger, C., Grover, P. L. and Sims, P. (1972), *Cancer Res.*, **32**, 716.
Martin, J. C. and Arhart, R. J. (1971), *J. Amer. Chem. Soc.*, **93**, 4327.
Mason, H. S. (1957), *Science*, **125**, 1185.
Masri, M. S., Lundin, R. E., Page, J. R. and Garcia, V. C. (1967), *Nature*, **215**, 753.
Matschiner, J. T., Bell, R. J., Anelotti, J. M. and Krauer, T. (1970), *Biochim. Biophys. Acta*, **201**, 309.
Mattocks, A. R. (1971), *Nature*, **232**, 478.
Maynert, E. W., Foreman, R. L. and Watabe, T. (1970), *J. Biol. Chem.*, **245**, 5234.
Miller, E. C. and Miller, J. A. (1967), *Proc. Soc. Exp. Biol. Med.*, **124**, 915.
Miller, J. A. (1970), *Cancer Res.*, **30**, 559.
Miller, J. A. and Miller, E. C. (1971), *J. Nat. Cancer Inst.*, **47**, v.
Nagata, C., Tagashira, Y., Kodama, M., Yoki, Y. and Oboshi, S. (1973), *Gann*, **24**, 277.
Nakatsugawa, T., Ishida, M. and Dahm, P. (1965), *Biochem. Pharmacol.*, **14**, 1853.
Neal, G. E. (1973), *Nature*, **244**, 432.
Neumann, H. G., Metzler, M. and Töpner, W. (1973), *Abstracts Second Meeting of the European Association of Cancer Research*, Heidelberg.
Newberne, P. M. and Butler, W. H. (1969), *Cancer Res.*, **29**, 236.
Newberne, P. M. and Rogers, A. E. (1973), *J. Nat. Cancer Inst.*, **50**, 439.
Newman, M. S. and Blum, S. (1964), *J. Amer. Chem. Soc.*, **86**, 5598.
Oesch, F. (1973), *Xenobiotica*, **3**, 305.
Oesch, F. and Daly, J. (1971), *Biochim. Biophys. Acta*, **227**, 692.
Oesch, F., Jerina, D. M. and Daly, J. W. (1971b), *Biochim. Biophys. Acta*, **227**, 685.
Oesch, F., Jerina, D. M., Daly, J. W. and Rice, J. M. (1973), *Chem. Biol. Inter.* **6**, 189.
Oesch, F., Kaubisch, N., Jerina, D. M. and Daly, J. W. (1971a), *Biochemistry*, **10**, 4858.
Ong, T. and de Serres, F. J. (1972), *Cancer Res.*, **32**, 1890.
Parke, D. V. (1968), *The biochemistry of foreign compounds*, International Series of Monographs in Pure and Applied Biology, Biochemistry Division, vol. 5, Pergamon Press.
Patterson, D. S. P. and Roberts, B. A. (1970), *Food Cosmet. Toxicol.*, **8**, 527.
Patterson, D. S. P. and Roberts, B. A. (1971), *Food Cosmet. Toxicol.* **9**, 829.
Patterson, D. S. P. and Roberts, B. A. (1972), *Food Cosmet. Toxicol.*, **10**, 501.
Peers, F. G. and Linsell, C. A. (1973), *Brit. J. Cancer*, **27**, 473.
Pitot, H. C. and Heidelberger, C. (1963), *Cancer Res.*, **23**, 1694.
Pohland, A. E., Cushmac, M. E. and Andrellos, P. J. (1968), *J. Assoc. Offic. Anal. Chemists*, **51**, 907.

Pong, R. S. and Wogan, G. N. (1971), *J. Nat. Cancer Inst.*, **47**, 585.
Ptashne, K. A. and Neal, R. A. (1972), *Biochemistry*, **11**, 3224.
Ptashne, K. A., Wolcott, R. M. and Neal, R. A. (1971), *J. Pharmacol. Exp. Ther.*, **179**, 380.
Pullman, A. and Pullman, B. (1955), *Adv. Cancer Res.*, **3**, 117.
Purchase, I. F. H. (1967), *Food Cosmet. Toxicol.*, **5**, 339.
Radomski, J. L. and Davidow, B. J. (1953), *J. Pharmacol. Exp. Ther.*, **107**, 266.
Rapaport, B. A. and Ts'O, P. O. P. (1966), *Proc. Nat. Acad. Sci.* **55**, 381.
Robbins, J. H. and Burk, P. G. (1973), *Cancer Res.* **33**, 929.
Sarasin, A. and Moulé, Y. (1973), *FEBS Lett.*, **32**, 347.
Sato, T., Fukuyama, T., Suzuki, T. and Yoshikawa, H. (1963), *J. Biochem.* (*Japan*), **53**, 23.
Schoental, R. (1970), *Nature*, **227**, 401.
Schoental, R. and Gibbard, S. (1972), *Brit. J. Cancer*, **26**, 504.
Schultzen, O. and Naunyn, B. (1867), *Arch. Anat. Physiol.*, 349.
Selkirk, J. K., Huberman, E. and Heidelberger, C. (1971), *Biochem. Biophys. Res. Commun.* **43**, 1010.
Sih, C. J. (1969), *Science*, **163**, 1297.
Sims, P. (1966), *Biochem. J.*, **98**, 215.
Sims, P. (1970), *Biochem. Pharmacol.*, **19**, 795.
Sims, P. (1971), *Biochem. J.*, **125**, 159.
Sims, P. (1972a), *Biochem. J.*, **130**, 27.
Sims, P. (1972b), *Xenobiotica*, **2**, 469.
Sims, P. (1973), *Biochem. J.*, **131**, 405.
Sims, P., Grover, P. L., Kuroki, T., Huberman, E., Marquardt, H., Selkirk, J. K. and Heidelberger, C. (1973), *Biochem. Pharmacol.*, **22**, 1.
Sims, P. and Grover, P. L. (1974), *Adv. Cancer Res.*, **20**, 165.
Sinnhuber, R. O., Lee, D. J., Wales, H. H., Landers, M. K. and Keyle, A. C. (1970), *Fed. Proc.* **29**, 568.
Smith, J. N. and Williams, R. T. (1950), *Biochem. J.*, **46**, 243.
Sobell, H. M., Jain, S. C., Sakore, T. D. and Nordman, C. E. (1971), *Nature New Biol.*, **231**, 200.
Sporn, M. B., Dingman, C. W., Phelps, H. L. and Wogan, G. N. (1966), *Science*, **151**, 1539.
Steyn, M., Pitout, M. J. and Purchase, I. F. H. (1971), *Brit. J. Cancer*, **25**, 291.
Stich, H. F. and San, R. H. C. (1973), *Proc. Soc. Exp. Biol. Med.*, **142**, 155.
Stoloff, L., Verrett, M. J., Dantzman, J. and Reynaldo, E. F. (1972), *Toxicol. Appl. Pharmacol.*, **23**, 385.
Swaisland, A. J., Grover, P. L. and Sims, P. (1973), *Biochem. Pharmacol.*, **22**, 1547.
Swenson, D. H., Miller, J. A. and Miller, E. C. (1973), *Biochem. Biophys. Res. Commun.* **53**, 1260.
Ts'O, P. O. P. and Lu, P. (1964), *Proc. Nat. Acad. Sci.*, **51**, 272.
Ullrich, V., Wolf, J., Amadori, E. and Staudinger, H. (1968), *Z. Physiol. Chem.*, **349**, 85.
Vesselinovitch, S. D., Mihailovitch, N., Wogan, G. N., Lombard, L. S. and Rao, K. V. N. (1972), *Cancer Res.*, **32**, 2289.
Wang, I. Y., Rasmussen, R. E. and Crocker, T. T. (1972), *Biochem. Biophys. Res. Commun.*, **49**, 1142.
Warwick, G. P. (1971), *Fed. Proc.* **30**, 1760.
Waterfall, J. F. and Sims, P. (1972), *Biochem. J.* **128**, 265.
Weisburger, J. H. and Weisburger, E. K. (1973), *Pharmacol. Rev.*, **25**, 1.
Wilkinson, A. T. S., Finlayson, D. G. and Morley, H. V. (1964), *Science*, **143**, 681.
Williams, R. T. (1959), *Detoxication mechanisms*, Chapman and Hall, London.

Wogan, G. N. (1969), *Prog. Exp. Tumor Res.* **11**, 134.
Wogan, G. N. and Newberne, P. M. (1967), *Cancer Res.* **27**, 2370.
Wogan, G. N. and Newberne, P. M. (1972), *Cancer Res.* **32**, 2058.
Wong, D. T. and Terriere, L. C. (1965), *Biochem. Pharmacol.*, **14**, 375.
Wurtz, A. (1859), *Ann. Chim. Phys.*, **55**, 400.
Yagi, H. and Jerina, D. M. (1973), *J. Amer. Chem. Soc.*, **95**, 243.
Yamagiwa, K. and Ichikawa, K. (1918), *J. Cancer Res.*, **3**, 1.
Yamamoto, S. and Bloch, K. (1970), *J. Biol. Chem.* **245**, 1670.

Note Added in Proof

Since this chapter was written, a number of papers have appeared describing other compounds which are converted metabolically to epoxides and the identification of new epoxide metabolites of compounds already included in this review. In particular, mention should be made of the polycyclic hydrocarbon diol-epoxides, metabolites with greater reactivity than K-region epoxides. Digests of the reaction products of the hydrocarbon diol-epoxides with nucleic acids gave similar chromatographic profiles to digests of nucleic acids isolated from hamster embryo cells exposed to the parent hydrocarbon or to exogenous DNA recovered from microsomal trapping experiments (Sims, P., Grover, P. L., Swaisland, A., Pal, K. and Hewer, A. (1974), *Nature*, **252**, 326).

Epoxide intermediates may also be formed during the metabolism of furosemide and other furan derivatives and of thiophene (Mitchell, J. R., Potter, W. Z., Hinson, J. A. and Jollow, D. G. (1974), *Nature*, **251**, 508).

Studies with radiolabelled aflatoxin B_1 *in vivo* indicated a greater binding of the carcinogen to liver nucleic acids in sensitive compared to resistant animal species, as well as a more rapid removal of DNA—aflatoxin B_1 conjugates from the former group (Garner, R. C. and Wright, C. M. (1975), *Chem. Biol. Inter.*, **11**, 123). Dietary modifications which reduce aflatoxin B_1 carcinogenicity were found to decrease the amount of carcinogen bound to nucleic acid in target tissues (Garner, R. C. (1975), *Biochem. Pharmacol.*, **24**, 1553). Two new metabolites of aflatoxin B_1 have recently been identified, aflatoxin Q, (Masri, M. S., Haddon, W. F., Lundin, R. E. and Hsieh, D. P. H. (1974), *J. Agr. Food Chem.*, **22**, 512) and aflatoxicol H_1 (Salhab, A. S. and Hsieh, D. P. H. (1975), *Res. Commun. Chem. Pathol. Pharmacol.*, **10**, 419); neither of these metabolites are as potent as aflatoxin B_1 in bioassay systems, probably because they are more polar than the parent compound.

CHAPTER 4

Clinical aspects of microsomal enzyme induction

J. Hunter and L. F. Chasseaud

INTRODUCTION*

Drugs and other foreign compounds enter the body through gastrointestinal, respiratory or cutaneous routes usually by a process of passive diffusion of which an important determinant is the degree of lipid solubility of the compound (Brodie, 1964; Schanker, 1964; Goldstein *et al*, 1968; Chasseaud, 1970; Brodie & Gillette, 1971; La Du *et al*, 1971; Levine, 1973). The same characteristics that enhance the absorption of compounds delay their excretion by the kidneys since lipid-soluble drugs in the glomerular filtrate are reabsorbed in the renal tubules (Schanker, 1964; Goldstein *et al.*, 1968; Chasseaud, 1970; Weiner, 1971) and could therefore, if unmodified, persist in the body. Metabolic pathways exist to convert drugs and other compounds into metabolites with physicochemical properties that favour more rapid excretion from the body in the bile and urine (Brodie & Maickel, 1962; Brodie & Reid, 1967). However, the metabolites formed may sometimes be more toxic or pharmacologically active than the parent compound, and metabolic processes are thus not necessarily directed towards detoxication or inactivation.

Most drugs are metabolized in the endoplasmic reticulum of liver cells (Table 1) (Gillette, 1966; Hutson, 1970; La Du *et al*, 1971; Brodie & Gillette, 1971) but metabolism can occur in other tissues as well, such as the lungs, kidneys, gastrointestinal tract and skin (Uehleke, 1969; Wattenberg & Leong, 1971). The endoplasmic reticulum of the liver cell is a network of submicroscopic lipoprotein tubules extending almost throughout the cytoplasm and existing in two main forms, rough where the tubules are studded with ribosomes and smooth from which ribosomes are absent (Palade & Siekevitz, 1956; Feinman *et al*, 1972). The rough endoplasmic reticulum is the main site of protein synthesis whereas the smooth endoplasmic reticulum is probably the more important site of drug metabolism (Fouts, 1961; Remmer & Merker, 1963; Holtzman *et al*, 1968). Disruption of the hepatocyte by homogenization techniques converts the endoplasmic reticulum into heterogeneous small vesicles called microsomes which may be separated from other cellular fractions by ultracentrifugation. Microsomes derived from the rough endoplasmic reticulum may be separated from those derived from the smooth, by centrifugation on discontinuous gradient systems (Fouts, 1961, 1971). The microsomal drug-metabolizing enzymes are membrane bound and are apparently nonspecific.

Many drugs, steroids, pesticides and other foreign compounds are metabolized by an NADPH-dependent microsomal enzyme system, the components of which appear to function as an integrated unit. The terminal oxygenase for this enzyme system is thought to be a carbon monoxide-binding cytochrome P-450 and its congeners (Estabrook, 1971) which

*Estimated errors of values quoted in this chapter are standard deviations unless otherwise stated.

Table 1 Drug metabolism in the liver (Parke, 1968; Gillette, 1971)

Metabolic pathways	Location of enzymes*
Oxidations	
Hydroxylation	ER
Dealkylation	ER
Epoxidation	ER
S- and N-Oxidation	ER
Desulphuration	ER
Dehalogenation	ER
Deamination	ER, MT
Alcohol oxidation	ER, CT
Aldehyde oxidation	CT
Reductions	
Aldehyde reduction	CT
Azoreduction	ER
Nitroreduction	ER, CT
Hydrolyses	
De-esterification	ER, CT
Deamidation	ER, CT
Conjugations	
Glucuronidation	ER
Sulphation	CT
Glutathione conjugation	CT
Methylation	CT
Acylation	CT

*ER = endoplasmic reticulum, CT = cytosol, MT = mitochondria.

incorporates one atom of oxygen, derived from molecular oxygen, into the substrate (RH) thus:

$$RH + NADPH + H^+ + O_2 \rightarrow ROH + NADP^+ + H_2O$$

This subject has been extensively reviewed in recent years (Goldstein *et al*, 1968; Gillette *et al*, 1969; Hutson, 1970, 1972; La Du *et al*, 1971; Fouts, 1971; Brodie & Gillette, 1971; Knoefel *et al*, 1972; Estabrook *et al*, 1973).

In 1954, Brown *et al* first discovered that in rats, certain dietary supplements, such as polycyclic hydrocarbons, increased the activity of a hepatic microsomal enzyme, aminoazo dye N-demethylase. Work showed that treatment of rats with certain carcinogenic polycyclic hydrocarbons, such as benzo[*a*]pyrene, dibenz[*a*,*h*]anthracene and 3-methylcholanthrene, rapidly induced the activities of several hepatic microsomal enzymes, such as that reducing the azo linkage and N-demethylating aminoazo dyes (Conney *et al*, 1956), that hydroxylating benzo[*a*]pyrene (Conney *et al*, 1957) and other drugs (Conney *et al*, 1959), and that ring-hydroxylating 2-acetylaminofluorene (Cramer *et al*, 1960). It was discovered independently (Remmer, 1958a, b) that barbiturates produced similar effects in rodents and reduced the sleeping time caused by a standard dose of hexobarbitone. Hepatic microsomes prepared from barbiturate-treated animals metabolized hexobarbitone more rapidly *in vitro*, and this increased enzyme activity was accompanied by proliferation of the smooth endoplasmic reticulum *in vivo* (Remmer & Merker, 1963, 1965; Fouts & Rogers, 1965). This phenomenon of increased enzyme activity caused by the administration of certain foreign compounds is now known as enzyme induction. It is due to the *de novo* synthesis of enzyme protein. Proliferation of the smooth endoplasmic reticulum in the liver is associated with increased hepatic cytochrome P-450 concentrations and an increased rate of drug or steroid metabolism. Enzyme induction has been the subject of many reviews (*inter alia* Burns, 1964; Conney, 1965, 1967, 1969a, 1971; Burns *et al*, 1965; Mannering, 1968, 1972; Remmer, 1969, 1972; Gelboin, 1971; Sher, 1971; Parke, 1972). From these early observations an extensive literature on the subject of enzyme induction has developed, much of it based on studies in laboratory animals and less on studies in humans. Although only the latter are discussed in this review, it is worth noting that supporting experimental data in animals almost invariably exists.

EFFECT OF ENZYME INDUCTION ON DRUG ACTION

During chronic administration of a drug, plasma and tissue concentrations of the drug and its metabolites may alter due to changes in the rates of elimination. Such adaptation to repeated dosing is of special importance clinically or during animal toxicity testing, but in both cases, it is often ignored or may go unnoticed. In animals, dramatic changes have resulted from the repeated administration of drugs and other foreign compounds, but frequently the route, conditions and dosage (usually relatively high), bear little relationship to those likely to be encountered for man. In man, the marked individual differences that occur in the rates of metabolism of many drugs (Brodie & Mitchell, 1973) is a further complicating feature such that in some cases therapeutically effective drug levels in the blood and tissues may never be reached (because of rapid metabolism), or accumulation occurs which leads to side effects (because of slow metabolism). These situations may be exaggerated in certain individuals by enzyme induction or inhibition. However, the list of compounds (Table 2) thought to produce enzyme induction or inhibition in man is relatively small. It is worth noting that many good inducers actually inhibit drug metabolism during the first few hours after administration (Mannering, 1968) and ignorance of this or poor choice of experimental conditions may lead to equivocal results.

The toxicity and pharmacological effects of a drug depend not only upon the properties of the drug itself, but also upon those of its metabolites. These effects are governed by the rates and manner in which the drug and its metabolites are absorbed, distributed and eliminated. Enzyme induction

Table 2 Some compounds that are enzyme inducers or inhibitors in man

Inducers*	Reference
Antipyrine	Breckenridge *et al* (1971)
Barbiturates	Cucinell *et al* (1965)
Carbamazepine	Hansen *et al* (1971b)
Cigarette smoke (polycyclic hydrocarbons)	Welch *et al* (1969)
o,p'-DDD (mitotane)	Bledsoe *et al* (1964)
DDT	Kolmodin *et al* (1969)
Diphenylhydantoin	Werk *et al* (1964)
Endrin	Hunter *et al* (1972a)
Ethanol	Misra *et al* (1971)
Eucalyptol	Jori *et al* (1970)
Glutethimide	Schmid *et al* (1964)
Griseofulvin	Catalano and Cullen (1966)
Lindane	Kolmodin-Hedman (1973)
Marijuana smoking	Lemberger *et al* (1971)
Medroxyprogesterone	Gordon *et al* (1971)
Meprobamate	Douglas *et al* (1963)
Nikethamide	Serini *et al* (1967)
Phenobarbitone	Conney (1969a)
Phenylbutazone	Chen *et al* (1962)
Rifampicin	Jezequel *et al* (1971)
Spironolactone	Huffman *et al* (1973)
Inhibitors†	
Ethanol	Rubin *et al* (1970)
Allopurinol	Vesell *et al* (1970)
Chloramphenicol	Christensen and Skovsted (1969)
Diethylstilboestrol	Sotaniemi *et al* (1973)
Disulfiram	Vesell *et al* (1971c)
Isoniazid	Kutt *et al* (1970)
Monoamine oxidase inhibitors	Sjöqvist (1965)
Nortriptyline	Vesell *et al* (1970)
Oral contraceptives	Carter *et al* (1974)
Prazepam	Vesell *et al* (1972)

*Additional references to these and other drugs are given throughout the text.
†The evidence for enzyme inhibition by some of these compounds is not strong and sometimes contradictory.

increases the rate of conversion of a drug to its metabolites. In many cases the metabolites are less therapeutically active or toxic than the parent compound, and consequently the extent and duration of drug action will be decreased. Good examples are the anticoagulant drugs (Conney, 1969b; Kazmier and Spittell, 1970). Treatment of patients with phenobarbitone, antipyrine or griseofulvin increased the rate of microsomal metabolism of certain coumarins whose anticoagulant effect was thereby reduced (Cucinell *et al*, 1965; Corn and Rockett, 1965; Catalano and Cullen, 1966; Robinson and MacDonald, 1966; Breckenridge *et al*, 1971). Relatively higher doses of anticoagulants are therefore required to produce an adequate therapeutic effect in patients concurrently receiving inducing drugs (Goss and Dickhaus, 1965). If the inducing agent is then withdrawn, dangerous levels of anticoagulation could result which may be sufficient to cause fatal haemorrhage (Avellaneda, 1955; Cucinell *et al*, 1966). If the metabolites are more therapeutically active or toxic than the parent compound, their action will be enhanced by enzyme induction (Gillette *et al*, 1974). Good examples in animals are carbon tetrachloride (Garner and McLean, 1969; Stenger, 1970), halothane (Stenger and Johnson, 1972) and paracetamol (Mitchell *et al*, 1973a, b).

Drugs are often simultaneously converted to both less-active and more-active metabolites, and there can occur a multiplicity of effects, which are sometimes opposing. Drugs that are poorly metabolized by microsomal enzymes are probably unaffected by enzyme induction, although such drugs may still have inducing properties—an example is barbitone (Burns *et al*, 1957). It must be appreciated that many drugs may increase the rate of their own metabolism as a result of enzyme induction. This is, however, only one factor in the development of tolerance to drugs, which can also arise when the rate of drug metabolism is unaltered (Butler *et al*, 1954). Thus enzyme induction or inhibition may modify, sometimes quite extensively, the duration and extent of drug effects. The clinical consequences of enzyme inhibition have been outlined recently (Longshaw, 1973) and enzyme inhibitors reviewed (Vesell and Passananti, 1973). Inhibition of drug metabolism may lead to potentially more dangerous situations because of the toxicity that could result from the accumulation of the drug in the body, as for example, during inhibition of diphenylhydantoin metabolism (Kutt, 1972). Unexpected results can be obtained when a drug previously administered to a patient inhibits the metabolism of the test drug even though the first drug is an enzyme-inducing agent. In the rat, for example, metabolism of other drugs may be impaired for up to six hours after a dose of phenobarbitone (Ernster and Orrenius, 1965). SKF 525-A inhibits the metabolism of other drugs and yet is itself an inducing agent (Anders and Mannering, 1966).

Drug interactions are now occurring more often as a result of increasing polypharmacy (Morrelli and Melmon, 1968; Prescott, 1969; Hartshorn, 1971; Swidler, 1971; Vesell, 1971; Brown, 1972; Avery, 1973; Morselli *et al*, 1974). It must be emphasized that drug interactions may be caused by factors such as altered absorption, distribution or excretion, as well as by enzyme induction or inhibition.

MICROSOMAL ENZYMES IN HUMAN LIVER

Direct assay of microsomal enzyme activities in the liver of man has been hampered by the difficulty in getting sufficient tissue with which to perform reliable measurements. Needle biopsy frequently yields only 20 mg or so of liver tissue, which is insufficient for the adequate preparation of microsomes. However, Billing and Black (1971) were able to obtain larger amounts of liver from patients undergoing abdominal surgery. The concentrations of cytochrome P-450 in apparently normal individuals taking no medication for a month prior to surgery were 12·2 ± 5·6 nmol per gram of liver (Black *et al*, 1974). In patients given phenobarbitone (180 mg daily for one week) prior to surgery, the concentrations of hepatic P-450 were 16·9 ± 7·4 nmol/g whereas in 24 patients taking a variety of other enzyme-inducing drugs yet higher concentrations of 20·7 ± 7·5 nmol/g were measured (Billing and Black, 1971); see also Table 14.

Workers in Remmer's group have since developed a method of estimating cytochrome P-450 in needle liver biopsy specimens without first preparing microsomes (Schoene *et al*, 1972). The concentrations of P-450 which were found in normal liver (10·8 ± 2·6 nmol/g) are close to those (10·6 ± 1·6 nmol/g) reported by May *et al* (1974) using a similar technique. Schoene *et al* (1972) found that the concentrations of P-450 were not reduced by 'mild' or 'moderate' viral hepatitis, although in seven patients with severe hepatitis or cirrhosis a reduction in concentrations was detected. These workers have also shown increased concentrations of cytochrome P-450 in patients taking anticonvulsant drugs or rifampicin. It has been shown that the hepatic concentrations of cytochrome P-450 in man are markedly less than those found in the rat (approximately 30 nmol/g). As the human liver, relative to bodyweight, is only half the size of the rat's, the relative differences in the total amounts of cytochrome P-450 available are considerable, and this has been suggested to be an important factor underlying the more rapid rate of drug metabolism generally enjoyed by rat (Remmer, 1970a). However, Kuntzman *et al* (1966a) have shown that in human liver the activities of certain microsomal drug-metabolizing enzymes may be as high as those in rat liver. The properties of cytochromes P-450 or b_5 in human liver are similar in some respects to those in rat or rabbit liver (Alvares *et al*, 1969). Also May *et al* (1974) related the concentrations of cytochrome P-450 in needle liver biopsy specimens to the plasma half-lives of quinine and antipyrine and were unable to find any correlation between the two. These findings together with data that have been obtained in animal investigations suggest that factors other than cytochrome P-450 concentrations are rate limiting in hepatic drug metabolism. Nelson *et al* (1971) showed that hepatic microsomal enzyme activities and P-450 concentrations may vary widely irrespective of whether liver was obtained from subjects who died from disease, drug overdose or accidental death.

A hepatic enzyme system which has been the subject of much study is UDP-glucuronyltransferase, which catalyses the conjugation with glucuronic acid of a large number of compounds (Dutton, 1966). In earlier studies, the fluorescent 4-methylumbelliferone was used as a substrate (Arias, 1962; di Toro *et al*, 1968). However, because of its importance in bilirubin metabolism, more recent investigators have studied the enzyme system using bilirubin itself as a substrate (Arias *et al*, 1969; Black and Billing, 1969; Black and Sherlock, 1970; Billing and Black, 1971). Preparations of apparently normal liver samples obtained at laparotomy conjugated 1·41 mg bilirubin per gram of liver per hour, and correspondingly larger amounts (see also Table 14) were metabolized by those taken from patients who were receiving phenobarbitone or other enzyme-inducing drugs (Billing and Black, 1971; Felsher *et al*, 1973). Using bilirubin as a substrate, low levels of the enzyme were reported to be present in various forms of unconjugated hyperbilirubinaemia, including Gilbert's syndrome (Arias *et al*, 1969; Black and Billing, 1969), but there was little, if any, increase after phenobarbitone pretreatment of these patients, despite reductions in the plasma-bilirubin concentrations (Arias *et al*, 1969; Black & Sherlock, 1970; Felsher *et al*, 1973; Black *et al*, 1974). Mulder (1970) has pointed out some of the pitfalls of enzymic assays of UDP-glucuronyltransferase. Enzyme activity may be considerably influenced by subsequent manipulations of the tissue such as prolonged homogenization (which may increase enzyme activity by exposing further binding sites), or detergents added to increase the sensitivity of the technique.

Microsomal enzyme activity has been reported to be low in the livers of animals at birth, rising to adult values during the course of a few weeks (Kato *et al*, 1964; Fouts and Adamson, 1959; Jondorf *et al*, 1959; Catz and Yaffee, 1968). Similar findings have been published with regard to human liver. Thus Lathe and Walker (1957) reported absent bilirubin conjugation in post-mortem neonatal human liver, and di Toro *et al* (1968) found that needle biopsy specimens of neonatal human liver had reduced capacity for conjugating 4-methylumbelliferone. This deficiency was suggested to be an important factor in the development of 'physiological jaundice' after birth. A similar inability to metabolize chloramphenicol has been put forward as the cause of the 'Gray syndrome' seen in infants receiving this drug (Weiss *et al*, 1960).

Other more recent studies have shown that the activities of microsomal drug-metabolizing enzymes in the foetal liver are lower than in the adult (Rane and Ackerman, 1972; Pelkonen *et al*, 1973; Rane *et al*, 1973; Juchau *et al*, 1973) and increase after birth (Yaffe and Juchau, 1974). However, the activities of some nonmicrosomal enzymes are apparently similar in adult or foetal liver (Chasseaud, 1973). Microsomes isolated from placenta at term (Meigs and Ryan, 1968) or earlier (Juchau *et al*, 1968) can also metabolize drugs as can certain foetal tissues (Juchau *et al*, 1972). Drug-metabolizing enzyme activity in the placenta seems to be low.

Enzyme-inducing agents increase the activities of microsomal enzymes when given directly to neonatal animals or when given to the lactating mothers (Fouts and Hart, 1965). Furthermore, enzyme activities are increased if the inducing agent is given to the mother in the latter stages of her pregnancy. In the rabbit, the drug is ineffective if given earlier than four days before birth. In humans phenobarbitone is effective in this way if given from the thirty-second week of pregnancy onwards (see page 173).

However, reports have recently appeared suggesting that the low microsomal enzyme activities previously cited for human foetal liver may be anomalous. Ackermann *et al* (1972) discovered that high activities of enzymes usually found in the microsomal fraction of adult liver were present in the nuclear fraction of foetal liver, and suggested that this was because of differences in the effects of homogenization on foetal and adult liver tissue resulting in inadequate separation of the various subcellular fractions. However, it is difficult to reconcile these findings with those of di Toro *et al* (1968) who found low conjugating capacity in homogenized neonatal human liver, when the subcellular fractions had not been separated.

DETECTION OF ENZYME INDUCTION IN MAN

Enzyme induction has been reported to occur in all mammalian species so far studied, although considerable interspecies differences may occur. Thus certain organochlorine pesticides increased drug metabolism in rats but not in mice (Conney, 1967; Abernathy *et al*, 1971). Nikethamide was found to increase pentobarbitone metabolism in rats, rabbits and mice, but not in guinea pigs (Brazda *et al*, 1965). Tolbutamide stimulates its own metabolism in rats but not in man (Conney, 1967; Redman and Prescott, 1973). There were species differences in the induction of microsomal haemoproteins and benzo[*a*]pyrene hydroxylase by phenobarbitone and 3-methylcholanthrene treatment (Alvares *et al*, 1970). Caution is obviously necessary before extending conclusions drawn from studies in one animal species to another.

While several procedures may be used for animals (Fouts, 1971), the detection of enzyme induction in man has proved difficult. The ideal way is to measure directly enzyme levels in hepatic tissue as was discussed earlier. However, there are many difficulties. Repeated liver biopsies cannot be justified and population surveys are impossible. The alternative use of post-mortem tissue may be unreliable because the enzymes involved often have a short half-life once outside the body (Nebert *et al*, 1969). Experiments with rabbit liver under the time-lag conditions occurring before human post-mortem tissue is available for assay showed that the activities of several of the microsomal drug-metabolizing enzymes had rapidly declined (Macleod *et al*, 1973). Human post-mortem liver may often be diseased or contain drug residues or may be obtained from geriatric subjects.

Many workers have attempted to assess enzyme induction in man by measuring the rates of elimination from the plasma, of drugs metabolized by liver microsomes. This approach is not ideal because it has been suggested on the basis of results obtained from controlled studies in twins, that genetic factors are more important than environmental factors in determining the rates of drug metabolism in man (Vesell, 1972a, b). Identical twins, even when living in different environments, still metabolize drugs at the same rate, demonstrating genetic control of drug metabolism. Drug metabolism is very similar in monozygotic twins, but often varies greatly in dizygotic twins (Table 3) and in the normal population (Sjöqvist and von Bahr, 1973). This

Table 3 Drug half-lives in identical and fraternal twins (adapted from Vesell *et al*, 1971b)

Twin	Half-life (hours)*		
	Bishydroxycoumarin	Antipyrine	Phenylbutazone
Identical			
1A	25	11	46
1B	25	11	50
2A	56	10	67
2B	56	10	70
3A	36	12	67
3B	34	12	67
4A	74	15	96
4B	72	15	96
5A	41	7	77
5B	43	7	70
6A	72	12	94
6B	69	13	98
7A	46	11	62
7B	44	11	62
Fraternal			
8A	45	15	175
8B	22	6	86
9A	47	7	55
9B	51	15	79
10A	35	5	50
10B	28	13	29
11A	7	12	62
11B	19	6	55
12A	25	15	67
12B	38	9	84
13A	67	8	70
13B	72	7	72
14A	41	8	46
14B	35	7	50

*Values calculated to the nearest whole number.

has been observed for drugs as different as antipyrine (Vesell and Page, 1969), alprenolol (Rawlins *et al*, 1974), nortriptyline (Alexanderson *et al*, 1969; Alexanderson and Sjöqvist, 1971), halothane (Cascorbi *et al*, 1971) and ethanol (Vesell *et al*, 1971a).

Thus in one series of patients receiving 75 mg of nortriptyline daily, a fiftyfold variation occurred in the steady-state plasma levels of the drug (Sjöqvist *et al*, 1968). Lesser variations, over threefold, have been observed in the steady-state plasma levels of diazepam and its bioactive metabolite nordiazepam in man (Berlin *et al*, 1972). Doubt has been expressed, however, that there is sufficient evidence that genetic factors are a more important determinant of microsomal drug metabolism than environmental factors (Fouts, 1973). Nevertheless, the evidence for certain drugs is well documented (Peters *et al*, 1965; Price-Evans, 1968; White and Price-Evans, 1968; Watson, 1969; La Du, 1971; Kutt, 1971; Peters and Levy, 1971; Hunter *et al*, 1974).

Ideally drug elimination needs to be determined before and after induction has taken place in man, an objective difficult to achieve except under carefully controlled conditions. The determination of drug elimination half-lives is often tedious involving the collection of several blood samples and their assay. Furthermore administration of drugs, such as antipyrine or phenylbutazone (Table 4) which are often used for these tests, carries a small but definite risk of hypersensitivity reactions (Goodman and Gilman, 1970).

Antipyrine has proved to be the most popular drug used for the evaluation of drug metabolism in man (Huffman *et al*, 1974) and animals (Welch *et al*, 1967) because it is little bound to plasma proteins, is distributed evenly in the total body water and is excreted after metabolism by the microsomal enzyme

Table 4 Typical baseline values (± S.D.) obtained for 'indicators' of hepatic enzyme activity

Indicator	Reference
Antipyrine half-life (h)	
14·1 ± 2·7 (n = 7)	Vesell *et al* (1971c)
15·0 ± 8·4 (n = 10)	Vesell *et al* (1971c)
12·7 ± 2·7 (n = 12)	Vesell *et al* (1972)
12·0 ± 3·5 (n = 61)	Ballinger *et al* (1972)
11·4 ± 3 (n = 8)	Huffman *et al* (1974)
12·5 ± 3·7 (n = 14)	Smith and Rawlins (1974)
11·7 ± 3·8 (n = 17)	Davis *et al* (1974b)
10·9 ± 1·5 (n = 16)	Lindgren *et al* (1974)
Phenylbutazone half-life (h)	
81 ± 15·7 (n = 18)	Poland *et al* (1970)
63·9 ± 11·7 (n = 12)	Kolmodin-Hedman (1973)
63·2 ± 21·7 (n = 15)	Smith and Rawlins (1974)
6β-Hydroxycortisol excretion (μg/24 h)	
400 (150–840, n = 14)	Werk *et al* (1964)
185 ± 72 (n = 18)	Poland *et al* (1970)
320 ± 160 (n = 14)	Ballinger *et al* (1972)
245 ± 108 (n = 10)	Smith and Rawlins (1974)
D-Glucaric-acid excretion (μmol/24 h)*	
12·0 ± 5·1 (n = 38)†	Hunter (1973)
15 ± 16 (n = 9)†	Smith & Rawlins (1974)
13·9 ± 4·9 (n = 24)†	Sotaniemi *et al* (1974)
34·3 ± 16 (n = 18)‡	Davis *et al* (1974a)

*D-Glucaric acid excretion may also be expressed as μmol/g creatinine (Hunter *et al*, 1972a). Variations in results for D-glucaric acid excretion arise because, in some cases, pure glucaro-1,4-lactone† was used as a standard and in other cases D-glucaric acid‡ was used, being converted to the corresponding lactone with only a 30% yield.

system. Antipyrine half-lives have been shown to correlate with phenylbutazone half-lives (Davies and Thorgeirsson, 1971a, b). Although it is unlikely that measurement of antipyrine half-lives (Table 4) could form a basis on which to adjust drug dosage regimens, it is worth exploring whether such measurements would be a useful means of highlighting cases of overt enzyme induction (or inhibition) or of gauging an individual's ability to oxidize drugs (Davies and Thorgeirsson, 1971a, b).

The plasma concentrations of *p,p'*-DDE, the principal metabolite of the dietary contaminant DDT, found in the body of most people, are lowered by enzyme-inducing drugs (Davies *et al*, 1969), and this reduction has also been used as an index of hepatic enzyme activity in man (Jager, 1970). However, the plasma concentrations of *p,p'*-DDE are usually low and changes may be difficult to detect. This approach may also be vitiated by excess exposure to DDT.

Determination of the change in the rate and extent of urinary excretion of an important drug metabolite may also be used to establish whether enzyme induction has occurred (Remmer, 1970a). Control of urinary pH may be necessary and complete urine collections are required. An example is the urinary excretion of 4-hydroxyantipyrine (Petruch *et al*, 1974).

An alternative to measurement of drug clearance is the determination of the plasma concentrations of an endogenous substance. Enzyme-inducing drugs lower plasma-bilirubin concentrations (Thompson *et al*, 1969a), which could therefore be measured as an indicator of hepatic enzyme activity (Sherlock, 1972). However, plasma-bilirubin concentrations are relatively low in normal subjects and changes are not easy to detect. Plasma-bilirubin concentrations decline after eating and may be affected by exercise; they also show diurnal variations (With, 1968). Thus plasma bilirubin is unreliable for the detection of enzyme induction.

The plasma levels of the enzyme γ-glutamyltranspeptidase rises in patients receiving enzyme-inducing drugs, such as anticonvulsants and hypnotics (Rosalki *et al*, 1971; Whitfield *et al*, 1973). The changes seen are less pronounced than changes in D-glucaric acid excretion (Davidson *et al*, 1974). However, as this increase may sometimes not occur until nearly two months after drug administration has started (Rosalki *et al*, 1971), it seems unlikely that it is closely related to enzyme induction which is usually evident within a few days. Furthermore, changes in the activities of this enzyme may be caused by liver disease (Szczeklik *et al*, 1961) and may occur in patients who are receiving no drugs whatsoever. Although changes in the levels of this enzyme following enzyme-inducing drugs are of general pharmacological interest, not enough is yet known of the underlying physiology, and it is not possible to regard measurement of this enzyme as a useful test for detecting enzyme induction in man. However, some encouragement may be obtained from a recent report that plasma γ-glutamyltranspeptidase activity was significantly correlated with urinary D-glucaric acid excretion in epileptic children ($n = 43$) receiving phenobarbitone alone or together with other anticonvulsants (Davidson *et al*, 1974).

The most satisfactory approach to date has been possibly the measurement of hepatic metabolites excreted in the urine. Two such substances which have been studied in some detail are 6β-hydroxycortisol and D-glucaric acid. 6β-Hydroxycortisol is a metabolite of cortisol produced by microsomal enzymes in the liver (see page 164). Only small amounts of 6β-hydroxycortisol are found in normal urine, but increased excretion has been detected following the administration of a number of drugs including diphenylhydantoin (Werk *et al*, 1964), phetharbital and other barbiturates (Kuntzman *et al*, 1968a), phenylbutazone (Kuntzman *et al*, 1966b), *o,p'*-DDD (Bledsoe *et al*, 1964), antipyrine (Breckenridge *et al*, 1971), and occupational exposure to organochlorine pesticides, such as DDT (Poland *et al*, 1970) and endrin (Jager, 1970). Thus measurement of 6β-hydroxycortisol excretion would appear to be an excellent way of detecting enzyme induction.

Unfortunately, 6β-hydroxycortisol assay is relatively difficult and time consuming and consequently its excretion has never received adequate critical evaluation as an index of enzyme induction. No direct comparison has apparently been made between 6β-hydroxycortisol excretion in animals and the activities of microsomal drug-metabolizing enzymes. Anomalous results have been reported, such as for example an increase in 6β-hydroxycortisol levels in the urine of normal volunteers after 7-days' administration of tricyclic antidepressants, but not after 28-days' administration (O'Malley *et al*, 1973). The range of normal values appears too wide (Table 4) to permit accurate separation of induced or normal subjects (Orme *et al*, 1972) unless large groups are studied.

D-Glucaric acid was first discovered in normal mammalian urine by Marsh (1963a) and is known to be an end-product of glucuronic-acid metabolism (Figure 3) in the liver of primates and guinea pigs. Its study is only relevant in these species since they are unable to biosynthesize ascorbic acid which with L-xylulose is another main product of the glucuronic acid pathway (see page 161). A considerable amount of work has now been done to understand the relationship of D-glucaric acid excretion (Table 4) with enzyme induction in man. D-Glucaric acid excretion has been shown to increase after the administration of many enzyme-inducing drugs (Table 5). Drugs which are excreted as glucuronides, but which are not enzyme-inducing agents apparently do not increase D-glucaric acid excretion (Aarts, 1968). The urinary excretion of D-glucaric acid has been shown to undergo a diurnal variation and is maximal in the late afternoon and evening; this is similar to diurnal variations observed in the activities of the drug-metabolizing enzymes in the livers of rats (Radzialowski and Bousquet, 1968). A similar diurnal variation has been noted in the content of smooth endoplasmic reticulum of rat hepatocytes (Chedid and Nair, 1972). Not surprisingly, D-glucaric acid excretion is diminished by fasting (Sotaniemi *et al*, 1974), as are the activities of microsomal enzymes (Marshall and McLean, 1969). Like the activities of many drug-metabolizing enzymes, D-glucaric acid excretion is low in neonates and increases with maturity

Table 5 Substances which increase urinary excretion of D-glucaric acid in man

Substance*	Reference
Aminopyrine	Aarts (1965)
Antipyrine	Davis *et al* (1974a)
Barbiturates	Hunter *et al* (1971a)
DDT	Hunter *et al* (1971d)
Diphenylhydantoin	Okada *et al* (1969)
Endrin (and related compounds)	Hunter *et al* (1972a)
Glutethimide	Greenwood *et al* (1973)
Methaqualone	Nayak *et al* (1974)
o,p' DDD	Hunter (1973)
Oral contraceptives	Mowat (1968)
Phenylbutazone	Aarts (1965)
Progesterone	Fahim *et al* (1969)
Rifampicin	Edwards *et al* (1974)
Spironolactone	Huffman *et al* (1973)

*D-glucaric acid excretion is not increased by the following which have not been reported to be enzyme inducers (Morgan and Roan, 1974): allopurinol, chlorpheniramine, cyclopentamine, hydrallazine, metapyrilene, methyldopa, phenylephrine, reserpine, saccharin, scopolamine, thyroid extract and α-tocopherol.

(Mowat, 1968). Unmedicated healthy persons of either sex apparently excrete D-glucaric acid in a highly consistent ratio to creatinine (March *et al*, 1974). The influence of varied diets on D-glucaric acid excretion does not appear to have been reported.

The quantity of D-glucaric acid excreted by epileptic subjects taking anticonvulsant drugs correlated directly with the dose of the drug taken. During a study of fifty four epileptic patients taking anticonvulsant drugs and normal controls, a highly significant correlation was found between D-glucaric acid excretion and the plasma-bilirubin concentrations (Hunter *et al*, 1971a). A significant correlation was found during studies of men engaged in the manufacture of organochlorine pesticides and control subjects with respect to D-glucaric acid excretion and the blood concentrations of *p,p'*-DDE (Hunter *et al*, 1972; Hunter, 1973). Both bilirubin and *p,p'*-DDE are metabolized by microsomal enzyme systems in man. Increased D-glucaric acid excretion follows within a few hours of barbiturate administration (Hunter, 1973), an interval consistent with the time of onset of enzyme induction (Ernster and Orrenius, 1965). Following treatment with organochlorine pesticides, increased excretion begins after a few days (Hunter, 1973; Sotaniemi *et al*, 1974). Recent work has shown that urinary D-glucaric acid determination is a reliable indicator of enzyme induction in patients on multiple-drug therapy, who excreted a mean of $37 \cdot 6 \pm 23 \cdot 1$ μmol/day ($n = 41$) compared to $13 \cdot 9 \pm 4 \cdot 9$ μmol/day ($n = 24$) by controls (Sotaniemi *et al*, 1974).

In guinea pigs which had received intraperitoneal doses of phenobarbitone (50 mg/kg) for up to five days, a significant correlation was found between the hepatic concentrations of cytochrome P-450 and the urinary excretion of D-glucaric acid 24 hours before the animals death ($n = 20$). A significant correlation between D-glucaric acid excretion and cytochrome P-450 was also found in guinea pigs which had received an inhibitor of protein synthesis to prevent enzyme induction by phenobarbitone (Hunter *et al*, 1973). Several studies have now been published concerning the relationship between D-glucaric acid and drug metabolism (Smith *et al*, 1972; Hunter *et al*, 1974; Davis *et al*, 1974a; Cunningham and Price-Evans, 1974). Not surprisingly, there is little direct correlation, for D-glucaric acid excretion is believed to reflect hepatic cytochrome P-450 concentrations (Hunter *et al*, 1973). Although changes in the activities of this and other enzymes may affect the rate of drug metabolism, drug metabolism is also dependent on many other factors, such as hepatic blood flow, drug uptake by the hepatocyte and biliary excretion. It must be remembered that experiments in which the rate of drug metabolism *in vivo* was compared to the concentrations of cytochrome P-450 in biopsy specimens of human hepatic tissue showed no significant correlation between the two (May *et al*, 1974). However, confusion on this point has crept even into the columns of *Lancet* where D-glucaric acid and 6β-hydroxycortisol excretion are considered unsatisfactory as indices of enzyme induction because they do not directly reflect individual rates of drug metabolism (*Lancet*, 1974). Only when other factors are kept constant do changes in the rates of drug metabolism reflect changes in hepatic enzyme activity, and under such conditions, a significant correlation has been observed between D-glucaric acid excretion and changes in the half-life of antipyrine (Hunter *et al*, 1974).

In earlier work, 24-hour urine collections were made for D-glucaric acid estimations, but this proved inconvenient, and more recently the concentrations of D-glucaric acid in urine have been related to that of creatinine, thus permitting enzyme induction to be assessed from single urine samples (Hunter *et al*, 1972a; Hunter, 1973).

ENZYME INDUCING AGENTS

More than two hundred drugs, pesticides, carcinogens and other chemicals have been discovered that induce hepatic microsomal enzymes in experimental animals (Conney, 1967). Several of these compounds are also known to produce enzyme induction in man (Table 2). Enzyme-inducing agents are structurally extremely diverse, and there is no apparent relationship between their action or structure and their ability to produce enzyme induction. However, most are lipid soluble at physiological pH. It is now believed that inducing agents are of at least two types, phenobarbitone being typical of one type and the carcinogenic polycyclic hydrocarbons of another. In general, phenobarbitone induces enzymes catalysing the metabolism of a much wider range of drugs than do the polycyclic hydrocarbons (Conney, 1967; Bousquet, 1970).

Recent studies have suggested that polycyclic hydrocarbons induce a different type of cytochrome P-450 from phenobarbitone (Sladek and Mannering, 1966, 1969; Lu *et al*, 1971), a conclusion supported by the different spectral properties of the reduced haemoprotein observed in the presence of ethyl isocyanide. Sladek and Mannering (1966) termed the new haemoprotein cytochrome P_1-450 and its existence has also been confirmed by others who have called it P-446 (Hildebrandt *et al*, 1968) or P-448 (Kuntzman *et al*, 1968b). Cytochrome P_1-450 appears to have less affinity for many drugs than does the normal form (Mannering, 1972). While it might be thought that polycyclic hydrocarbons induce mainly the metabolism of those compounds producing a Type-II spectral change (Imai and Sato, 1966) with microsomes whereas phenobarbitone induces the metabolism of both Type-I and Type-II substrates (see Remmer, 1972), this does not appear to be true.

The time interval between drug administration and the onset of enzyme induction varies somewhat according to the nature of the enzyme-inducing agent involved. D-Glucaric acid excretion in man increases very rapidly following the administration of barbiturates, and reaches a maximum in less than 24 hours (Hunter, 1973). Enzyme induction has been detected in rats given phenobarbitone after a similarly short interval (Ernster and Orrenius, 1965). After the cessation of barbiturate therapy, D-glucaric acid excretion returned to normal in approximately seven days (Hunter *et al*, 1971a). After exposure to organochlorine pesticides, however, enzyme induction appears to develop much more slowly. No increase in D-glucaric acid excretion was detected until several weeks had passed in one patient with adrenal carcinoma treated with *o,p'*-DDD (Hunter, 1973). As organochlorine pesticides are excreted very slowly from the body, the enzyme induction they produce is long lasting (Thompson *et al*, 1969b).

Phenobarbitone

Of the enzyme inducers known, phenobarbitone has probably been the most extensively studied (Cucinell, 1972). Like phenobarbitone, other barbiturates are also potent inducers. Barbitone, although hardly metabolized *in vivo*, is apparently an effective enzyme inducer (Burns *et al*, 1957).

After treatment for two months with phenobarbitone (120 mg), epileptic patients metabolized diphenylhydantoin (300 mg) more rapidly, since plasma drug concentrations (± standard error) fell from $11{\cdot}4 \pm 1{\cdot}6$ μg/ml ($n = 10$) to $3{\cdot}7 \pm 0{\cdot}7$ μg/ml ($n = 7$) (Cucinell *et al*, 1965). Similar results were reported by Buchanan and Sholiton (1972) who observed a threefold decline in diphenylhydantoin blood levels in subjects treated with phenobarbitone for 28 days, and by Morselli *et al* (1971) who showed that inclusion of phenobarbitone in diphenylhydantoin anticonvulsant therapy, lowered diphenylhydantoin-plasma levels. These levels returned to the original values when the barbiturate was withdrawn, but this was sometimes accompanied by side effects (Morselli *et al*, 1971). In another study, the serum half-lives of diphenylhydantoin measured before (12·5 h, $n = 12$) and after (8·5 h, $n = 12$) phenobarbitone treatment of human subjects were significantly different (Kristensen *et al*, 1969). Less differences between the plasma-drug concentrations in a group ($n = 37$) of patients taking diphenylhydantoin alone (9·5 ± 4·4 μg/ml) and in a group ($n = 44$) taking diphenylhydantoin and phenobarbitone together (8·1 ± 3·9 μg/ml) led Kutt *et al* (1969) to conclude that commonly used doses of phenobarbitone would cause unpredictable effects on plasma diphenylhydantoin levels. These effects, however, would be of small clinical significance in the majority of patients, a conclusion which can also be drawn from the studies of Buchanan and Sholiton (1972). Similarly, although it was suggested that a dose of phenobarbitone as low as 1 mg/kg/day would depress serum-diphenylhydantoin levels in epileptic children (Garrettson and Dayton, 1970), these results were contradicted by a separate study which showed that there was no apparent difference in diphenylhydantoin blood levels or in seizure control when the drug alone was given to epileptic children, or together with phenobarbitone (Buchanan and Allen, 1971). An explanation for these contradictions may be that in some cases the subjects studied were already almost maximally induced by the existing (diphenylhydantoin) therapy. For example, plasma-lidocaine levels were lower after an intravenous dose (2 mg/kg) to epileptic patients pretreated with phenobarbitone or diphenylhydantoin than in control subjects. Additional phenobarbitone treatment did not produce further reduction of plasma lidocaine levels in the epileptics suggesting that they were already maximally induced by their normal therapy (Heinonen *et al*, 1970). The effects of phenobarbitone on anticoagulant therapy are more obvious, and it is known that concurrent administration of phenobarbitone would require increases of the daily maintenance dosage of anticoagulants, such as bishydroxycoumarin (Cucinell *et al*, 1965; Goss and Dickhaus, 1965). A survey of numerous cases concluded that the withdrawal of enzyme-inducing drugs, such as phenobarbitone, may have contributed to some cases of fatal haemorrhage occurring during continued anticoagulant treatment (MacDonald and Robinson, 1968). The need for frequent prothrombin determinations, particularly during changes in the prescribed therapy, is obvious, so that anticoagulant dosage may be readjusted to avoid the risk of severe haemorrhage due to increases in anticoagulant blood levels (Kazmier and Spittell, 1970; Sigell and Flessa, 1970). In a randomized crossover study with healthy subjects, treatment for 3-week periods with sedative-hypnotic drugs enhanced the plasma clearance of warfarin although prothrombin time was only altered by two of the drugs (Table 6) (MacDonald *et al*, 1969).

Davis *et al* (1974b) have listed drugs whose pharmacological activity is affected by barbiturates and those drugs affecting barbiturate pharmacological activity. If patients have been receiving barbiturates for more than 4 to 7

Table 6 Changes in plasma-warfarin clearances produced by sedative–hypnotics (from MacDonald *et al*, 1969)

Inducing agent and dose	Mean plasma-warfarin half-life (h ± S.E.)
Phenobarbitone* (120 mg)	29·1 ± 3·1
Glutethimide* (1 g)	28·5 ± 2·9
Chloral betaine (1·74 g)	38·2 ± 3·8
None	52·4 ± 6·2

*These drugs lowered prothrombin times.

days, which is usually sufficient to induce microsomal enzymes, and a second drug is added to the therapeutic regimen, then the dose of the second drug necessary to produce the desired therapeutic effect might have to be increased in relation to the degree of induction produced by the barbiturate. Cessation of barbiturate therapy then should be followed by an appropriate reduction in the dosage of the second drug. The interactions caused by concomitant barbiturate therapy are at their most significant when the second drug has a very low therapeutic index for toxic and other side effects, e.g. warfarin (Davis *et al*, 1974b) and other anticoagulants whose plasma levels and elimination half-lives are decreased after pretreatment with barbiturates (Dayton *et al*, 1961; Corn, 1966; van Dam and Gribnau-Overkamp, 1967).

Steady-state concentrations of digitoxin fell by about 50% when this drug was administered concurrently with phenobarbitone and reverted to control values when the barbiturate was discontinued. Treatment of digitalized patients for eight weeks with phenobarbitone lowered the digitoxin-plasma elimination half-life, e.g. from 7·8 days to 4·5 days, and increased the proportion of polar drug metabolites excreted in the urine (Solomon and Abrams, 1972). Curry *et al* (1970) noted that concomitant phenobarbitone administration to mental patients resulted in lowered blood-chlorpromazine levels, presumably with increased amounts of chlorpromazine glucuronides excreted in the urine (Forrest *et al*, 1970), and a return to psychotic symptoms (Curry *et al*, 1970). The metabolism of phenylbutazone in man is apparently under genetic control, but is probably enhanced by phenobarbitone administration, particularly in those subjects who metabolize phenylbutazone more slowly, as implied by a relatively long plasma elimination half-life (Whittaker and Price-Evans, 1970). The use of enzyme-inducing drugs in treating hepatic dysfunction has been suggested by the work of Levi *et al* (1968) who showed that the relatively longer plasma half-life (± S.E.M.) of phenylbutazone in patients with liver disease was shortened from

100 ± 10 h ($n = 34$) to $54{\cdot}3 \pm 5$ h ($n = 61$) by phenobarbitone pretreatment (90 mg/day for 3 days). However, this approach has not been extensively explored possibly because of reports that in cirrhotic patients, for example, the activities of microsomal drug-metabolizing enzymes do not seem to be markedly reduced (Maxwell *et al*, 1972a). On the other hand, a recent comparative study of meperidine pharmacokinetics showed that the overall first-order elimination rate constant decreased from $0{\cdot}672\ h^{-1}$ in normal subjects to $0{\cdot}242\ h^{-1}$ in cirrhotics, apparently because of impaired hepatic drug-metabolizing activity (Klotz *et al*, 1974). Also, Prescott and Wright (1973) demonstrated that paracetamol metabolism was impaired in patients with liver damage.

Pharmacokinetic studies in cancer patients with apparently normal renal and hepatic function, demonstrated that treatment with phenobarbitone for ten days increased the rate of formation of metabolites of cyclophosphamide, but did not greatly affect the total amount formed. Thus, although cyclophosphamide is biotransformed to bioactive metabolite(s) by a hepatic microsomal enzyme system, it was thought unlikely that phenobarbitone treatment would modify cyclophosphamide efficacy to a significant extent (Jao *et al*, 1972). Detection of higher blood levels of griseofulvin in control subjects ($n = 8$) than in those treated with phenobarbitone ($n = 8$) for three days led to the conclusion that the biotransformation of griseofulvin was enhanced by the barbiturate (Busfield *et al*, 1963). However, the demonstration that the elimination kinetics of orally administered griseofulvin were unaffected by intravenous phenobarbitone was taken as evidence that the lowering of plasma griseofulvin levels produced by oral phenobarbitone was due to impaired absorption and not enzyme induction (Riegelman *et al*, 1970). These studies show that it is inadvisable to conclude that enzyme induction (or inhibition) has occurred merely on the basis of changes in the plasma-drug elimination half-life. The latter change is, however, often the first clue (figure 1) that should then be supported with additional experimentation. Enhanced fenoprofen elimination from the plasma of human subjects following phenobarbitone pretreatment has been ascribed to enzyme induction (Helleberg *et al*, 1974). In reporting that patients treated with barbiturates or certain other compounds metabolized cortisol to 6β-hydroxycortisol more extensively, Conney (1969a) argued that drug therapy may result in alterations in the proportions and rates at which endogenous substrates (hormones) are produced, with consequential changes in physiological function. Thus phenobarbitone treatment enhanced the urinary excretion of 6β-hydroxycortisol by schizophrenics (Burstein and Klaiber, 1965). Excretion of this metabolite is also greater during pregnancy (Cucinell, 1972).

Phenobarbitone administration may also result in the reduction of the body burden of environmental contaminants, particularly persistant substances like some organochlorine compounds. Serum concentration of *p,p'*-DDE (a metabolite of environmentally occurring DDT) were lower in those

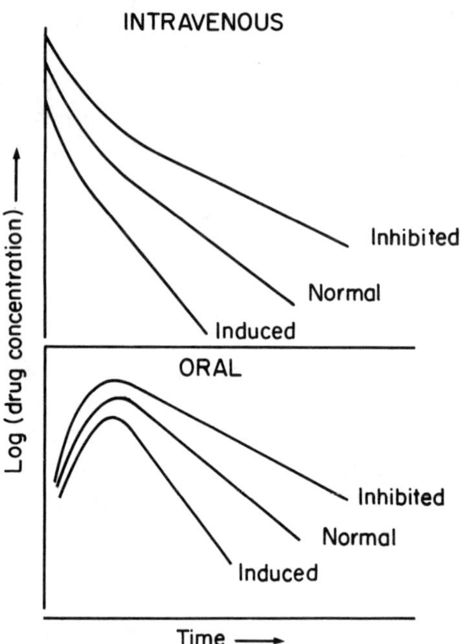

Figure 1 Effect of hepatic enzyme induction and inhibition on the plasma concentrations of a hypothetical drug (adapted from Rowland, 1972)

Table 7 Effect of phenobarbitone and other drugs in reducing the body burden of *p,p*-DDE, a metabolite of DDT (from Watson *et al*, 1972)

Drug regimen	Serum concentrations of *p,p*-DDE (ng/ml ± S.D.)
None ($n = 46$)	31·2 ± 18.6
Phenobarbitone ($n = 8$)	6·8 ± 5·4
Diphenylhydantoin ($n = 5$)	5·3 ± 6·8
Phenobarbitone and diphenylhydantoin ($n = 15$)	1·6 ± 1·0
Tranquillizers and sedatives ($n = 28$)	16·6 ± 21·0

patients taking drugs, such as phenobarbitone, than in those control patients taking no drugs at all; see Table 7 (Davies *et al*, 1969; Watson *et al*, 1972).

Other Barbiturates and Hypnotics

The increased rates of drug biotransformation caused by barbiturate therapy probably partly accounts for the tolerance which develops to such agents with prolonged use. Maximal induction could be expected to occur following chronic exposure to high doses of such drugs, taken during barbiturate dependence. Thus patients on barbiturates for periods ranging from 1 to 20 years eliminated antipyrine from the plasma with a half-life of $5{\cdot}3 \pm 1{\cdot}2$ h ($n = 8$). After a 7-day withdrawal period, antipyrine half-lives were still low ($6{\cdot}8 \pm 1{\cdot}6$ h) but reverted to control levels (11·3 h) in those patients who remained drug-free. The urinary output of 6β-hydroxycortisol was higher in barbiturate-dependent patients (1000 μg/day) than in controls (320 μg/day), whereas the output of 17-hydroxycorticosteroids was similar from both groups (Ballinger *et al*, 1972).

Twenty-one days' treatment of human subjects ($n = 7$) with amylobarbitone lowered antipyrine plasma half-lives from $11{\cdot}9 \pm 3{\cdot}2$ h to $6{\cdot}9 \pm 1{\cdot}2$ h (O'Malley *et al*, 1973), showing that this barbiturate was also a potent inducer of drug metabolizing enzymes. Due to enzyme induction, the hypnotic drugs amylobarbitone, secobarbitone, dichloralphenazone (a molecular complex of chloral hydrate and antipyrine), but not nitrazepam, caused a fall in plasma-warfarin concentrations and altered anticoagulant control. Dichloralphenazone acted as an inducer because of the antipyrine component, not the chloral hydrate (hypnotic) component. Plasma-antipyrine half-life was correlated with the percentage fall in plasma-warfarin levels in five patients administered dichloralphenazone (Breckenridge and Orme, 1971; Breckenridge, 1971).

It has been reported that withdrawal of chloral hydrate from a patient receiving bishydroxycoumarin resulted in raised plasma levels of the anticoagulant and a fatal haemorrhage (Cucinell *et al*, 1966). Chloral hydrate was considered to have acted as an enzyme inducer and its withdrawal resulted in a slowing of drug metabolism and an increase in drug-plasma levels leading to a prolongation of the prothrombin time. However, currently chloral hydrate is considered not to be an enzyme-inducing agent (Breckenridge *et al*, 1971). Decreased plasma warfarin half-life after chloral hydrate administration was thought to be due to displacement of warfarin from protein-binding sites caused by trichloroacetic acid, a metabolite of chloral hydrate. Enzyme induction by the latter was probably not the cause (Sellers and Koch-Weser, 1970). These authors concluded that the clinical problem encountered when warfarin and chloral hydrate are administered together would be potentiation, not reduction of the hypoprothrombinaemic action of warfarin as would occur after enzyme induction. Other studies in patients suggested that the interaction between warfarin and chloral hydrate would not be of clinical significance under certain conditions of treatment (Griner *et al*, 1971).

Quinalbarbitone administration (100 mg/night for 33 days) reduced the steady-state plasma-warfarin concentrations in patients on anticoagulant therapy by almost 65%. A dose–response relationship was demonstrable since in one patient the plasma-warfarin half-life was reduced from a control value of 53·1 h to 42·3, 21·7 and 24·4 h respectively after repeated dosage of 100, 200 and 300 mg/day of the barbiturate. Maximal enzyme induction in this subject had been achieved with the 200 mg/day dosage regimen (Breckenridge *et al*, 1973). Treatment with secobarbitone and amobarbitone for 21 days reduced the plasma elimination half-life of warfarin and the prothrombin time whereas similar treatment with the tranquillizer chlordiazepoxide and the diuretic chlorothiazide had no effect. The overall plasma drug half-life measured was 41·2 h. This value is intermediate to that (36·3 ± 3·5 h, $n = 12$) recently measured by a more specific high-pressure liquid-chromatographic method and that reported using (55·9 ± 8·4 h, $n = 12$) the less specific fluorimetric method (Vesell and Shively, 1974).

Studies in humans showed that the decreased response to warfarin obtained during heptabarbitone administration was due only to induction of the warfarin-metabolizing enzyme system and not to effects on the blood-coagulation process (Levy *et al*, 1970). A similar conclusion may be drawn from related studies with bishydroxycoumarin (O'Reilly and Levy, 1970), except that the barbiturate had the added effect of diminishing the absorption of orally administered bishydroxycoumarin (Aggeler and O'Reilly, 1969). This was suggested by the more pronounced effects obtained when the anticoagulant was given orally than when it was given intravenously (Table 8).

Patients receiving the hypnotic drug *Mandrax* (methaqualone: diphenhydramine, 10:1 w/w) eliminated antipyrine more rapidly (half-life 6·2 ± 2·0 h, $n = 3$) than normal subjects would; see Table 4 (Ballinger *et al*, 1972). Treatment of normal subjects with therapeutic doses of methaqualone resulted in a threefold increase of urinary D-glucaric acid excretion (Nayak *et al*, 1974). After 18-days' treatment of human subjects with the nonhypnotic barbiturate phetharbital, the urinary excretion of 6β-hydroxycortisol increased from 186 μg/day to 481 μg/day, whereas 17-hydroxycorticosteroid excretion was unaffected. In parallel experiments, phetharbital was shown to induce cortisol 6β-hydroxylase activity in the hepatic microsomes of guinea pigs (Kuntzman *et al*, 1968).

Table 8 Effect of heptabarbitone on the response to bishydroxycoumarin (from Aggeler and O'Reilly, 1969)

Drug treatment	Prothrombin response (units)*	Bishydroxycoumarin plasma half-life (h ± S.D.)
Oral bishydroxycoumarin†		
Controls	41·7 ± 17·0	81·6 ± 23·5
Heptabarbitone treated	18·0 ± 9·4	51·4 ± 21·0
Intravenous bishydroxycoumarin‡		
Controls	36·1 ± 15·1	100·2 ± 33·0
Heptabarbitone treated	24·0 ± 12·4	75·2 ± 27·8

*Area under the curve.
†$n = 10$.
‡$n = 7$.

Diphenylhydantoin

For effective therapy, blood levels of diphenylhydantoin of 10–20 μg/ml are generally required while levels exceeding 20 μg/ml may lead to side effects. Thus alteration of diphenylhydantoin blood levels by other drugs due to induction or inhibition of drug-metabolizing enzymes (Kutt, 1971) may be clinically important (Kradjan, 1974). At clinical dosages, diphenylhydantoin does not appear profoundly to induce its own metabolism (Kutt, 1971) although the activities of hepatic drug-metabolizing enzymes are increased (Remmer *et al*, 1973). In patients, diphenylhydantoin blood levels may remain stable for relatively long periods (Kutt, 1971). The plasma-elimination half-life in man varies at least sixfold: a mean value is 22 h (Arnold and Gerber, 1970).

Studies in children showed that additional therapy with diphenylhydantoin during phenobarbitone treatment resulted in increased plasma levels of the barbiturate, implying diminished elimination of the barbiturate. The resulting clinical improvement was apparently not related to the higher barbiturate levels, but to diphenylhydantoin therapy (Morselli *et al*, 1971). The plasma half-life of a test dose of antipyrine was significantly reduced from $10{\cdot}0 \pm 3{\cdot}4$ to $6{\cdot}1 \pm 1{\cdot}6$ h in epileptic subjects ($n = 8$) treated with diphenylhydantoin, and the urinary excretion of 4-hydroxyantipyrine was also increased (Petruch *et al*, 1974) suggesting that administration of the anticonvulsant had induced drug hydroxylation. Decreased serum dicoumarol (bishydroxycoumarin) levels after patients had also been treated with diphenylhydantoin was ascribed to enzyme induction and not to diminished absorption of the anticoagulant or its displacement from protein-binding sites (Hansen *et al*, 1971a).

There have been reports that diphenylhydantoin therapy significantly increased the cortisol-secretion rate due to increased formation and elimination of 6β-hydroxycortisol. The plasma-cortisol half-life was decreased (Reynolds and Mirkin, 1973). However, no adverse effects associated with changes in cortisol production have been observed (Werk *et al*, 1971). Excretion of 6β-hydroxycortisol may be increased by up to tenfold in normal subjects or patients administered diphenylhydantoin for several weeks. Excretion of 17-ketosteroids or 17-hydroxycorticosteroids was apparently not significantly affected (Werk *et al*, 1964). Neonates exposed to anticonvulsant drugs *in utero* did not show enhanced 6β hydroxylation of cortisol possibly because of the already considerable 6β-hydroxylation of cortisol characteristic of the neonate (Reynolds and Mirkin, 1973). Six weeks treatment of patients with diphenylhydantoin (3 to 5 mg/kg/day) significantly enhanced the plasma clearance of a single intravenous dose of tritium-labelled cortisol and the urinary excretion of 6β-hydroxycortisol (Choi *et al*, 1971). The influence of diphenylhydantoin on calcium and folate metabolism is discussed later (see pages 165 and 168).

Other Drugs

Several other enzyme inducers in man are known that have been less extensively reported (Table 2). Pretreatment of human subjects for up to 11 days with oral doses of phenylbutazone resulted in lowered plasma concentrations of intravenously administered aminopyrine and increased concentrations of the corresponding metabolite, 4-aminoantipyrine (Chen *et al*, 1962).

The clearances of the anticoagulants warfarin (Corn, 1966) and bishydroxycoumarin (van Dam and Gribnau-Overkamp, 1967) were enhanced by pretreatment of humans with glutethimide. The rate of antipyrine metabolism was accelerated by glutethimide treatment of uremic patients. The magnitude of the reduction in antipyrine half-life correlated with the initial half-life. Thus, the higher the initial half-life, the greater the degree of induction. The plasma clearance of antipyrine was not impaired in these uremic subjects; see Table 9 (Lichter *et al*, 1973). Glutethimide may also induce its own metabolism since patients tolerant to the drug metabolized it more rapidly than normal subjects (Schmid *et al*, 1964). Meprobamate can apparently stimulate its own metabolism, as subjects receiving the drug for 30 days produced a greater proportion of urinary hydroxymeprobamate than those receiving a single dose (Douglas *et al*, 1963).

Table 9 Plasma antipyrine half-life in normal, induced and uremic subjects (from Lichter *et al*, 1973)

Subjects	Half-life (h)
Control ($n = 11$)	10·8
Uremic ($n = 6$)	10·3
Uremic after induction ($n = 6$) with glutethimide	7·0

The decrease in concentrations of diazepam in the plasma of a few patients after one to six weeks therapy together with other evidence suggested that diazepam might induce its own metabolism (Kanto *et al*, 1974). It is likely, however, that evidence of self-induction by drugs, such as diazepam, which can exhibit considerable intersubject variations in plasma concentrations would be harder to obtain unless large numbers of subjects were studied.

After at least nine days treatment with carbamazepine, human subjects metabolized an intravenous dose of diphenylhydantoin more rapidly: serum diphenylhydantoin half-lives fell from 10·6 to 6·4 h. Carbamazepine treatment also reduced the serum half-life of warfarin (Hansen *et al*, 1971b). Tricyclic antidepressants administered for 28 days caused a small, but significant decrease in plasma antipyrine half-lives from 11·7 ±2·9 h ($n = 30$) to 10·1 ±2·2 h ($n = 29$) (O'Malley *et al*, 1973).

The antituberculosis drug rifampicin is a powerful enzyme-inducing agent in man and it induces its own metabolism, the plasma elimination half-life of rifampicin being shorter after repeated administration of the drug (Acocella *et al*, 1971; Curci *et al*, 1972; Nitti *et al*, 1973; Virtanen and Tala, 1974). Other studies showed that the smooth endoplasmic reticulum and the activities of microsomal drug-metabolizing enzymes were increased in the livers (biopsy samples) of patients treated with rifampicin (Jezequel *et al*, 1971; Remmer *et al*, 1973). Rifampicin has been reported to increase the rate of cortisol metabolism (Edwards *et al*, 1974) and tolbutamide metabolism (Syvälahti *et al*, 1974) in man.

Treatment of healthy human subjects with spironolactone, an aldosterone antagonist, for two weeks produced a significant decrease in the plasma-antipyrine half-life from 12·4 to 7·6 h ($n = 8$) due to the increased rate of formation of the 4-hydroxy metabolite but not the 3-hydroxymethyl metabolite of antipyrine. Urinary excretion of 6β-hydroxycortisol was increased from 152 μg/day to 292 μg/day (Huffman *et al*, 1973).

That anaesthetists excreted an intravenous dose of ^{14}C-halothane more rapidly than pharmacists was ascribed to possible enzyme induction in the former group due to occupational exposure (Cascorbi *et al*, 1970). Nevertheless, genetic factors were held to be more important in determining the metabolism of halothane than environmental ones (Cascorbi *et al*, 1971). The importance of enzyme induction in anaesthesia has been surveyed (Brown, 1973). The reduction in serum antibiotic half-lives from $2{\cdot}06 \pm 0{\cdot}30$ h to $1{\cdot}47 \pm 0{\cdot}55$ h, observed after repeated dosing of normal subjects with cefazolin may have been due to the drug inducing its own metabolism (Welling *et al*, 1974).

Oral Contraceptives

Oestrogen-containing oral contraceptives have been reported to increase the urinary excretion of D-glucaric acid (Mowat, 1968), a property shared by progesterone (Fahim *et al*, 1969). This suggests that they may be enzyme-inducing agents. Paradoxically, however, it has been reported that subjects taking oral contraceptives, showed a decrease in the rate of drug metabolism (O'Malley *et al*, 1972). Oestrogens and progesterone are known to be competitive inhibitors of drug metabolism in animals (Tephly and Mannering, 1968), and it seems probable that this effect outweighs the enzyme induction produced. Other competitive inhibitors of drug metabolism, notably SKF 525-A and piperonyl butoxide, have also been shown in animals to produce enzyme induction (Anders and Mannering, 1966; Wagstaff and Short, 1971). A similar state of enzyme induction masked by inhibition of drug metabolism caused by steroids seems likely to occur in pregnancy (Hunter *et al*, 1972b) where the excretion of both D-glucaric acid (Marsh, 1963a) and 6β-hydroxycortisol (Cucinell, 1972) is increased.

Ethanol

It has been known for many years that the oxidation of ethanol *in vivo* is mediated by alcohol dehydrogenase, an apparently noninducible enzyme located in hepatic cytosol (von Wartburg and Rothlisberger, 1961; von Wartburg, 1971). More recently it has been shown that the oxidation of ethanol is also carried out by an inducible microsomal enzyme (Lieber and deCarli, 1968; von Wartburg, 1971), but the importance of this enzyme, known as M.E.O.S., has been questioned (Caldwell and Sever, 1974).

Alcohol administration to human volunteer subjects, alcoholics or non-alcoholics causes proliferation of the smooth endoplasmic reticulum (Iseri *et al*, 1966; Feinman *et al*, 1972) as shown by electron microscopy (Lane and Lieber, 1972); drug-metabolizing enzymes are induced and drugs are therefore cleared more rapidly from the plasma. Thus the alcoholic, when sober, has an increased tolerance to certain drugs (Kater *et al*, 1969a); when intoxicated, however, alcoholics are more susceptible to the action of various drugs (Misra *et al*, 1971) because of inhibition of drug metabolism by alcohol.

Apparently, two thirds of the ethanol in the body is oxidized by alcohol dehydrogenase and the remainder by the microsomal enzyme system, but during intoxication the relative amounts metabolized by the latter enzyme system may increase (Lieber *et al*, 1971). Thus the increased resistance of alcoholics, when sober, to drug action can be explained not only by central nervous system adaptation, but also by an increase in microsomal drug-metabolizing enzyme activity, leading to more rapid drug clearance from the body. Effects of simultaneous alcohol and drug administration can be explained not only by an additive (or synergistic) effect on the central nervous system, but also by the short-term inhibition of microsomal drug-metabolizing enzymes, resulting in delayed drug detoxication and clearance. Thus, moderate ethanol consumption reduced the clearance of meprobamate and pentobarbitone, presumably because of competition between ethanol and the other drugs for hepatic biotransformation (Misra *et al*, 1970). Clearance of ethanol and these drugs was accelerated after daily administration of ethanol to healthy subjects for one month: the plasma elimination half-life of meprobamate (± S.E.) was reduced from $13{\cdot}7 \pm 1{\cdot}0$ to $8{\cdot}2 \pm 0{\cdot}3$ h and that of pentobarbitone from $35{\cdot}1 \pm 6{\cdot}1$ to $26{\cdot}3 \pm 4{\cdot}4$ h (Misra *et al*, 1971). A notorious ethanol–drug interaction is that occurring between alcohol and chloral hydrate (Sellers *et al*, 1972).

Heavy drinkers metabolize phenobarbitone (Rubin and Lieber, 1968) and tolbutamide (Kater *et al*, 1969a) more rapidly, and these and other studies (Table 10) have implied that the accelerated drug clearance caused by alcohol is clinically important because it may cause problems in adjusting alcoholic patients to the correct drug therapy. However, the amount of alcohol necessary to elicit effects in these cases is large and about a third of the total dietary calories must apparently be supplied as ethanol. Alcohol

Table 10 Influence of alcohol on the clearance of drug from the plasma (from Kater *et al*, 1969a, b)

Drug	Alcoholics*	Non-alcoholics*
Tolbutamide (i.v.)†	165·4 ± 33·5 min (n = 31)	350·6 ± 130·6 min (n = 13)
Warfarin (p.o)†	26·5 ± 13·3 h (n = 15)	41·1 ± 19·2 h (n = 11)
Diphenylhydantoin (p.o)†	16·3 ± 6·8 h (n = 15)	23·5 ± 11 h (n = 76)

*Results ± S.D.
†Intravenous (i.v.) or oral (p.o.) routes.

may be eliminated more rapidly by subjects treated with enzyme-inducing drugs, as has been suggested by studies in asthmatics who displayed more rapid clearance of intravenously infused ethanol from their blood than control subjects (Sotaniemi *et al*, 1972). Beckett (1970) has reported that regular heavy alcohol drinkers are able to metabolize alcohol faster than moderate or occasional drinkers.

Organochlorine Compounds

There is currently much concern over the possible harmful effects of environmental pollution by chemicals, such as the pesticide DDT. These substances, which can find their way into food via the soil, water and air, have been shown to increase the activity of hepatic microsomal drug-metabolizing enzymes in laboratory animals, often at concentrations much lower than those producing toxicity. However, most experiments which demonstrate the enzyme-inducing properties of chemicals present in the environment involve the administration of relatively large doses to animals. The environmental exposure of the human population is considerably less and its effects are thus more difficult to assess, particularly in the absence of suitably sensitive methods. This has led to speculative and alarmist extrapolation of animal data to man, such as the statement, 'In animals the level of DDT which starts to cause enzyme induction is 1 mg/kg of food (1 ppm) or a single dose of 1 mg/kg bodyweight. At these dose levels the DDT content of the body fat reaches about 10 ppm. In England DDT levels in food are about one thirtieth of a dose that would induce enzymes in rats, but human body fat levels of DDT averaged 3 ppm in 1965 reaching 8 ppm in some individuals. In other words we live on the verge of induction by DDT' (McLean, 1972). There is of course no evidence whatsoever to suggest that the concentrations of DDT in fat necessary to produce enzyme induction in man is the same as it is in the rat.

Although the use of DDT is now curtailed in Europe and the U.S.A., but not in Africa or Asia, it, together with organochlorine compounds like dieldrin, continue to form part of man's dietary intake (Fishbein, 1974). Since the initial report that the spraying of an animal room with chlordane led to enzyme induction in animals (Hart *et al*, 1963; Fouts, 1965), there have been a few studies of such compounds in man. Kolmodin *et al* (1969) found that the rate of antipyrine metabolism was significantly greater in men engaged in organochlorine-pesticide manufacture than in control subjects, although the overlap in antipyrine half-lives between the two groups was considerable: in exposed workers, the half-life was $7{\cdot}7 \pm 2{\cdot}6$ h ($n = 26$) and in controls the half-life was $13{\cdot}1 \pm 7{\cdot}5$ h ($n = 33$). In a similar study, it was shown that the concentrations of DDT-related substances in the serum and fat (gluteal fat biopsy) of DDT-factory workers exceeded those in a control population by twenty or thirtyfold. The serum half-life of phenylbutazone ($65{\cdot}5 \pm 3{\cdot}5$ h, $n = 18$) was 19% lower, and the urinary excretion of 6β-hydroxycortisol (291 ± 36 μg/day, $n = 18$) was 57% higher in the factory workers (Poland *et al*, 1970; Conney *et al*, 1971). These increases were relatively small in relation to the individual differences which might have been dependent on genetic factors, or even unknown environmental factors. Furthermore no correlation existed between the phenylbutazone half-life and the daily 6β-hydroxycortisol excretion, nor between either of these and the body burden of DDT and its metabolites. Large individual differences were observed in another study which compared phenylbutazone plasma half-lives in control subjects ($63{\cdot}9 \pm 11{\cdot}7$ h, $n = 12$) to those ($51{\cdot}5 \pm 14{\cdot}8$ h, $n = 14$) occupationally exposed to lindane by skin contact and inhalation (Kolmodin-Hedman, 1973).

Studies in patients receiving anticonvulsant therapy have shown that the concentrations of the DDT metabolite, *p,p'*-DDE present in blood and adipose tissue were lowered (Table 11). Thus drug therapy can influence the body burden of persistent compounds like DDT (Davies *et al*, 1969; Davies *et al*, 1972; Edmundson *et al*, 1972; Davies and Edmundson, 1972). Conve-

Table 11 Influence of enzyme-inducing drugs on the body burden of DDE (from Davies *et al*, 1969, 1972)

Subjects and treatment	Mean blood level (ppb) of DDE	Mean fat level (ppm) of DDE
Healthy controls ($n = 199$)	9·1	—
Outpatients on drugs for more than 3 months		
Phenobarbitone ($n = 28$)	3·5	—
Diphenylhydantoin ($n = 18$)	1·9	—
Both drugs together ($n = 31$)	1·7	—
General population ($n = 90$)	—	5·5
Inpatients on phenobarbitone and/or diphenylhydantoin ($n = 7$)	—	0·09
Inpatients not on anticonvulsant drugs	—	2·08

nient methods for estimating enzyme induction caused by environmental agents are those which determine the excretion of a hepatic metabolite, such as D-glucaric acid or 6β-hydroxycortisol. The usefulness of these methods has been demonstrated during studies made on workers engaged in the manufacture of the cyclodiene pesticides, endrin, aldrin and its epoxide dieldrin, at Pernis in Holland. Hunter *et al* (1972a) studied forty six workmen of whom seven were office staff never directly exposed to pesticides as the office and production areas were about a kilometer apart. D-Glucaric acid excretion by these seven subjects was not elevated, being similar to that by twenty one control subjects studied in Britain (figure 2). Five of the fourteen men employed in the plant area where aldrin and dieldrin alone were produced had D-glucaric acid excretion above normal limits but not significantly so. Men employed in the manufacture of endrin alone, however, excreted the most D-glucaric acid (figure 2) and nearly all of the thirteen examined excreted more D-glucaric acid than did controls ($P < 0{\cdot}01$): four men with normal excretion had worked with endrin for less than two years. The remaining group of workers examined ($n = 12$) were exposed to aldrin, dieldrin and endrin. In nine of these subjects, D-glucaric acid excretion increased similarly to workers exposed to endrin alone (figure 2). These findings were in agreement with those of Jager (1970) who found increased

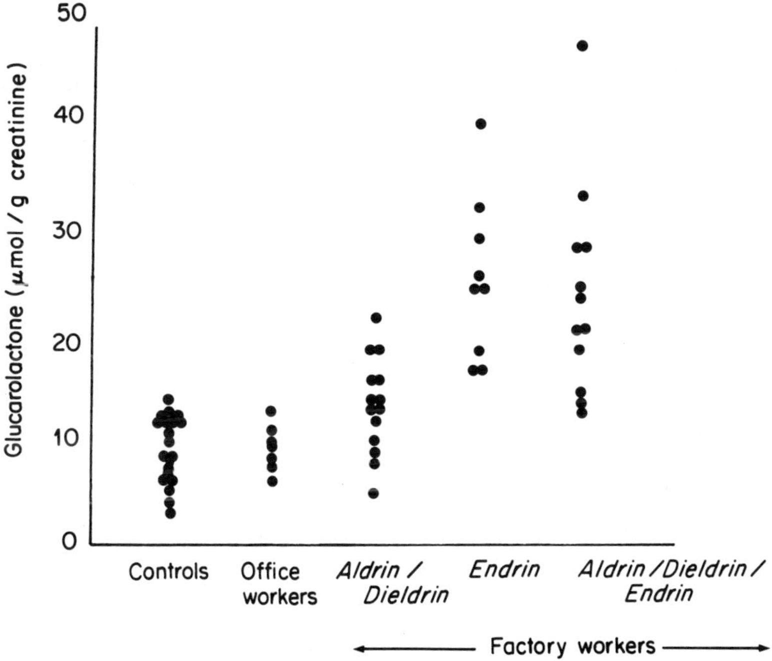

Figure 2 D-Glucaric acid excretion by subjects exposed to cyclodiene organochlorine pesticides and by control subjects (from Hunter *et al*, 1972a)

urinary excretion of 6β-hydroxycortisol by endrin workers, but not by those manufacturing aldrin and dieldrin, despite the large concentrations of dieldrin present in the blood. These men had been much more exposed to the pesticides than the general population. The mean concentration of dieldrin in the blood of the workers studied by Hunter *et al* (1972a) was 0·026 μg/ml, and was much greater than that in the blood of the general population of southern England, which in 1968 was 0·0009 μg/ml (Robinson and Roberts, 1969). Thus it seems unlikely that environmental exposure of the general population to dieldrin and aldrin at the current levels is sufficient to produce enzyme induction. Endrin is rapidly metabolized in the body and was not detected in the blood of any of the workers studied. It is therefore not possible to compare absolutely the exposure to endrin of workers and of the general population. Endrin is particularly useful for pest control on cotton, tobacco, maize and sugar cane, but as yet, no study has been made of possible enzyme induction in populations in areas, such as India and the lower Mississippi, where the use of endrin has been extensive.

Cigarette Smoking

Epidemiological studies have suggested that cigarette smoking can cause lung cancer (Stocks, 1970; Steinfeld, 1971) although this has been difficult to demonstrate in laboratory animals, possibly because the appropriate animal model or smoke-delivery system are unavailable. Cigarette smoke contains carcinogenic polycyclic hydrocarbons, such as benzo[*a*]pyrene, as do exhaust gases and smoked or grilled food. Recent studies have demonstrated that cigarette smoking induces drug metabolism or drug-metabolizing enzymes, particularly the microsomal enzyme system that has been loosely named aryl hydrocarbon hydroxylase (AHH). AHH can be induced readily in extrahepatic tissues.

Benzo[*a*]pyrene hydroxylase and aminoazo dye N-demethylase activities were much higher in the placentae of women who smoked during pregnancy than in non-smokers (Table 12) (Welch *et al*, 1969; Jacobson *et al*, 1974). There was a twentyfivefold variation in the activity of placental benzo[*a*]pyrene hydroxylase in women who smoked a similar number (20) of cigarettes, and this variability may be related to individual differences in enzyme induction or to the amount of cigarette smoke inhaled (Welch *et al*, 1969). Another study showed that smoking during pregnancy induced the activity of placental benzo[*a*]pyrene hydroxylase by severalfold when measured at term. This enzyme was not, however, detected in foetal or neonatal (33 weeks) liver, (Juchau, 1971). There was negligible hydroxylating activity in the placenta during the first trimester of pregnancy (Juchau, 1971), a period during which many teratogens are known to exert their effects. Significantly higher levels of placental AHH activity at term were detected in women who were cigarette smokers (31 ± 39 units/mg protein, $n = 17$) than in those who were non-smokers ($6{\cdot}7 \pm 6{\cdot}2$ units/mg protein, $n = 51$),

Table 12 Effect of cigarette smoking during pregnancy on placental enzyme activity (from Welch *et al*, 1969)

Subjects	Cigarettes smoked daily during pregnancy	Enzyme activity (mean and range)
Non-smokers (n = 17)	0	< 100*
Smokers (n = 8)	10–30	1005* (275–2168)
Smokers (n = 9)	10–40	9715* (4206–23205)
Non-smokers (n = 17)	0	< 1†
Smokers (n = 17)	10–40	6† (1–21)

*Hydroxybenzo[*a*]pyrene formed (ng/g/h).
†3-Methyl-4-aminoazobenzene formed (μg/g/h).

(Nebert *et al*, 1969). Presumably in these cases, induction was caused by the polycyclic hydrocarbons present in cigarette smoke. Placental and foetal drug metabolism and their induction have been well reviewed (Pelkonen and Kärki, 1973a; Yaffee and Juchau, 1974). Tobacco smoking was thought to induce nicotine metabolism as indicated by the lower recoveries of smoked or intravenously administered nicotine in the acid urine of smokers (Beckett and Triggs, 1967). Later experiments appeared to be less conclusive (Beckett *et al*, 1971), but the pattern of nicotine metabolism in man has been confirmed to be altered by smoking (Gorrod and Jenner, 1974).

Clinical data has suggested that the metabolism of commonly prescribed benzodiazepines may be more rapid in smokers than in non-smokers and similarly the latter group required larger doses of propoxyphene for effective analgesia (Boston Collaborative Drug Surveillance Program, 1973a, b). In Canada, Keeri-Szanto and Pomeroy (1971) used pentazocine as a supplementary drug in patients undergoing nitrous-oxide anaesthesia and found that smokers and city dwellers required significantly more nitrous oxide than did non-smokers or country dwellers; possibly the metabolism of supplementary pentazocine had been induced by exposure to polycyclic hydrocarbons in smoke. Peak plasma levels of phenacetin at two hours were significantly lower in average smokers ($0{\cdot}48 \pm 0{\cdot}28$ μg/ml, $n = 9$) than in non-smokers ($2{\cdot}24 \pm 0{\cdot}73$ μg/ml, $n = 9$) after a 900 mg oral dose. Ratio of plasma metabolites as total N-acetyl-*p*-aminophenol (paracetamol) and phenacetin were higher in smokers than in non-smokers (Pantuck *et al*, 1974) indicating enhanced metabolism of phenacetin to paracetamol in smokers. Mitchell (1972), however, found that smoking did not significantly influence the rate of warfarin metabolism.

There may be a positive but not direct relationship between the toxicity caused by polycyclic hydrocarbons and the presence of the aryl hydrocarbon hydroxylase (AHH) enzyme system. Thus an oxidative metabolic pathway exists in human placenta at term that is probably important for maintaining the appropriate hormonal balance for normal foetal development. In altering this balance, enzyme-inducing polycyclic hydrocarbons (and other compounds) may contribute to the alleged disadvantages that are attendant with the babies of smoking mothers. AHH currently attracts much attention and has been suggested as a useful means for screening the general population for susceptibility to cancers caused by cigarette smoke (Conney, 1973) because of the report that susceptibility to bronchogenic carcinoma was associated with higher levels of inducible AHH activity in cultured human lymphocytes (Kellerman *et al*, 1973). The induction *in vitro* of AHH by 3-methylcholanthrene in cultured lymphocytes was correlated with AHH activity in pulmonary alveolar macrophages from the same individuals (Cantrell and Busbee 1973), but the activity of the latter did not relate to the extent of cigarette smoking. Pulmonary alveolar macrophages obtained from smokers had elevenfold higher AHH activities than those from non-smokers (Cantrell *et al*, 1973) suggesting that pollution may play a smaller role in the supply of carcinogenic polycyclic hydrocarbons to the lungs than does smoking. AHH is widely distributed and has been studied in tissues as diverse as human neonatal foreskin (Alvares *et al*, 1973) and in human peripheral blood monocytes (Bast *et al*, 1974). Polycyclic hydrocarbons causing enzyme induction have been reviewed (Gelboin, 1967), but it is not clear whether enzyme induction by a particular compound enhances carcinogenicity or reduces it (Falk, 1971).

PHYSIOLOGICAL EFFECTS OF ENZYME INDUCTION

Administration of enzyme-inducing agents may produce some considerable physiological changes. Some of these changes afford an increased rate of drug metabolism; others stem from the effect of increased microsomal enzyme activity on endogenous compounds.

Liver Weight

Liver weight is increased in animals treated with enzyme-inducing agents (Conney *et al*, 1960; Remmer and Merker, 1963; Conney, 1967), and may be associated with an increase in the size and numbers of the hepatocytes (Preis *et al*, 1966). In man, however, there is no reported clinical enlargement of the liver in patients taking enzyme-inducing drugs. Hunter *et al* (1971b), employing a scintiscan technique for measuring hepatic volume, found no volume increase in patients with Gilbert's syndrome during daily treatment with phenobarbitone (60 mg) or phetharbital (600 mg). Enzyme-inducing drugs increase the rate of growth of regenerating as well as of normal liver in animals (Gershbein, 1966) by stimulating mitosis (Conney *et al*, 1960; Goodman and Gilman, 1970; Burger and Herdson, 1966). By using a thermocouple implanted in the liver, Ohnhaus *et al* (1971) demonstrated an increase in hepatic blood flow in rats after phenobarbitone or antipyrine administration, but not after benzo[*a*]pyrene.

Bile Flow

Increased bile flow which was not accompanied by an increased output of bile salts (Berthelot *et al*, 1970) has been reported to occur after phenobarbitone administration to rats (Roberts and Plaa, 1967; Klaassen, 1969; Berthelot *et al*, 1970), but not after other enzyme inducers (Klaassen, 1969) indicating that enzyme induction and increases in bile flow are probably unrelated. The effects of phenobarbitone on bile flow and bile constitution have been studied in monkeys using an elegant device that allows diversion of all or part of the biliary stream (Redinger and Small, 1973). Phenobarbitone administration caused an increase in bile flow by promoting the output of bile salts and of the bile salt-independent fraction. The phospholipid content of bile increased, but as cholesterol production had been unaffected, the relative concentrations of cholesterol decreased. Bile-acid synthesis was stimulated by phenobarbitone administration even when the enterohepatic circulation of bile salts had not been interrupted. The observation that cholesterol concentrations were lowered suggests that phenobarbitone could be used to treat cholesterol gallstones but the results of Redinger and Small (1973) have yet to be confirmed by others.

Glucuronic-acid Pathway

Increased excretion of L-xylulose in a patient with essential pentosuria after the administration of drugs was first reported by Margolis (1929). This was confirmed by Enklewitz and Lasker (1935) who found that administration of antipyrine, aminopyrine and borneol, also produced this effect, but that a polysaccharide, gastric mucin, did not. As well as L-xylulose, increased D-glucuronic acid excretion in the urine was also detected, and it was shown that the oral administration of D-glucuronic acid elevated urinary L-xylulose concentrations. Thus the increased excretion of L-xylulose was linked to the glucuronic-acid pathway by this early work.

Shortly afterwards, urinary L-ascorbic acid excretion in rats was also shown to be increased by a number of dietary substances, including a lipid found in alfalfa meal and several terpenes, such as carvone, piperitone and α- and β-ionone (Longenecker *et al*, 1939). Several terpenes are now known to be enzyme-inducing agents (Parke and Rahman, 1969). Certain drugs then in use, including barbiturates and antipyrine, were found to have the same stimulatory effect (Longenecker *et al*, 1940). Although D-glucaric acid was not identified in the urine until 1963 (Marsh, 1963a), it was in the same year that its excretion by rats was shown to increase after treatment with barbitone and chloretone (Marsh and Reid, 1963). Increased excretion of D-glucaric acid by man after drug administration was demonstrated by Aarts

(1965) and by Okada *et al* (1969). The latter also found increased serum concentrations of D-glucaric acid.

Most information on the stimulation of the glucuronic-acid pathway (figure 3) by drugs has come from the study of L-ascorbic acid, for it has provided a convenient means of investigating ascorbate biosynthesis. Increased urinary ascorbic-acid excretion was shown to be a result of increased ascorbate biosynthesis by Burns *et al* (1954), when they used ascorbic acid-1-^{14}C to determine the body pool and daily synthesis rate (both expressed in terms of 100 g bodyweight) of this compound in rats. In control animals the body pool was 10·7 mg/100 g, whereas in animals which had been given chloretone or pentobarbitone it was greater, 19·2 and 19·6 mg/100 g respectively. Similarly, the daily turnover rate of ascorbate was increased from 2·6 mg/100 g to 21·5 and 11·6 mg/100 g respectively. Conney *et al* (1961) extended this work and showed that the body pool of ascorbate in rats treated with 3-methylcholanthrene rose to 22·5 mg/100 g and the turnover rate to 19·0 mg/100 g. Ascorbate turnover increased as well as excretion from 2·2 mg/100 g daily in normal rats to 11·3, 11·9 and 9·2 mg/100 g respectively in rats which had received chloretone, 3-methylcholanthrene or pentobarbitone.

The body pool of D-glucaric acid was measured in guinea-pigs by Aarts (1968). In controls the mean value was found to be 0·38 μmol. This was less than the daily excretion by the animals studied, which averaged 0·48 μmol. After barbitone administration to guinea-pigs of a similar size, the daily excretion rose to 3·2 μmol per day. In view of the relatively small size of the body pool in the controls, it seems likely that increased D-glucaric acid excretion is the result of increased biosynthesis.

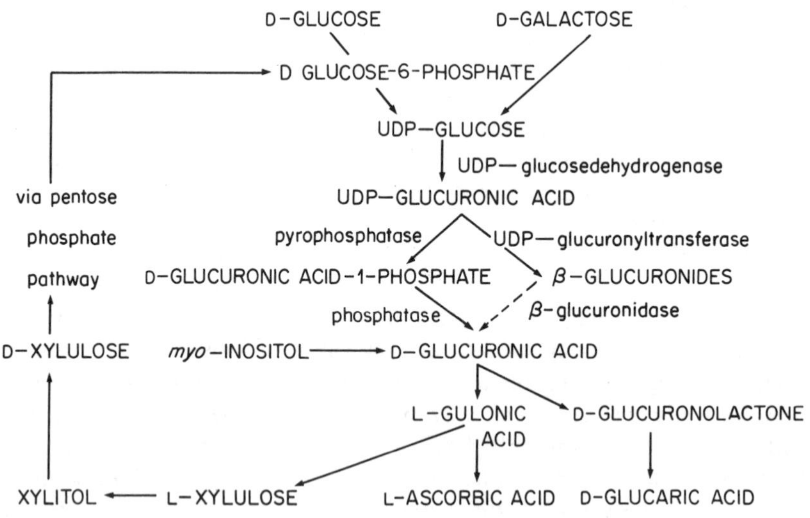

Figure 3 Glucuronic-acid pathway in the rat

Although many enzymes of the glucuronic-acid pathway (figure 3) are found in the kidney (Hänninen, 1968), the liver is the site of increased ascorbate biosynthesis. Burns *et al* (1960) showed that the levels of ascorbate increased in the blood after treatment with chloretone, even in rats in which the kidneys had previously been removed. The concentrations of ascorbate increase in the liver (but not in testes, brain or muscle), after chloretone administration, nor is this response abolished by nephrectomy (Burns *et al*, 1960; Martin, 1961). Similarly, increased hepatic concentrations of D-glucaric acid were found following barbitone administration to rats (Aarts, 1968), although the effect of nephrectomy has not been examined. However, as levels of glucuronolactone dehydrogenase, the final enzyme in the biosynthesis of D-glucaric acid, are much lower in the kidney than in the liver, especially in man (Marsh, 1963b), it seems highly probable that increased D-glucaric acid synthesis, like ascorbate biosynthesis, occurs in the liver.

Free D-glucuronic acid may also appear in the urine in varying amounts after drug administration (Enklewitz and Lasker, 1935; Longenecker *et al*, 1940). As this is an intermediate compound in the pathway (figure 3) and most of it is further metabolized, it would not be a reliable index of the metabolic activity of the pathway. The amount appearing in the urine probably depends largely on the permeability of the hepatocytes. Despite considerable effort, the mechanism by which drugs stimulate the glucuronic-acid pathway remains unknown. Although UDP–glucuronyltransferase is the only microsomal enzyme system in the relevant part of the pathway between UDP–glucose and D-glucuronic acid (figure 3) which is increased in activity after administration of the same substances that stimulate glucuronic-acid synthesis, this does not necessarily mean that its activity is the rate-limiting stage in the pathway.

Bilirubin Metabolism

Bilirubin is formed at sites of red-cell catabolism, including the liver, spleen and bone marrow. A microsomal haemoxygenase (Tenhunen *et al*, 1969) is responsible for converting haem to biliverdin (a precursor of bilirubin) and is increased in activity by phenobarbitone. Unconjugated bilirubin is transported to the liver bound to albumin. In the hepatic cytosol, two anionic binding proteins (designated Y and Z) have been shown to take up bilirubin and sulphobromophthalein (Levi *et al*, 1969) and are closely related to the proteins taking up cortisol (Morey and Litwack, 1969) and certain carcinogens (Ketterer *et al*, 1967). They may be involved in the hepatic uptake of certain drugs and even in the biotransformation of some drugs. Phenobarbitone administration is thought to increase hepatic concentrations of the Y protein but not the Z (Levi *et al*, 1969) and this may be a factor in the increased hepatic uptake of bilirubin which occurs after this drug (Black *et al*, 1974). Once in the hepatocyte, bilirubin is conjugated with glucuronic acid by the phenobarbitone-inducible UDP–glucuronyltransferase as previously described. Thus, although phenobarbitone causes increased haem catabolism and consequently increased bilirubin formation, it also increases hepatic uptake and conjugation of bilirubin and bile flow, leading on balance to a reduction in plasma bilirubin concentrations (Thompson *et al*, 1969a).

Corticosteroid Metabolism

Corticosteroids are endogenous substrates for microsomal drug-metabolizing enzymes. Under normal conditions, cortisol is metabolized in the liver (by nonmicrosomal enzymes) to compounds such as tetrahydrocortisol and tetrahydrocortisone, which are then conjugated with glucuronic acid and excreted in the urine as 17-hydroxycorticosteroids (Mattingly, 1968). Werk *et al* (1964) have shown that in man, treatment with diphenylhydantoin was associated with changes in the excretion of cortisol: the urinary excretion of 17-hydroxycorticosteroids diminished, and there was increased production of a polar metabolite, 6β-hydroxycortisol, which is considered to reflect increased microsomal drug metabolism (see page 141).

Enzyme-inducing drugs have been demonstrated to increase the activity of an enzyme system in guinea-pig microsomes which hydroxylates cortisol in the 6 position (Kuntzman *et al*, 1968a), and cortisol elimination through formation of 6β-hydroxycortisol appears more rapid than by the usual pathway. A number of drugs known to increase the 6β-hydroxylation of cortisol in man have also been discovered to lead to clinical improvement in patients with Cushing's syndrome; these include *o,p'*-DDD (Bledsoe *et al*, 1964; Southren *et al*, 1966), diphenylhydantoin (Werk *et al*, 1966) and phetharbital (Southren *et al*, 1969). In subjects with apparently normal adrenal function, cortisol production rates were increased by diphenylhydantoin (Werk *et al*, 1971), anticonvulsants (Hunter, 1974) and rifampicin (Edwards *et al*, 1974). Presumably this is because increased cortisol metabolism is compensated by increased ACTH release.

The action of other steroids may be influenced by microsomal enzyme inducers as, for example, during the dexamethasone suppression test, which is a screening test for the suppressibility of the hypothalamo-pituitary axis. In normal subjects, the expected level of plasma cortisol after dexamethasone (2 mg the previous night) should be less than 6 μg/100 ml (Mattingly, 1968). Increased dexamethasone metabolism may occur in patients taking diphenylhydantoin (Jubiz *et al*, 1970) or phenobarbitone (Brooks *et al*, 1972) and so reduce the effect of the steroid. This may be relevant to abnormalities of dexamethasone suppression tests reported in psychiatric patients (Carroll *et al*, 1968; Carroll and Davies, 1970). After a 2-mg dose of dexamethasone, severely depressed patients were found not to have normally suppressed plasma 11-hydroxycorticosteroid levels: this abnormal response became less marked as the patients depression improved. However, most of the depressed patients studied were receiving amylobarbitone. As a group the depressives needed larger amounts of amylobarbitone during the initial testing period than they did before discharge (Carroll *et al*, 1968). It seems likely that the amylobarbitone (a potent inducer) may have been the true cause of the abnormalities observed in dexamethasone response.

Patients with intact adrenals are able to compensate for the increased catabolism of corticosteroids caused by microsomal enzyme-inducing drugs, but difficulties may arise if, for any reason, the availability of these steroids is limited. Brooks *et al* (1972) have shown that the condition of adrenocorticosteroid-dependent patients deteriorated when phenobarbitone was administered as a sedative, and was associated with an increased rate of clearance of the steroids from the plasma. Edwards *et al* (1974) recently described a patient with Addison's disease who, despite replacement doses of adrenal steroids which would normally be considered adequate, suffered an Addisonian crisis when rifampicin was added to his antituberculous medication, an observation confirmed by Maisey *et al* (1974). Again increased cortisol metabolism was demonstrated as a result of enzyme induction by rifampicin.

Sex-hormone Metabolism

The hepatic microsomal hydroxylases that metabolize drugs and endogenous steroids have similar properties (Conney, 1971). Steroid hormones are potent competitive inhibitors of the drug hydroxylases (Conney, 1967). In animals, inducers of drug metabolism, such as phenobarbitone, also induce the hydroxylation of testosterone (Conney and Klutch, 1963; Conney and Schneidman, 1964), oestrogens (Welch *et al*, 1971) and progesterone (Conney *et al*, 1966). Stimulation of the hydroxylation of several steroids by hepatic microsomal enzymes caused by phenobarbitone administration is associated *in vivo* with an accelerated metabolism and decreased physiological effects of these steroids (Levin *et al*, 1974).

Reports of the effects of enzyme-inducing drugs on sex-hormone metabolism in man are as yet few. However, amenorrhoea has been described in patients taking anticonvulsant drugs and this could be caused by increased metabolism of oestrogens. A similar mechanism could underlie the problems, such as increased incidents of breakthrough bleeding, which occurred in patients with tuberculosis who were taking oral contraceptives and receiving concurrent therapy with rifampicin (Reimers and Jezek, 1971). Similar effects have been described in epileptic patients (Mumford, 1974).

Vitamin-D Metabolism

Abnormalities of plasma-calcium levels in epileptic subjects have been recorded for many years (Griffiths, 1934), but reports of elevated levels of alkaline phosphatase in the plasma of epileptic subjects taking anticonvulsant drugs (Wright, 1965; Vas and Parsonage, 1967) were puzzling until Kruse (1968) and later others (Dent *et al*, 1970; Biasini, 1971; Schaefer *et al*, 1972) reported cases of rickets or osteomalacia developing in such patients. A survey (Richens and Rowe, 1970) of a colony of epileptic patients showed that 23% had hypocalcaemia and 29% had raised plasma alkaline-phosphatase levels and that there was a significant correlation between the plasma levels of calcium and the total dose of anticonvulsant drugs taken by the patients. As vitamin D is essential for the normal absorption of calcium and phosphorus from the intestine, it was suggested that these changes might be a result of hepatic enzyme induction increasing the rate of metabolism of vitamin D to inactive products. Evidence supporting this hypothesis was put forward by Hunter *et al* (1971c) who found a similar incidence of hypocalcaemia among a group of epileptic children. In these patients, there was a significant relationship between serum-calcium levels and urinary D-glucaric acid excretion. Further studies have confirmed that greater D-glucaric acid excretion was related to lower serum-calcium levels in epileptic patients; Table 13 (Latham *et al*, 1973).

It is now known that vitamin D3 (cholecalciferol), the main form of the vitamin in man, is converted in the liver to 25-hydroxycholecalciferol which has greater antirachitic activity, and this in turn is converted in the kidneys to 1,25-dihydroxycholecalciferol, the most active form of the vitamin known (Lawson *et al*, 1971). The main circulating form of vitamin D3 in man is believed to be 25-hydroxycholecalciferol, concentrations of which are lower in the serum of epileptics (Stamp *et al*, 1972; Hahn *et al*, 1972b). Administration of fairly small doses of 25-hydroxycholecalciferol will correct the biochemical abnormalities of calcium metabolism found in these patients (Stamp *et al*, 1972; Hunter, 1974), which are comparatively resistant to vitamin D3 itself (Borgstedt *et al*, 1972). The patients also respond to ultra-violet light therapy (Dent *et al*, 1970).

Table 13 Relationship between anticonvulsant therapy of epileptic patients, serum-calcium levels and D-glucaric acid excretion (from Latham *et al*, 1973)

Drug (mean dose)	Serum calcium* (mg/100 ml)	Urinary D-glucaric acid* (μmol/24 h)
Pheneturide (550 mg)	9·05 ± 0·37	360 ± 143
Primidone (835 mg)	9·15 ± 0·42	289 ± 155
Diphenylhydantoin (290 mg)	9·18 ± 0·42	247 ± 200
Phenobarbitone (135 mg)	9·22 ± 0·43	248 ± 216

*Appropriate range of normal values were 9·0–10·5 mg/100 ml and <25 μmol/24 h respectively.

Investigations into the cause of 'anticonvulsant osteomalacia' in epileptic patients had produced conflicting results. The elimination of vitamin D from the plasma was reported to be increased in these subjects (Hahn *et al*, 1972a), but this could not be confirmed by Hunter *et al* (1975). Although the plasma concentrations of 25-hydroxycholecalciferol are reduced in many epileptic subjects (Hahn *et al*, 1972b), Silver *et al* (1974) found that the production of this metabolite in rats was increased when the animals were given phenobarbitone. These workers also found that the biliary excretion of radioactively labelled vitamin D was increased in phenobarbitone-treated rats, but that the total faecal excretion of radioactivity was no different from controls.

However, recent work in man has resolved many of these apparent inconsistencies. Studies on the clearance of radioactively labelled cholecalciferol from the plasma of normal subjects and epileptics revealed that the rate of metabolism of the parent vitamin was dependent largely on the plasma concentrations of 25-hydroxycholecalciferol, which reflects total body stores of the vitamin. If the rate of cholecalciferol clearance was plotted against the plasma 25-hydroxycholecalciferol concentrations, then it was found that epileptic subjects eliminated the vitamin more quickly than did controls; figure 4 (Hunter *et al*, 1975). In the United States, anticon-

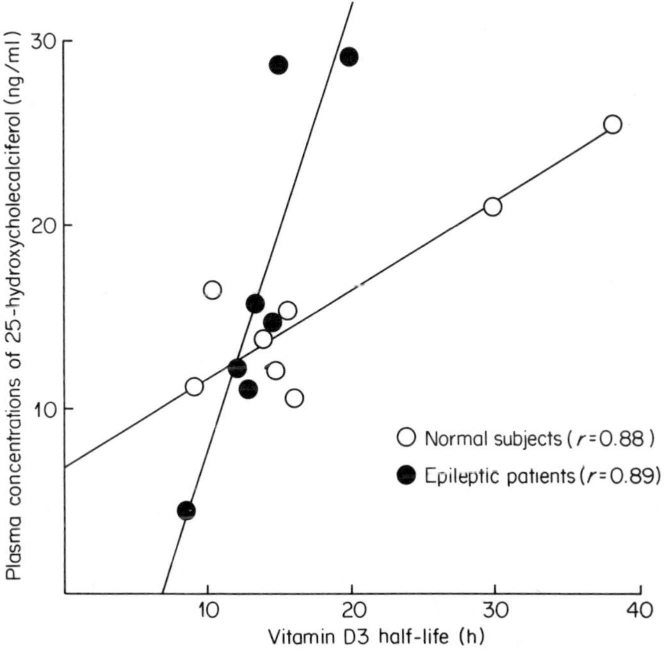

Figure 4 Relationship between the plasma concentrations of 25-hydroxycholecalciferol and plasma-elimination half-life of vitamin D3 (cholecalciferol) in epileptic patients and normal subjects (from Hunter *et al*, 1975).

vulsant osteomalacia appears to be uncommon, and reports have appeared of large surveys in which no epileptic patients were found to have hypocalcaemia (Livingston and Berman, 1973). This is probably a result of the deliberate fortification of foodstuffs with vitamin D, which provides a large daily intake of 2000–3000 I.U. (American Academy of Pediatrics, 1963). Lifshitz and MacLaren (1973), who also studied epileptic patients in the United States, found that rickets occurred in non-ambulant patients who were confined indoors, and it seems likely that lack of exposure to sunlight may have been an important factor in the development of this condition. As many adults in northwest England have a dietary vitamin-D intake of only 30–60 I.U. daily (Lumb *et al*, 1971) and as exposure to sunlight in Britain is less extensive, it is perhaps not surprising that anticonvulsant osteomalacia appears more commonly on this side of the Atlantic.

Folate Metabolism

Anaemia occurring after treatment with anticonvulsant drugs has been recognized to be due to folate deficiency but the underlying mechanism is unknown. It has been suggested that malabsorption of folate occurs (Meynell, 1966) possibly due to alkalinization of the upper small intestine (Benn *et al*, 1971), although other work (Rosenberg *et al*, 1968; Doe *et al*, 1971) does not confirm this view nor the theory that diphenylhydantoin inhibits the intestinal conjugases which convert dietary folic-acid precursors (polyglutamate) to the monoglutamate forms that are absorbed (Baugh and Krumdieck, 1969; Houlihan *et al*, 1972). The evidence for malabsorption of folic acid is therefore conflicting (Reynolds, 1972).

Many of the commonly used anticonvulsant drugs (Reynolds, 1968; Reynolds *et al*, 1969) which lead to folate deficiency are powerful enzyme-inducing agents thus suggesting that enzyme induction might be implicated in this deficiency (Richens and Waters, 1971). Initially this seemed improbable, for folic acid is water soluble and hence unlikely to be a substrate for microsomal enzymes. Baylis *et al* (1971), however, reported that administration of folic acid to folate-deficient epileptics reduced the steady-state concentrations of diphenylhydantoin in their blood, an observation that raised the possibility that folic acid might be involved in microsomal drug hydroxylations. Thus if microsomal hydroxylation reactions were increased as a result of enzyme induction, folic-acid stores might become depleted. This suggestion is still unproven. However, Maxwell *et al* (1972b) found a significant correlation between the degree of enzyme induction, as represented by D-glucaric acid excretion, and the concentrations of folic acid in both the serum and erythrocytes of epileptic children. Latham *et al* (1973) later reported that of a group of drugs (pheneturide, primidone, diphenylhydantoin and phenobarbitone), those which apparently caused the most enzyme induction (again measured by D-glucaric acid excretion) also produced the greatest reduction in serum-folate levels in epileptic patients.

In rats, administration of phenobarbitone or diphenylhydantoin has been shown to cause induction of the enzymes, glutamate formiminotransferase and methylenetetrahydrofolate dehydrogenase, involved in tetrahydrofolate metabolism (Spray and Burns, 1972). In some, but not all, animals treated with phenobarbitone there was a significant decrease in the concentration of serum folate. In those treated with diphenylhydantoin, there was a significant decrease in the hepatic concentrations of folate. Enzyme induction as a cause of folate deficiency would also provide a satisfactory explanation for folate depletion which may accompany treatment with other drugs such as oral contraceptives (Shojania *et al*, 1968; Streiff, 1970); the latter may also increase hepatic microsomal enzyme activity (Mowat, 1968).

Vitamin-K Treatment

Disorders connected with vitamin-K treatment have been observed in babies born to mothers taking anticonvulsant drugs (Mountain *et al*, 1970; Davies, 1970). No evidence exists as to the pathogenesis of this vitamin deficiency, but since vitamin K is a lipid-soluble vitamin, it may be worth investigating the role of enzyme induction.

Haem Biosynthesis

The precipitation of attacks of porphyria by drugs such as barbiturates is not a true example of microsomal enzyme induction. The induction of mitochondrial δ-aminolaevulinic acid synthetase, which is the initial and probable rate-limiting enzyme in porphyrin biosynthesis (Granick and Urata, 1963; Tschudy *et al*, 1965), is now thought to be a secondary effect of increased haem biosynthesis and not a direct effect of the drug itself on the enzyme (Marver, 1969).

Thyroid Status

That thyroid status might influence drug metabolism was suggested by the studies of Brunk *et al* (1974) and of Eichelbaum *et al* (1974) who showed that antipyrine half-lives ($\pm$ S.E.M.) were shorter ($7{\cdot}9 \pm 1{\cdot}0$ h) than control values (about 12 h) in hyperthyroid patients and greater ($17{\cdot}3 \pm 1{\cdot}1$ h) in hypothyroid patients. When thyroid function was corrected, the antipyrine half-lives returned to control values. There was a significant correlation between thyroid dysfunction (serum-thyroxine concentrations) and antipyrine half-lives (Eichelbaum *et al*, 1974). Similar results have been obtained by others (Vesell and Passananti, 1973).

THERAPEUTIC VALUE OF ENZYME INDUCTION

As hepatic microsomal enzymes are responsible for the metabolism of many different drugs and endogenous substances, hepatic enzyme induction is potentially of value in therapeutics by modifying the extent and duration of action of these drugs and endogenous substances. Indeed, some attempts have also been made to increase the activity of extrahepatic enzymes, by administration of drugs producing hepatic enzyme induction. However, Sherwood *et al* (1971), found that phenobarbitone did not induce glucose-6-phosphate dehydrogenase in the erythrocytes of subjects deficient in the enzyme, while Applegarth and Dunn (1972) were unable to increase the serum levels of the lysosomal enzyme, N-acetyl hexosaminidase, in a child with a variant of Tay-Sach's disease (Sandhoff *et al*, 1968) despite administering phenobarbitone (60 mg/day) for more than a year. A notable example of the induction of an extrahepatic enzyme system is the influence of smoking on placental aryl hydrocarbon hydroxylase (AHH) activity (Table 12) in pregnant women. There is no evidence to date that enzyme-inducing drugs will prove of therapeutic value in the induction of enzymes not located principally in the liver, and it is only in the management of unconjugated hyperbilirubinaemia that deliberate induction of hepatic enzymes has become standard clinical practice.

Unconjugated Hyperbilirubinaemia

Unconjugated hyperbilirubinaemia can arise by several different mechanisms (see review by Fleishner and Arias, 1970). One of the most important is increased catabolism of haemoglobin, as occurs in the haemolytic disease of the new-born. Ineffective erythropoiesis may be one of the mechanisms leading to the so-called 'shunt' hyperbilirubinaemia. Certain compounds, notably flavaspidic acid and bunamiodyl can produce unconjugated hyperbilirubinaemia by interfering with the uptake of bilirubin by the hepatocytes. Although no clinical condition has so far been described in which abnormalities of the hepatic bilirubin carrier proteins Y and Z have been proven, varying degrees of deficiency of the conjugating enzyme bilirubin UDP–glucuronyltransferase (Heirwegh *et al*, 1973) may produce three overlapping syndromes of hyperbilirubinaemia (Arias *et al*, 1969). However, drug glucuronidation is not necessarily impaired in hyperbilirubinaemic subjects (Levy and Ertel, 1971).

In the Crigler–Najjar syndrome type I, bilirubin UDP–glucuronyltransferase is completely absent and bile only contains traces of bile pigments: the plasma-bilirubin concentration usually exceeds 20 mg/100 ml and kernicterus is thus frequent. In the Crigler–Najjar syndrome type II, the enzyme levels are reduced and bile contains pigments. Jaundice is less severe and kernicterus is rare. In Gilbert's syndrome, a mild deficiency of the enzyme produces a slight increase in plasma-bilirubin concentrations, usually less than 5 mg/100 ml and no other abnormalities occur (Gilbert *et al*, 1907; Fleishner and Arias, 1970).

Phenobarbitone treatment has been shown to be effective in conditions where glucuronyltransferase activity is reduced but not absent, such as in the Crigler–Najjar syndrome type II (Crigler and Gold, 1966; Arias *et al*, 1969; Kreek and Sleisenger, 1968) and in Gilbert's syndrome, (Whelton *et al*, 1968; Black and Sherlock, 1970; Hunter *et al*, 1971b). Phenobarbitone treatment of two adult siblings with lifelong unconjugated hyperbilirubinaemia lowered serum bilirubin within 12 to 36 h after a large dose (390 mg/day). In one subject, for example, serum-bilirubin levels decreased from 8·0 to 0·3 mg/100 ml in 22 days (Kreek and Sleisenger, 1968). Two-weeks' treatment of patients suffering from Gilbert's syndrome, with phenobarbitone (180 mg/day) produced a considerable decrease in serum-bilirubin concentrations, in some cases to normal levels (Billing and Black, 1971; Black *et al*, 1974). Mean plasma concentrations of bilirubin in patients with Gilbert's syndrome were lowered to normal levels within one week by treatment with phenobarbitone or glutethimide. The results indicated that both accelerated hepatic bilirubin clearance and reduced plasma-bilirubin turnover contributed to the observed reduction in plasma-bilirubin concentrations (Blaschke *et al*, 1974).

The mechanism by which phenobarbitone decreases plasma-bilirubin concentrations is presumably that of induction of bilirubin UDP–glucuronyltransferase (Table 14), and although no correlation has been observed between hepatic bilirubin UDP–glucuronyltransferase activity and cytochrome P-450 concentrations in patients, phenobarbitone pretreatment has resulted in increases in both parameters (Black *et al*, 1973). Blaschke *et al* (1974) have observed a linear relationship between hepatic bilirubin clearance and bilirubin UDP–glucuronyltransferase activity in most cases in man. However, induction of this enzyme has been demonstrated in only a few patients (Black *et al*, 1974) whilst other workers found that although the enzyme was induced by phenobarbitone in some subjects, it was not induced in patients suffering from Gilbert's syndrome (Felsher *et al*, 1973). It is possible that other mechanisms may also be involved, since phenobarbitone has been shown to increase the concentrations of the hepatic bilirubin-

Table 14 Effect of enzyme inducers on hepatic bilirubin conjugation and cytochrome P-450 concentrations in patients (from Billing and Black, 1971)

Treatment for one week	Bilirubin conjugated (mg/g liver/h)†	Cytochrome P-450 concentrations (nmol/g liver)†
No drugs ($n = 26$)	1·41 ± 0·68	12·2 ± 5·0
Phenobarbitone ($n = 28$)	2·03 ± 0·88*	16·87 ± 7·4
Other drugs (e.g. glutethimide) ($n = 24$)	3·0 ± 1·2**	20·7 ± 7·5

†Level of significance.
*$P < 0{\cdot}01$.
**$P < 0{\cdot}001$.

carrier protein Y, but not Z (Levi *et al*, 1969) and is known to increase liver size and bile flow (Roberts and Plaa, 1967; Klaassen, 1969; Berthelot *et al*, 1970). A further mechanism which has been suggested is inhibition of the hydrolysis of bilirubin glucuronide by β-glucuronidase. However, Felsher *et al.* (1973) found no change in β-glucuronidase activity in liver samples obtained from normal subjects, patients with hepatitis and those with Gilbert's syndrome, even after phenobarbitone treatment.

The therapeutic use of phenobarbitone in ameliorating the degree of jaundice associated with unconjugated hyperbilirubinaemia is now well established, but its use in Gilbert's syndrome is still debatable. The symptoms of this syndrome are nonspecific and patients often complain of vague abdominal pains, nausea and general malaise. It remains to be established whether reduction of plasma-bilirubin levels improves these symptoms. The situation is further complicated because phenobarbitone may produce drowsiness which some patients are unable to tolerate. In a double-blind trial of phenobarbitone and phetharbital in the management of Gilbert's syndrome, Hunter *et al* (1971b) found that although both drugs consistently reduced the concentrations of plasma bilirubin, there was no correlation between the concentrations of plasma bilirubin and the symptoms of which the patient complained, and that furthermore, only four out of eleven patients noticed any improvement in their symptoms, which could have been due to a placebo effect. As family surveys have shown, many patients exist in whom there are slight elevations of plasma bilirubin without any obvious symptoms, and it seems likely that the symptoms associated with Gilbert's syndrome may be due to an anxiety state. The current view is that treatment of mild unconjugated hyperbilirubinaemia is unnecessary unless the degree of jaundice is such as to produce social embarrassment.

Although kernicterus is believed to be rare in the Crigler–Najjar syndrome type II (Arias *et al*, 1969), treatment with enzyme-inducing drugs in these patients reduces jaundice and may produce a valuable cosmetic effect. Reports exist of the value of phenobarbitone (Crigler and Gold, 1966; Arias *et al*, 1969) and phetharbital (Hunter *et al*, 1971b). Thompson *et al* (1969b) in attempting to overcome the problem of sleepiness produced by phenobarbitone, treated one patient with the organochlorine pesticide DDT. This compound is stored in body fat and only slowly released, hence maintaining enzyme induction and thereby low plasma-bilirubin concentrations long after dosage had ended. The patient received DDT for six months and the plasma-bilirubin concentrations remained at less than 1 mg/100 ml for a further year.

Neonatal Hyperbilirubinaemia

Phenobarbitone is effective in reducing hyperbilirubinaemia associated with haemolytic anaemia (Matsuda and Takase, 1969), and it may be particularly valuable in the treatment of neonates with severe rhesus incompatability. The administration of phenobarbitone to the severely jaundiced neonate reduces plasma-bilirubin levels and may remove the need for exchange transfusions (Yaffe *et al*, 1966; Yeung and Field, 1969). The drug has also been administered to the mother during the last weeks of pregnancy to reduce significantly the plasma-bilirubin concentrations in the infant at birth (Maurer *et al*, 1968; Ramboer *et al*, 1969; Jouppila and Suonio, 1970). Thus, treatment of pregnant mothers with phenobarbitone for at least two weeks resulted in lowered ($2{\cdot}7 \pm 0{\cdot}4$ mg/100 ml) serum-bilirubin concentrations (± S.E.) in their offspring when compared with untreated controls, viz $5{\cdot}9 \pm 0{\cdot}5$ mg/100 ml (Maurer *et al*, 1968). Similar data were obtained in a retrospective survey of the serum-bilirubin concentrations in the newborn infants of epileptic mothers treated with phenobarbitone (Trolle, 1968). A controlled clinical trial showed that phenobarbitone treatment was effective in lowering the serum-bilirubin concentrations of low birth-weight Negro neonates (Valdes *et al*, 1971). The studies of Yeung and Field (1969) showed that the need for exchange transfusions in Chinese neonates with moderate jaundice (bilirubin 10–20 mg/100 ml) was greatly diminished by phenobarbitone treatment.

Further evidence of the enzyme-inducing properties of ethanol is the report that controlled treatment of near-term or term patients with more than 100 g of ethanol (in saline) by intravenous infusion reduced serum-bilirubin levels by about twofold in the corresponding infants during the third to fifth days of life compared to infants of untreated patients or those treated with less ethanol (Waltman *et al*, 1969). An earlier report suggested that promazine, pethidine or chlorpromazine given to mothers during labour did not influence serum-bilirubin concentrations (McDonald *et al*, 1964).

Even though severe unconjugated jaundice during the neonatal period may cause kernicterus, there has been much criticism of the use of phenobarbitone in pregnant women or in infants probably because the full implications (Behrman and Fisher, 1970) such as concomitant induction of steroid metabolism, are not known. Not all workers have shown a significant reduction in serum-bilirubin concentrations when compared to controls, although phenobarbitone may have been administered to neonates even within eight hours of birth (Ramboer *et al*, 1969), probably because enzyme induction takes three or four days to develop. Phenobarbitone given to the pregnant woman in the last weeks of pregnancy can be very effective in reducing neonatal serum-bilirubin levels, but it may also depress the infant's respiration after delivery and a bleeding tendency has been reported in babies born to epileptic mothers taking anticonvulsant drugs (Mountain *et al*, 1970; Davies, 1970). While it is therefore probably unjustified to give phenobarbitone to all pregnant women it is even more difficult to identify the foetus at risk to whom treatment might be valuable. Phenobarbitone has, however, been shown to be of great value for the prevention of hyperbilirubinaemia in neonates with glucose-6-phosphate dehydrogenase deficiency (Meloni *et al*, 1973). Many workers claim that phototherapy (Hodgman and Schwartz, 1970; Valdes *et al*, 1971; Martin, 1974) or early feeding (Davies, 1969) may be a safer means of reducing plasma-bilirubin concentrations in British infants, and exchange transfusion remains the corner-stone of the treatment of this condition.

Conjugated Hyperbilirubinaemia

Phenobarbitone is ineffective in reducing serum-bilirubin levels where extrahepatic biliary obstruction exists. It has been claimed, however, that doses of 120–240 mg daily may reduce serum-bilirubin levels and relieve itching in primary biliary cirrhosis (Admirand and Bauer, 1971), possibly by increasing bile flow (see page 161). A similar mechanism may be the reason for the fall in plasma-bilirubin concentrations observed in children with intrahepatic biliary atresia, after phenobarbitone treatment (Sharp and Mirkin, 1972). However, in both these conditions, the reduction of plasma bilirubin is often only slight and the progress of the underlying pathological condition remains unaffected.

Treatment of Other Conditions

It seems likely that many of the clinical effects of the so-called adrencorticolytic drugs in man are due as much to their ability to cause hepatic enzyme induction as to any effects they may exert on the synthesis of hormones in the adrenals. Most of the initial effect of *o,p'*-DDD (mitotane) in ameliorating the clinical and biochemical consequences of Cushing's syndrome is mediated through increased hepatic metabolism of cortisol (Bledsoe *et al*, 1964), and it is not until after several weeks' treatment that any fall in cortisol secretion can be detected (Southren *et al*, 1966). Treatment with *o,p'*-DDD resulted in increased excretion of 6β-hydroxycortisol by patients suffering from Cushing's syndrome (Southren *et al*, 1966). Less clear-cut results were obtained during similar studies in cancer patients (Fukushima *et al*, 1971). Other enzyme inducers shown to produce clinical improvement in patients with Cushing's syndrome include diphenylhydantoin (Werk *et al*, 1966) and barbitone (Southren *et al*, 1969). As *o,p'*-DDD causes considerable nausea and vomiting, it would probably be worth evaluating DDT as an alternative.

Other examples of the use of enzyme induction in the treatment of endocrinological disease are few. Medroxyprogesterone–acetate administration causes increased activity of testosterone A-ring reductase in human liver, which may be the reason for its effectiveness in conditions, such as male precocious puberty, where there is increased production of testosterone (Gordon *et al*, 1971). It has been common practice for many years to treat patients with thyrotoxicosis with a barbiturate as a sedative; this may have the unsuspected advantage of increasing hepatic metabolism of thyroxine (Larsen *et al*, 1970). Treatment with enzyme-inducing agents could be employed to accelerate the rate of metabolism and thus the elimination of unwanted foreign compounds from the body. So far, it has only been used to increase the elimination of organochlorine pesticides, such as dieldrin (Jager, 1970).

TOXICOLOGICAL ROLE OF ENZYME INDUCTION

Enzyme inducers, such as phenobarbitone, may modify the toxicological effects, both short-term and long-term, produced by foreign compounds. As far as the effects on man are concerned the evidence is generally indirect, being obtained from animal experiments.

A pertinent example of increased drug toxicity in the rat following enzyme induction is that of paracetamol, since the results are probably relevant to man (Wright and Prescott, 1973). In therapeutic doses, paracetamol does not produce liver damage, but overdose may result in acute hepatic necrosis (Clark *et al*, 1973), which is now thought to be caused by a toxic metabolite (possibly an N-hydroxy derivative, as was suggested by Boyland and Chasseaud (1969) for the related analgesic phenacetin) produced by microsomal enzymes. Animals receiving enzyme inducers apparently produce more of this toxic metabolite, while those receiving enzyme inhibitors, such as piperonyl butoxide, produce less. The toxic metabolite is probably conjugated with glutathione, an endogenous nucleophilic tripeptide which protects cellular constituents (Chasseaud, 1973), before excretion. Following paracetamol overdose, the amounts of the toxic metabolite produced are presumably sufficiently large to exhaust hepatic stores of glutathione (or saturate protective glutathione S-transferases), and this then allows the metabolite to react with important cellular constituents to produce hepatic necrosis. Administration of other nucleophilic agents, such as cysteamine, reduces both liver-glutathione depletion and the subsequent necrosis (Mitchell *et al*, 1973a, b; Jollow *et al*, 1973; Potter *et al*, 1973). It is possible that cysteamine could be of benefit to patients suffering from paracetamol overdosage (Prescott *et al*, 1974; Mitchell *et al*, 1974).

Many enzyme-inducing agents can enhance their own metabolism as well as that of other drugs. Where prolonged treatment with a drug results in a decrease of its action, a phenomenon known as tolerance, enzyme induction may be suspected, but is not always the cause. Tolerance to barbitone arises even though this drug is hardly metabolized (Burns *et al*, 1957), and tolerance to phenobarbitone has been shown to occur without changes in rates of metabolism (Butler *et al*, 1954); the mechanism is possibly one of adaptation of the central nervous system. Changes in the central nervous system are believed to underlie the increased sensitivity of cirrhotics to chlorpromazine, and in these patients hepatic metabolism of chlorpromazine was not found to be abnormal (Maxwell *et al*, 1972a).

Although some substances, such as polycyclic hydrocarbons, which cause enzyme induction are carcinogens, there is no evidence that the two properties are related (Conney *et al*, 1959). Nonetheless the possible relationship between enzyme induction and carcinogenesis is intriguing. The polycyclic hydrocarbons, representative of one group of inducers, act on fewer biotransformations than, for example, phenobarbitone which is representative of another group of inducers. It has long been known that in experimental animals, administration of polycyclic hydrocarbons, such as 3-methylcholanthrene, can reduce the carcinogenic effect of such compounds as 3-methyl-4-dimethylaminoazobenzene (Meechan *et al*, 1953) or 2-acetylaminofluorene (Miyaji *et al*, 1953), an effect now presumed to be the result of a stimulation of hepatic metabolism to noncarcinogenic metabolites (Conney *et al*, 1956; Cramer *et al*, 1960). However, this information has not proved to be prophylactically applicable (with noncarcinogenic inducers), for in most human cancers, the carcinogen responsible is unknown, and furthermore, some substances, such as carbon tetrachloride, dimethylnitrosamine (Magee, 1965) and the polycyclic hydrocarbons (see chapter 3), are metabolized by microsomes to substances that are probably active carcinogens. Also tumours may appear long after exposure to the carcinogenic agent has ceased.

Until recently, it has been assumed that hydroxylation of polycyclic hydrocarbons *in vivo* enhances their elimination and reduces their carcinogenicity. Thus Schlede *et al* (1970) found that pretreatment of rats with benzo[*a*]pyrene, 3-methylcholanthrene or 7,12-dimethylbenz[*a*]anthracene stimulated the disappearance of subsequent doses of radioactively labelled benzo[*a*]pyrene and reduced the concentrations of this compound in various tissues. However, other studies suggest that this view may be an oversimplification. Using foetal cells in culture, Gelboin *et al* (1972) found that a microsomal hydroxylase system did indeed convert most carcinogens to weak or noncarcinogenic metabolites. The toxicity of the polycyclic hydrocarbons to the cells was nevertheless related to the presence of the hydroxylating enzymes, since inhibition of enzyme activity coincided with a reduction in the toxic effects of 7,12-dimethylbenz[*a*]anthracene. The formation of covalent bonds between benzo[*a*]pyrene and DNA, an event observed frequently for carcinogens (Gelboin, 1969), was catalysed by the microsomal enzyme system. 7,8-Benzoflavone which inhibited the microsomal enzyme system, also inhibited skin tumorigenesis caused by 7,12-dimethylbenz[*a*]anthracene. It is apparent that the relationship between microsomal hydroxylation and polycyclic-hydrocarbon carcinogenesis is far from simple.

Up to the present there has been little study of enzyme induction by drugs in relation to carcinogenesis. However, cell divisions stimulated by such drugs may be of potential importance, since partial hepatectomy (and consequential cell replication) renders the tissue more susceptible to the carcinogenicity of certain compounds (Hollander and Bentvelzen, 1968; Chernozemski and Warwick, 1970). In mice, certain enzyme-inducing compounds, including dieldrin and DDT (Walker *et al*, 1973), griseofulvin (Epstein *et al*, 1967) and phenobarbitone (Thorpe and Walker, 1973), have been found to increase the incidence of neoplasia in the liver, (possibly by influencing oncogenic viruses present there). Such an effect has not been found in other species including dogs, rats (Walker *et al*, 1969) or monkeys (A. S. Wright, personal communication, 1973). As some mice strains are particularly susceptible to tumours (*British Medical Journal*, 1972), it seems likely that the effects of phenobarbitone, DDT and griseofulvin, on this species may be of limited consequence to man. However, much further work is needed before this conclusion can be cheerfully accepted. In man, a large scale survey of post-mortem findings from epileptic subjects who had received anticonvulsant drugs for many years (Clemmesen *et al*, 1974) was interpreted as revealing no increase of neoplasia except in the brain. (It must be remembered that brain tumours frequently cause fits). However, the interpretation of this finding has already been attacked by Schneiderman (1974) who interprets Clemmesen's data differently and suggests that the incidence of tumours of the liver may be greater than should be expected. The relationship between enzyme induction and carcinogenesis seems likely to prove a fruitful field for further research.

CONCLUSIONS

Modern medicine is serviced by a large number of therapeutically effective drugs, and it is often deemed necessary to use several of these concurrently. This situation has led to numerous adverse drug reactions or interactions for which one explanation is that of altered biotransformation due to enzyme induction or inhibition.

Clinically significant drug interactions may be expected to occur, (*i*) if large doses of potentially interacting drugs are administered, (*ii*) if these drugs are taken together, (*iii*) if these drugs are administered to patients with renal or hepatic dysfunction, and (*iv*) if the drugs are dosed on a chronic basis (Avery, 1973). Optimum dosage schedules are achieved by suitable adjustment of the dose and dosage interval and need to be modified in the light of the drug interaction mediated through enzyme induction or inhibition. Many interactions are not mediated through altered biotransformation although this has often become a favoured explanation on the basis of limited evidence. Sometimes altered absorption (Rowland, 1972) or altered protein binding (Anton and Solomon, 1972) may explain an interaction, and more than one mechanism may be operating. Like differences in bioavailability (Chasseaud and Taylor, 1974), enzyme induction can be expected to be clinically more important when it involves drugs having a low therapeutic index.

In establishing criteria that determine whether or not a particular drug is a microsomal enzyme inducer, Remmer (1970b) suggested the following: (*i*) Lipophilicity—good enzyme inducers are extremely lipid soluble, e.g. DDT. Lipid solubility is probably a necessary property for uptake into the endoplasmic reticulum. A recent study of a series of barbiturates in rats suggested that a certain degree of lipid solubility was one of several determinants of a compound's ability to induce microsomal drug-metabolizing enzymes (Pelkonen and Kärki, 1973b). (*ii*) Metabolism by cytochrome P-450—enzyme inducers are usually metabolized by the cytochrome P-450 enzyme system. (iii) Drug dosage—induction is usually dose dependent. (*iv*) Hepatic drug concentrations—relatively high concentrations of drug must be present in the liver for a sufficient length of time. Although those criteria may appear self-evident, it is by no means certain that they apply in all cases. The latter three criteria are closely inter-related properties dependent on the drug being localized in the endoplasmic reticulum.

Exposure to certain pesticides has been shown to influence drug metabolism, but the humans at risk are likely to be those involved in the usage of large amounts of such materials. In this connection, the studies of Conney *et al* (1971) are relevant since they showed that the plasma antipyrine half-lives in humans were unaffected by the administration of piperonyl butoxide (a pesticide synergist and inhibitor of insect and mammalian microsomal enzymes) at dosages judged to be much greater than usual exposure levels. This also may be an example of species differences, the inhibitory effect of piperonyl butoxide possibly being weak in humans. Future work may reveal other endogenous substances or metabolic pathways affected by enzyme induction, and the beneficial effects of induction, as in the treatment of hyperbilirubinaemia with phenobarbitone, must be balanced against the risk, for example, of causing vitamin-D deficiency. The implications of enzyme induction in chemical carcinogenesis remain to be established. The relative importance of genetic or environmental influence on drug metabolism will continue to be debated (Smith and Rawlins, 1973) and hopefully studies of the role of age, sex, disease, nutritional status, etc (Bousquet, 1970; Conney *et al*, 1974) will not be neglected.

Knowledge of enzyme induction has grown rapidly in recent years and in doing so, has helped to explain many clinical observations. It seems likely that studies of the relationship of hepatic and extrahepatic enzyme activity to pathological conditions such as cancer, will provide some of the more exciting advances in the years to come.

REFERENCES

Aarts, E. M. (1965), *Biochem. Pharmacol.*, **14**, 359.

Aarts, E. M. (1966), *Biochem. Pharmacol.*, **15**, 1469.

Aarts, E. M. (1968), *Ph. D. Thesis*, University of Nijmegen.

Abernathy, C. O., Hodgson, E. and Guthrie F. E. (1971), *Biochem. Pharmacol.*, **20**, 2385.

Ackermann, E., Rane, A. and Ericsson, J. L. E. (1972), *Clin. Pharmacol. Ther.*, **13**, 652.

Acocella, G., Pagani, V., Marchetti, M., Baroni, G. C. and Nicolis, F. B. (1971), *Chemotherapy*, **16**, 356.

Admirand, W. A. and Bauer, K. (1971), *J. Clin. Invest.* **50**, 1*a*.

Aggeler, P. M. and O'Reilly, R. A. (1969), *J. Lab. Clin. Med.*, **74**, 229.

Alexanderson, B., Price-Evans, D. A. and Sjöqvist, F. (1969), *Brit. Med. J.*, **4**, 764.

Alexanderson, B. and Sjöqvist, F. (1971), *Ann. NY Acad. Sci.*, **179**, 739.

Alvares, A. P., Kappas, A., Levin, W. and Conney, A. H. (1973), *Clin. Pharmacol. Ther.*, **14**, 30.
Alvares, A. P., Schilling, G. and Levin, W. (1970), *J. Pharmacol. Exp. Ther.*, **175**, 4.
Alvares, A. P., Schilling, G., Levin, W., Kuntzman, R., Brand, L. and Mark, L. C. (1969), *Clin. Pharmacol. Ther.*, **10**, 655.
American Academy of Pediatrics (1963), *Pediat.*, **31**, 512.
Anders, M. W. and Mannering, G. J. (1966), *Mol. Pharmacol.*, **2**, 341.
Anton, A. H. and Solomon, H. M. (ed.) (1972), *Ann. NY Acad. Sci.*, **226**.
Applegarth, D. A. and Dunn, H. G. (1972), *New Engl. J. Med.*, **287**, 148.
Arias, I. M. (1962), *J. Clin. Invest.*, **41**, 2233.
Arias, I. M., Gartner, L. M., Cohen, M., Ben-Ezzer, J. and Levi, A. J. (1969), *Amer. J. Med.*, **47**, 395.
Arnold, K. and Gerber, N. (1970), *Clin. Pharmacol. Ther.*, **11**, 121.
Avellaneda, M. (1955), *Medicina (Buenos Aires)*, **15**, 109.
Avery, G. S. (1973), *Drugs*, **5**, 187.
Ballinger, B., Browning, M., O'Malley K. and Stevenson, I. H. (1972), *Brit. J. Pharmacol.*, **45**, 638.
Bast, jr. R. C., Whitlock, jr. J. P., Miller, H., Rapp, H. J. and Gelboin, H. V. (1974), *Nature*, **250**, 664.
Baugh, C. M. and Krumdieck, C. L. (1969), *Lancet*, **2**, 519.
Baylis, E. M., Crowley, J. M., Preece, J. M., Sylvester, P. E. and Marks, V. (1971), *Lancet*, **1**, 62.
Beckett, A. H. (1970), in Porter, R. and Birch, J. (ed.), *Chemical influences on behaviour*, p. 89, Churchill, London.
Beckett, A. H., Gorrod, J. W. and Jenner, P. (1971), *J. Pharm. Pharmacol.*, **23**, 62S.
Beckett, A. H. and Triggs, E. J. (1967), *Nature*, **216**, 587.
Behrman, R. E. and Fisher, D. E. (1970), *J. Pediat.*, **76**, 945.
Benn, A., Swan, C. H. J., Cooke, W. T., Blair, J. A., Matty, A. J. and Smith, M. E. (1971), *Brit. Med. J.*, **1**, 148.
Berlin, A., Siwers, B., Agurell, S., Hiort, A., Sjöqvist, F. and Strom, S. (1972), *Clin. Pharmacol. Ther.*, **13**, 733.
Berthelot, P., Erlinger, S., Dhumeaux, D. and Preaux, A.-M. (1970). *Amer. J. Physiol.*, **219**, 809.
Biasini, G. C. (1971), *Minerv. Pediat.*, **23**, 1798.
Billing, B. H. and Black, M. (1971), *Ann. NY Acad. Sci.*, **179**, 403.
Black, M. and Billing, B. H. (1969), *New Engl. J. Med.*, **280**, 1266.
Black, M., Fevery, J., Parker, D., Jacobson, J., Billing, B. H. and Carson, E. R. (1974), *Clin. Sci. Mol. Med.*, **46**, 1.
Black, M., Perrett, R. D. and Carter, A. E. (1973), *J. Lab. Clin. Med.*, **81**, 704.
Black, M. and Sherlock, S. (1970), *Lancet*, **1**, 1359.
Blaschke, T. F., Berk, P. D., Rodkey, F. L., Scharschmidt, B. F., Collison, H. A. and Waggoner, J. G. (1974), *Biochem. Pharmacol.*, **23**, 2795.
Bledsoe, T., Island, D. P., Ney, R. L. and Liddle, G. W. (1964), *J. Clin. Endocrinol. Metab.*, **24**, 1303.
Borgstedt, A. D., Brysen, M. F., Young, L. W. and Forbes, G. B. (1972), *J. Pediat.*, **81**, 9.
Boston Collaborative Drug Surveillance Program (1973a), *Clin. Pharmacol. Ther.*, **14**, 259.
Boston Collaborative Drug Surveillance Program (1973b), New Engl. J. Med., **288**, 277.
Bousquet, W. F. (1970), in Swarbrick, J. (ed.), *Current concepts in the pharmaceutical sciences: Biopharmaceutics*, p. 143, Lea & Febiger, Philadelphia.
Boyland, E. and Chasseaud, L. F. (1969), *Adv. Enzymol.*, **32**, 173.
Brazda, F. G., Heidingsfelder, S. and Martin, M. (1965), *Comp. Biochem. Physiol.*, **14**, 239.
Breckenridge, A. (1971), *Acta Pharmacol. Toxicol.*, **29** (suppl. 3), 225.

Breckenridge, A. and Orme, M. (1971), *Ann. NY Acad. Sci.*, **179**, 421.
Breckenridge, A., Orme, M. L'E., Thorgeirsson, S. S., Davies, D. S. and Brooks, R. V. (1971), *Clin. Sci. Mol. Med.*, **40**, 351.
Breckenridge, A., Orme, M. L'E., Davies, L., Thorgeirsson, S. S. and Davies, D. S. (1973), *Clin. Pharmacol. Ther.*, **14**, 514.
British Medical Journal (1972), **1**, 261.
Brodie, B. B. (1964), in Binns, T. B. (ed.), *Absorption and distribution of drugs*, p. 16, Livingstone, Edinburgh.
Brodie, B. B. and Gillette, J. R. (ed.) (1971), *Handbook of experimental pharmacology*, vol. 28 (parts 1 and 2), Springer-Verlag, Berlin.
Brodie, B. B. and Maickel, R. D. (1962), *Proc. First Int. Pharmacol. Meet.*, **6**, 299, Pergamon Press, Oxford.
Brodie, B. B. and Mitchell, J. R. (1973) in Davies, D. S. and Prichard, B. N. C. (ed.), *Biological effects of drugs in relation to their plasma concentrations*, p. 1, Macmillan, London.
Brodie, B. B. and Reid, W. D. (1967), *Fed. Proc.*, **26**, 1062.
Brooks, S. M., Werk, E. E., Ackerman, S. J., Sullivan, I. and Thrasher, K. (1972), *New Engl. J. Med.*, **286**, 1125.
Brown, jr., B. R. (1973), *Anesthesiology*, **39**, 178.
Brown, R. R., Miller, J. A. and Miller, E. C. (1954), *J. Biol. Chem.*, **259**, 211.
Brown, S. S. (1972) in Hathway, D. E. (ed.), *Foreign compound metabolism in mammals*, vol. 2, p. 456, Chemical Society, London.
Brunk, S. F., Combs, S. P., Miller, J. D., Delle, M. and Wilson, W. R. (1974), *J. Clin. Pharmacol.*, **14**, 271.
Buchanan, R. A. and Allen, R. J. (1971), *Neurology*, **21**, 866.
Buchanan, R. A. and Sholiton, L. J. (1972), in Woodbury, D. M., Penry, J. K. and Schmidt, R. P. (ed.), *Antiepileptic drugs*, p. 181, Raven Press, New York.
Burger, P. C. and Herdson, P. B. (1966), *Amer. J. Pathol.*, **48**, 793.
Burns, J. J. (1964), *Amer. J. Med.*, **37**, 327.
Burns, J. J., Conney, A. H., Dayton, P. G., Evans, C., Martin, G. R. and Taller, D. (1960), *J. Pharmacol. Exp. Ther.*, **129**, 132.
Burns, J. J., Cucinell, S. A., Koster, R. and Conney, A. H. (1965), *Ann. NY Acad. Sci.*, **123**, 273.
Burns, J. J., Evans, C. and Trousof, N. (1957), *J. Biol. Chem.*, **227**, 785.
Burns, J. J., Mosbach, E. H. and Schulenberg, S. (1954), *J. Biol. Chem.*, **207**, 679.
Burstein, S. and Klaiber, E. L. (1965), *J. Clin. Endocrinol. Metab.*, **25**, 293.
Busfield, D., Child, K. J., Atkinson, R. M. and Tomich, E. G. (1963), *Lancet*, **2**, 1042.
Butler, T. C., Mahaffee, C. and Waddell, W. J. (1954), *J. Pharmacol. Exp. Ther.*, **111**, 425.
Caldwell, J. and Sever, P. S. (1974), *Clin. Pharmacol. Ther.*, **16**, 737.
Cantrell, E. and Busbee, D. (1973), *Life Sci.*, **13**, 1649.
Cantrell, E. T., Warr, G. A., Busbee, D. L. and Martin, R. R. (1973), *J. Clin. Invest.*, **52**, 1881.
Carroll, B. J. and Davies, B. (1970), *Brit. Med. J.*, **1**, 789.
Carroll, B. J., Martin, F. I. R. and Davies, B. (1968), *Brit. Med. J.*, **3**, 285.
Carter, D. E., Goldman, J. M., Bressler, R., Huxtable, R. J., Christian, C. D. and Heine, M. W. (1974), *Clin. Pharmacol. Ther.*, **15**, 22.
Cascorbi, H. F., Blake, D. A. and Helrich, M. (1970), *Anesthesiology*, **32**, 119.
Cascorbi, H. F., Vesell, E. S., Blake, D. A. and Helrich, M. (1971), *Clin. Pharmacol. Ther.*, **12**, 50.
Catalano, P. M. and Cullen, S. I. (1966), *Clin. Res.*, **14**, 266.
Catz, C. and Yaffe, S. J. (1968), *Pediat. Res.*, **2**, 361.
Chasseaud, L. F. (1970), in Hathway, D. E. (ed.), *Foreign compound metabolism in mammals*, vol. 1, p. 1, Chemical Society, London.

Chasseaud, L. F. (1973), *Drug Metab. Rev.*, **2**, 185.

Chasseaud, L. F. and Taylor, T. (1974), *Ann. Rev. Pharmacol.*, **14**, 35.

Chedid, A. and Nair, V. (1972), *Science*, **175**, 176.

Chen, W., Vrindten, R. A., Dayton, P. G. and Burns, J. J. (1962), *Life Sci.*, **2**, 35.

Chernozemski, I. N. and Warwick, G. B. (1970), *Cancer Res.*, **30**, 2685.

Choi, Y., Thrasher, K., Werk jr., E. E. Sholiton, L. J. and Olinger, C. (1971), *J. Pharmacol. Exp. Ther.*, **176**, 27.

Christensen, L. K. and Skovsted, L. (1969), *Lancet*, **2**, 1397.

Clark, R., Borirakchanyavat, V., Davidson, A. R., Thompson, R. P. H., Widdop, B., Goulding, R. and Williams, R. (1973), *Lancet*, **1**, 66.

Clemmesen, J., Fuglsang-Frederiksen, V. and Plum, C. M. (1974), *Lancet*, **1**, 705.

Conney, A. H. (1965), *Proc. Second Int. Pharmacol. Meet.*, **4**, 277, Pergamon Press, Oxford.

Conney, A. H. (1967), *Pharmacol. Rev.*, **19**, 317.

Conney, A. H. (1969a), *J. Mond. Pharm.*, **12**, 186.

Conney, A. H. (1969b), *New Engl. J. Med.*, **280**, 653.

Conney, A. H. (1971), in LaDu, B. N., Mandel, H. G. and Way E. L. (ed.), *Fundamentals of drug metabolism and drug disposition*, p. 253, Williams and Wilkins, Baltimore.

Conney, A. H. (1973), *New Engl. J. Med.*, **289**, 971.

Conney, A. H., Bray, G. A., Evans, C. and Burns, J. J. (1961), *Ann. NY Acad. Sci.*, **92**, 115.

Conney, A. H., Craven, B., Kuntzman, R. and Pantuck E. J. (1974), in Theorell, T., Dedrick, R. L. and Condliffe, P. G. (ed.), *Pharmacology and pharmacokinetics*, p. 147, Plenum Press, New York.

Conney, A. H., Davison, C., Gastel, R. and Burns, J. J. (1960), *J. Pharmacol. Exp. Ther.*, **130**, 1.

Conney, A. H., Gillette, J. R., Inscoe, J. K., Trams, E. G. and Posner, H. S. (1959), *Science*, **130**, 1478.

Conney, A. H., Jacobson, M., Levin, W., Schneidman, K. and Kuntzman, R. (1966), *J. Pharmacol. Exp. Ther.*, **154**, 310.

Conney, A. H. and Klutch, A. (1963), *J. Biol. Chem.*, **238**, 1611.

Conney, A. H., Miller, E. C. and Miller, J. A. (1956), *Cancer Res.* **16**, 450.

Conney, A. H., Miller, E. C. and Miller, J. A. (1957), *J. Biol. Chem.*, **228**, 753.

Conney, A. H. and Schneidman, K. (1964), *J. Pharmacol. Exp. Ther.*, **146**, 225.

Conney, A. H., Welch, R., Kuntzman, R., Chang, R., Jacobson, M., Munro-Faure, A. D., Peck, A. W., Bye, A., Poland, A., Poppers, P. J., Finster, M. and Wolff, J. A. (1971), *Ann. NY Acad. Sci.*, **179**, 155.

Corn, M. (1966), *Thromb. Diath. Haemorrh.*, **16**, 606.

Corn, M. and Rockett, J. F. (1965), *Med. Ann. D. C.*, **34**, 578.

Cramer, J. W., Miller, J. A. and Miller, E. C. (1960), *J. Biol. Chem.*, **235**, 250.

Crigler jr., J. F. and Gold, N. I. (1966) *J. Clin. Invest.* **45**, 998.

Cucinell, S. A. (1972), in Woodbury, D. M., Penry, J. K. and Schmidt, R. P. (ed.) *Antiepileptic drugs*, p. 319, Raven Press, New York.

Cucinell, S. A., Conney, A. H., Sansur, M. and Burns, J. J. (1965), *Clin. Pharmacol. Ther.*, **6**, 420.

Cucinell, S. A., Odessky, L., Weiss, M. and Dayton, P. G. (1966), *J. Amer. Med. Ass.*, **197**, 366.

Cunningham, J. L. and Price-Evans, D. A. (1974), *Eur. J. Clin. Pharmacol.*, **7**, 387.

Curci, G., Bergamini, N., Delli Veneri, F., Ninni, A. and Nitti, V. (1972), *Chemotherapy*, **17**, 373.

Curry, S. H., Davis, J. M., Janowsky, D. S. and Marshall, J. H. L. (1970), *Arch. Gen. Psychiat.*, **22**, 209.

Davidson, D. C., McIntosh, W. B. and Ford, J. A. (1974), *Clin. Sci. Mol. Med.*, **47**, 279.
Davies, D. S. and Thorgeirrson, S. S. (1971a), *Acta Pharmacol. Toxicol.*, **29**, suppl. 3, 181.
Davies, D. S. and Thorgeirrson, S. S. (1971b), *Ann. NY Acad. Sci.*, **179**, 411.
Davies, J. E. and Edmundson, W. F. (1972) in Davies, J. E. and Edmundson, W. F. (ed.), *Epidemiology of DDT*, p. 109, Futura Publishing, New York.
Davies, J. E., Edmundson, W. F., Carter, C. H. and Barquet, A. (1969), *Lancet*, **2**, 7.
Davies, J. E., Edmundson, W. F., Carter, C. H. and Barquet, A. (1972), in Davies, J. E. and Edmundson, W. F. (ed.), *Epidemiology of DDT*, p. 85, Futura Publishing, New York.
Davies, P. A., (1969), *Lancet*, **2**, 273.
Davies, P. P. (1970), *Lancet*, **1**, 413.
Davis, J. M. Sekerke, J. and Janowsky, D. S. (1974b), *Drug Intell. Clin. Pharm.*, **8**, 120.
Davis, M., Simmons, C. J., Dordoni, B. and Williams, R. (1974a), *Brit. J. Clin. Pharmacol.*, **1**, 253.
Dayton, P. G., Tarcan, Y., Chenkin, T. and Weiner, W. (1961), *J. Clin. Invest.*, **40**, 1797.
Dent, C. E., Richens, A., Rowe, D. J. F. and Stamp, T. C. B. (1970), *Brit. Med. J.*, **4**, 69.
Di Toro, R., Lupi, L. and Ansanelli, V. (1968), *Nature*, **219**, 265.
Doe, W. F., Hoffbrand, A. V., Reed, P. I. and Scott, J. M. (1971), *Brit. Med. J.*, **1**, 669.
Douglas, J. F., Ludwig, B. J. and Smith, N. (1963), *Proc. Soc. Exp. Biol. Med.*, **112**, 436.
Dutton, G. J. (ed.) (1966), *Glucuronic acid: free and combined. Chemistry, biochemistry, pharmacology and medicine*, Academic Press, New York.
Edmundson, W. F., Davies, J. E., Maceo, A. and Morgade, C. (1972), in Davies, J. E. and Edmundson, W. F. (ed.), *Epidemiology of DDT*, p. 93, Futura Publishing, New York.
Edwards, O. M., Courtenay-Evans, R., Galley, J., Hunter, J. and Tait, A. J. (1974), *Lancet*, **2**, 549.
Eichelbaum, M., Bodem, G., Gugler, R., Schneider-Deters, C. and Dengler, H. J. (1974), *New Engl. J. Med.*, **290**, 1040.
Enklewitz, M. and Lasker M. (1935), *J. Biol. Chem.*, **110**, 443.
Epstein, S. S., Andrea, J., Joshi, S. and Mantel, N., (1967), *Cancer Res.*, **27**, 1900.
Ernster, L. and Orrenius, S. (1965), *Fed. Proc.*, **24**, 1190.
Estabrook, R. W. (1971), in Brodie, B. B. and Gillette, J. R. (ed.), *Handbook of experimental pharmacology*, vol. 28 (part 2), p. 264, Springer-Verlag, Berlin.
Fahim, M. S., Hall, D. G. and Fahim, Z. (1969), *Amer. J. Obstet. Gynecol.*, **105**, 124.
Falk, H. L. (1971), *Prog. Exp. Tumor Res.*, **14**, 105.
Feinman, L., Rubin, E. and Lieber, C. S. (1972), in Orlandi, F. and Jezequel, A. M. (ed.), *Liver and drugs*, p. 41, Academic Press, New York.
Felsher, B. F., Craig, J. R. and Carpio, N. (1973), *J. Lab. Clin. Med.*, **81**, 829.
Fishbein, L. (1974), *Chromatog. Rev.*, **18**, 177.
Fleishner, G. and Arias, I. M. (1970), *Amer. J. Med.*, **49**, 576.
Forrest, F. M., Forrest, I. M. and Serra, M. T. (1970), *Biol. Psychiat.*, **2**, 53.
Fouts, J. R. (1961), *Biochem. Biophys. Res. Commun.* **6**, 373.
Fouts, J. R. (1965), *Proc. Second Int. Pharmacol. Meet.*, **4**, 261, Pergamon Press, Oxford.
Fouts, J. R. (1971), in Schwartz, A. (ed.), *Methods in pharmacology*, vol. 1, p. 287, Appleton-Century-Crofts, New York.
Fouts, J. R. (1973), *Drug Metab. Disposition*, **1**, 380.
Fouts, J. R. and Adamson, R. H. (1959), *Science*, **129**, 897.
Fouts, J. R. and Hart, L. G. (1965), *Ann. NY Acad. Sci.*, **123**, 245.

Fouts, J. R. and Rogers, L. A. (1965), *J. Pharmacol. Exp. Ther.*, **147**, 112.
Fukushima, D. K., Bradlow, H. L. and Hellman, L. (1971), *J. Clin. Endocrinol. Metab.*, **32**, 192.
Garner, R. C. and McLean, A. E. M. (1969), *Biochem. Pharmacol.*, **18**, 645.
Garrettson, L. K. and Dayton, P. G. (1970), *Clin. Pharmacol. Ther.*, **11**, 674.
Gelboin, H. V. (1967), *Adv. Cancer Res.*, **10**, 1.
Gelboin, H. V. (1969), *Cancer Res.*, **29**, 1272.
Gelboin, H. V. (1971), in Brodie, B. B. and Gillette, J. R. (ed.), *Handbook of experimental pharmacology*, vol. 28, part 2, p. 431, Springer-Verlag, Berlin.
Gelboin, H. V., Kinoshita, N. and Wiebel, F. J. (1972), *Fed. Proc.* **31**, 1298.
Gershbein, L. L. (1966), *Cancer Res.*, **26**, 1905.
Gilbert, A., Lereboullet, P. and Herscher, M. (1907), *Bull. Soc. Med. Hop. Paris*, **24**, 1203.
Gillette, J. R. (1966), *Adv. Pharmacol.*, **4**, 219.
Gillette, J. R. (1971), *Ann. NY Acad. Sci.*, **179**, 43.
Gillette, J. R., Conney, A. H., Cosmides, G. J., Estabrook, R. W., Fouts, J. R. and Mannering, G. J., (ed.) (1969), *Microsomes and drug oxidations*, Academic Press, New York.
Gillette, J. R., Mitchell, J. R. and Brodie, B. B. (1974), *Ann. Rev. Pharmacol.*, **14**, 271.
Goldstein, A., Aronow, L. and Kalman, S. M. (1968), *Principles of drug action*, Harper and Row, New York.
Goodman, L. S. and Gilman, A. (1970), *The pharmacological basis of therapeutics*, 4th ed., MacMillan, London.
Gordon, G. G., Altman, K., Southren, A. L. and Olivo, J. (1971), *J. Clin. Endocrinol., Metab.* **32**, 457.
Gorrod, J. W. and Jenner, P. (1975), *Essays in toxicology*, **6**, 35.
Goss, J. E. and Dickhaus, D. W. (1965), *New Engl. J. Med.*, **273**, 1094.
Granick, S. and Urata, G. (1963), *J. Biol. Chem.*, **238**, 821.
Greenwood, R. H., Prunty, F. T. G. and Silver, J. (1973), *Brit. Med. J.* **1**, 643.
Griffiths, G. M. (1934), *J. Neurol. Psychopathol.*, **15**, 29.
Griner, P. F., Raisz, L. G., Rickles, F. R., Wiesner, P. J. and Odoroff, C. L. (1971), *Ann. Intern. Med.*, **74**, 540.
Hahn, T. J., Birge, S. J., Scharp, C. R. and Avioli, L. V. (1972a), *J. Clin. Invest.*, **51**, 741.
Hahn, T. J., Hendin, B. A., Scharp, C. R. and Haddad, J. G. (1972b), *New Engl. J. Med.*, **287**, 900.
Hänninen, O. (1968) *Ann. Acad. Sci. Fenn., Series A II Chemica*, 142.
Hansen, J. M., Siersboek-Nielsen, K., Kristensen, M., Skovsted, L. and Christensen, L. K. (1971a), *Acta Med. Scand.*, **189**, 15.
Hansen, J. M., Siersboek-Nielsen, K. and Skovsted, L. (1971b), *Clin. Pharmacol. Ther.*, **12**, 539.
Hart, L. G., Shultice, R. W. and Fouts, J. R. (1963), *Toxicol. Appl. Pharmacol.*, **5**, 371.
Hartshorn, E. A. (1971), *Handbook of drug interactions*, Hamilton Press, Hamilton.
Heinonen, J., Takki, S. and Jarho, L. (1970), *Acta Anaesthesiol. Scand.*, **14**, 89.
Heirwegh, K. P. M., Meuwissen, J. A. T. P. and Fevery, J. (1973), *Adv. Clin. Chem.*, **16**, 239.
Helleberg, L., Rubin, A., Wolen, R. L., Rodda, B. E., Ridolfo, A. S. and Grubber jr., C. N. (1974), *Brit. J. Clin. Pharmacol.*, **1**, 371.
Hildebrandt, A., Remmer, H. and Estabrook, R. W. (1968), *Biochem. Biophys. Res. Commun.*, **30**, 607.
Hodgman, J. E. and Schwartz, A. (1970), *Amer. J. Dis. Child*, **119**, 473.
Hollander, C. F. and Bentvelzen, P. (1968), *J. Nat. Cancer Inst.*, **41**, 1303.
Holtzman, J. L., Gram, T. E., Gigon, P. L. and Gillette, J. R. (1968), *Biochem. J.*, **110**, 407.

Houlihan, C. M., Scott, J. M., Boyle, P. H. and Weir, D. G. (1972), *Gut*, **13**, 189.
Huffman, D. H., Shoeman, D. W., Pentikäinen, P. and Azarnoff, D. L. (1973), *Pharmacology*, **10**, 338.
Huffman, D. H., Shoeman, D. W. and Azarnoff, D. L. (1974), *Biochem. Pharmacol.*, **23**, 197.
Hunter, J., Maxwell, J. D., Carrella, M., Stewart, D. A. and Williams, R. (1971a), *Lancet*, **1**, 572.
Hunter, J., Maxwell, J. D., Stewart, D. A., Parsons, V. and Williams, R. (1971c), *Brit. Med. J.*, **4**, 202.
Hunter, J., Maxwell, J. D., Stewart, D. A., Williams, R., Robinson, J. and Richardson, A. (1971d), *Gut*, **12**, 970.
Hunter, J., Thompson, R. P. H., Rake, M. O. and Williams, R. (1971b), *Brit. Med. J.*, **2**, 497.
Hunter, J., Maxwell, J. D., Stewart, D. A., Williams, R., Robinson, J. and Richardson, A. (1972a), *Nature*, **237**, 399.
Hunter, J., Maxwell, J. D. and Williams, R. (1972b), in *Eighth Symposium on Advanced Medicine*, p. 243, Pitman Medical, London.
Hunter, J. (1973), *MD Thesis*, University of Cambridge.
Hunter, J., Maxwell, J. D., Stewart, D. A. and Williams, R. (1973), *Biochem. Pharmacol.*, **22**, 743.
Hunter, J. (1974), *J. Roy. Coll. Phycns.*, **8**, 163.
Hunter, J., Burnham, W. R., Chasseaud, L. F. and Down, W. H. (1974), *Biochem. Pharmacol.*, **23**, 2480.
Hunter, J., Spencer, R., Davie, M. W. J., Chalmers, T. M. and Kodicek, E. (1975), submitted for publication.
Hutson, D. H. (1970) in Hathway, D. E. (ed.), *Foreign compound metabolism in mammals*, vol. 1, p. 314, Chemical Society, London.
Hutson, D. H. (1972), in Hathway, D. E. (ed.), *Foreign compound metabolism in mammals*, vol. 2, p. 328, Chemical Society, London.
Imai, Y. and Sato, R. (1966), *Biochem. Biophys. Res. Commun.*, **22**, 620.
Iseri, O. A., Lieber, C. S. and Gottlieb, L. S. (1966), *Amer. J. Pathol.*, **49**, 593.
Jacobson, M., Levin, W., Poppers, P. J., Wood, A. W. and Conney, A. H. (1974), *Clin. Pharmacol. Ther.*, **16**, 701.
Jager, K. W. (1970), *Aldrin, Dieldrin, Endrin and Telodrin: an epidemiological and toxicological study of long term occupational exposure*, Elsevier, Amsterdam.
Jao, J. Y., Jusko, W. J. and Cohen, J. L. (1972), *Cancer Res.*, **32**, 2761.
Jezequel, A. M., Orlandi, F. and Tenconi, L. T. (1971), *Gut*, **12**, 984.
Jollow, D. J., Mitchell, J. R., Potter, W. Z., Davis, D. C., Gillette, J. R. and Brodie, B. B. (1973), *J. Pharmacol. Exp. Ther.*, **187**, 195.
Jondorf, W. R., Maickel, R. P. and Brodie, B. B. (1959), *Biochem. Pharmacol.*, **1**, 352.
Jori, A., Bianchetti, A., Prestini, P. E. and Garattini, S. (1970), *Eur. J. Pharmacol.*, **9**, 362.
Jouppila, P. and Suonio, S. (1970), *Ann. Clin. Res.*, **2**, 209.
Jubiz, W., Meikle, A. W., Levinson, R. A., Mizutani, S., West, C. D. and Tyler, F. H. (1970), *New Engl. J. Med.*, **283**, 11.
Juchau, M. R. (1971), *Toxicol. Appl. Pharmacol.*, **18**, 665.
Juchau, M. R., Lee, Q. H., Louviaux, G. L., Symms, K. G., Krasner, J. and Yaffe, S. J. (1973) in Boréus, L. O. (ed.), *Fetal pharmacology*, p. 321, Raven Press, New York.
Juchau, M. R., Niswander, K. R. and Yaffe, S. J. (1968), *Amer. J. Obstet, Gynecol.*, **100**, 348.
Juchau, M. R., Pedersen, M. G. and Symms, K. G. (1972), *Biochem. Pharmacol.*, **21**, 2269.

Kanto, J. Iisalo, E., Lehtinen, V. and Salminen, J. (1974), *Psychopharmacologia*, **36**, 123.
Kater, R. M. H., Roggin, G., Tobon, F., Zieve, P. and Iber, F. L. (1969b), *Amer. J. Med. Sci.*, **258**, 35.
Kater, R. M. H., Tobon, F. and Iber, F. L. (1969a), *J. Amer. Med. Ass.*, **207**, 363.
Kato, R., Vassanelli, P., Frontino, G. and Chiesara, E. (1964), *Biochem. Pharmacol.*, **13**, 1037.
Kazmier, F. J. and Spittell, J. A. (1970), *Mayo Clin. Proc.*, **45**, 249.
Keeri-Szanto, M. and Pomeroy, J. R. (1971), *Lancet*, **1**, 947.
Kellermann, G., Shaw, C. R. and Luyten-Kellerman, M. (1973), *New Eng. J. Med.*, **289**, 934.
Ketterer, B., Ross-Mansell, P. and Whitehead, J. K. (1967), *Biochem. J.*, **103**, 316.
Klaassen, C. D. (1969), *J. Pharmacol. Exp. Ther.*, **168**, 218.
Klotz, U., McHorse, T. S., Wilkinson, G. R. and Schenker, S. (1974), *Clin. Pharmacol. Ther.*, **16**, 667.
Knoefel, P. K., Huang, K. C., Klingele, H. O., LeFevre, P. G., Scharff, T. G. and Westphal, U. F. (1971), *Absorption, distribution, transformation and excretion of drugs*, C. C. Thomas, Springfield.
Kolmodin-Hedman, B. (1973), *Eur. J. Clin. Pharmacol.* **5**, 195.
Kolmodin, B., Azarnoff, D. L. and Sjöqvist, F. (1969), *Clin. Pharmacol. Ther.*, **10**, 638.
Kradjan, W. A. (1974), *Drug Intell. Clin. Pharm.*, **8**, 462.
Kreek, M. J. and Sleisenger, M. H. (1968), *Lancet*, **2**, 73.
Kristensen, M., Hansen, J. M. and Skovsted, L. (1969), *Acta Med. Scand.*, **185**, 347.
Kruse, R. (1968), *Monatsschr. Kinderheilkd.*, **116**, 378.
Kuntzman, R., Jacobson, M. and Conney, A. H. (1966b), *Pharmacologist*, **8**, 195.
Kuntzman, R., Jacobson, M., Levin, W. and Conney, A. H. (1968a), *Biochem. Pharmacol.*, **17**, 565.
Kuntzman, R., Levin, W., Jacobson, M. and Conney, A. H. (1968b), *Life Sci.*, **7**, 215.
Kuntzman, R., Mark, L. C., Brand, L., Jacobson, M., Levin, W. and Conney, A. H. (1966a), *J. Pharmacol. Exp. Ther.*, **152**, 151.
Kutt, H. (1971), *Ann. NY Acad. Sci.*, **179**, 704.
Kutt, H. (1972), in Woodbury, D. M., Penry, J. K. and Schmidt, R. P. (ed.), *Antiepileptic drugs*, p. 169, Raven Press, New York.
Kutt, H., Brennan, R., Dehejia, H. and Verebely, K. (1970), *Amer. Rev. Resp. Dis.*, **101**, 377.
Kutt, H., Haynes, J., Verebely, K. and McDowell, F. (1969), *Neurology*, **19**, 611.
La Du, B. N. (1971), in La Du, B. N., Mandel, H. G. and Way, E. L. (ed.), *Fundamentals of drug metabolism and drug disposition*, p. 308, Williams and Wilkins, Baltimore.
La Du, B. N., Mandel, H. G. and Way, E. L. (ed.) (1971), *Fundamentals of drug metabolism and drug disposition*, Williams and Wilkins, Baltimore.
Lancet, (1974) **1**, 790.
Lane, B. P. and Lieber, C. S. (1966), *Amer. J. Pathol.*, **49**, 593.
Larsen, P. R., Atkinson, A. J., Wellman, H. N. and Goldsmith, R. E. (1970), *J. Clin. Invest.*, **49**, 1266.
Latham, A. N., Millbank, L., Richens, A. and Rowe, D. J. F. (1973), *J. Clin. Pharmacol.*, **13**, 337.
Lathe, G. H. and Walker, M. (1957), *Biochem. J.*, **67**, 9P.
Lawson, D. E. M., Fraser, D. R., Kodicek, E., Morris, H. R. and Williams, D. H. (1971), *Nature*, **230**, 228.
Lemberger, L., Tamarkin, N. R., Axelrod, J. and Kopin, I. J. (1971), *Science*, **173**, 72.
Levi, A. J., Gatmaitan, Z. and Arias, I. M. (1969), *J. Clin. Invest.*, **48**, 2156.

Levi, A. J., Sherlock, S. and Walker, D. (1968), *Lancet*, **1**, 1275.
Levin, W., Welch, R. M. and Conney, A. H. (1974), *J. Pharmacol. Exp. Ther.*, **188**, 287.
Levine, R. R. (1973), *Pharmacology: drug actions and reactions*, Little, Brown and Co, Boston.
Levy, G. and Ertel, I. J. (1971), *Pediat.*, **47**, 811.
Levy, G., O'Reilly, R. A., Aggeler, P. M. and Keech, G. M. (1970), *Clin. Pharmacol. Ther.*, **11**, 372.
Lichter, M., Black, M. and Arias, I. M. (1973), *J. Pharmacol. Exp. Ther.*, **187**, 612.
Lieber, C. S. and DeCarli, L. M. (1968), *Science*, **162**, 917.
Lieber, C. S., Rubin, E. and DeCarli, L. M. (1971), in Kissin, B. and Begleiter, H. (ed.), *The biology of alcoholism*, vol. 1, p. 263, Raven Press, New York.
Lifshitz, F. and MacLaren, N. K. (1973), *J. Pediat.*, **83**, 612.
Lindgren, S., Collste, P., Norlander, B. and Sjöqvist, F. (1974), *Eur. J. Clin. Pharmacol.*, **7**, 381.
Livingston, S. and Berman, W. (1973), *J. Pediat.*, **82**, 347.
Longenecker, H. E., Fricke, H. H., King, C. G. (1940), *J. Biol. Chem.*, **135**, 497.
Longenecker, H. E., Musulin, R. R., Tully, R. H. and King, C. G. (1939), *J. Biol. Chem.*, **129**, 445.
Longshaw, R. N. (1973), *Drug Intell. Clin. Pharm.*, **7**, 263.
Lu, A. Y. H., Kuntzman, R., West, S. and Conney, A. H. (1971), *Biochem. Biophys. Res. Commun.*, **42**, 1200.
Lumb, G. A., Mawer, E. B. and Stanbury, S. W. (1971), *Amer. J. Med.*, **50**, 421.
MacDonald, M. G. and Robinson, D. S. (1968), *J. Amer. Med. Ass.*, **204**, 97.
MacDonald, M. G., Robinson, D. S., Sylwester, D. and Jaffe, J. J. (1969), *Clin. Pharmacol. Ther.*, **10**, 80.
MacLeod, S. M., Renton, K. W. and Eade, N. R. (1973), *Chem.–Biol. Inter.*, **7**, 29.
Magee, P. N. (1965), *Proc. Second Int. Pharmacol. Meet.*, **4**, 343, Pergamon Press, Oxford.
Maisey, D. N., Brown, R. C. and Day, J. L. (1974), *Lancet*, **2**, 896.
Mannering, G. J. (1968), in Tedeschi, D. H. and Tedeschi, R. E. (ed.), *Importance of fundamental principles in drug evaluation*, p. 105, Raven Press, New York.
Mannering, G. J. (1972), in Woodbury, D. M., Penry, J. K. and Schmidt, R. P. (ed.), *Antiepileptic drugs*, p. 23, Raven Press, New York.
March. J., Turner, W. J. Shanley, J. and Field, J. (1974), *Clin. Chem.* **20**, 1155.
Margolis, J. I. (1929), *Amer. J. Med. Sci.*, **177**, 348.
Marsh, C. A. (1963a), *Biochem. J.*, **86**, 77.
Marsh, C. A. (1963b), *Biochem. J.*, **87**, 82.
Marsh, C. A. and Reid, L. M. (1963), *Biochim. Biophys. Acta.* **78**, 726.
Marshall, W. F. and McLean, A. E. M. (1969), *Biochem. Pharmacol.*, **18**, 153.
Martin, G. R. (1961), *Ann. NY Acad. Sci.*, **92**, 141.
Martin, J. R. (1974), *N.Z. Med. J.*, **79**, 1022.
Marver, H. S. (1969), in Gillette, J. R., Conney, A. H., Cosmides, G. J., Estabrook, R. W., Fouts, J. R. and Mannering, G. J. (ed.), *Microsomes and drug oxidations*, p. 495, Academic Press, New York.
Matsuda, I. and Takase, A. (1969), *Lancet*, **2**, 1006.
Mattingly, D. (1968), in Baron, D. N., Compston, N. and Dawson, A. M. (ed.), *Recent advances in medicine*, 15th ed., p. 125, Churchill, London.
Maurer, H. M., Wolff, J. A., Finster, M., Poppers, P. J., Pantuck, E., Kuntzman, R. and Conney, A. H. (1968), *Lancet*, **2**, 122.
Maxwell, J. D., Carrella, M., Parkes, J. D., Williams, R., Mould, G. P. and Curry, S. H. (1972a), *Clin. Sci.*, **43**, 143.
Maxwell, J. D., Hunter, J., Stewart, D. A., Ardeman, S. and Williams, R. (1972b), *Brit. Med. J.*, **1**, 297.

May, B., Helmstaedt, D., Büstgens, L. and McLean, A. (1974), *Clin. Sci. Mol. Med.*, **46**, 11P.
McDonald, R., Shaw, M. and Craig, C. (1964), *Brit. Med. J.*, **1**, 677.
McLean, A. E. M. (1972), *Medicine*, **1**, 331.
Meigs, R. A. and Ryan, K. J. (1968), *Biochim. Biophys. Acta.*, **165**, 476.
Meloni, T., Cagnazzo, G., Dore, A. and Cutillo, S. (1973), *J. Pediat.*, **82**, 1048.
Meynell, M. J. (1966), *Lancet*, **1**, 487.
Meechan, R. J., McCafferty, D. E. and Jones, R. S. (1953), *Cancer Res.*, **13**, 802.
Misra, P. S., Gang, H., Rubin, E. and Lieber, C. S. (1970), *Clin. Res.*, **18**, 341.
Misra, P. S., Lefèvre, A., Ishii, H., Rubin, E. and Lieber, C. S. (1971), *Amer. J. Med.*, **51**, 346.
Mitchell, A. A. (1972), *New Engl. J. Med.*, **287**, 1153.
Mitchell, J. R., Jollow, D. J., Potter, W. Z., Gillette, J. R. and Brodie, B. B. (1973a), *J. Pharmacol. Exp. Ther.*, **187**, 185.
Mitchell, J. R., Jollow, D. J., Potter, W. Z., Gillette, J. R. and Brodie, B. B. (1973b), *J. Pharmacol. Exp. Ther.*, **187**, 211.
Mitchell, J. R., Thorgeirsson, S. S., Potter, W. Z., Jollow, D. J. and Keiser, H. (1974), *Clin. Pharmacol. Ther.*, **16**, 676.
Miyaji, T., Moskowski, L. I., Senoo, T., Ogata, M., Odo, T., Kawai, K., Sayama, Y., Ishida, J. and Matsuo, H. (1953), *Gann*, **44**, 281.
Morey, K. S. and Litwack, G. (1969), *Biochemistry*, **8**, 4813.
Morgan, D. P. and Roan, C. C. (1974), *Arch. Environ. Health*, **29**, 14.
Morrelli, H. F. and Melmon, K. L. (1968), *Calif. Med.* **109**, 380.
Morselli, P. L., Garattini, S. and Cohen, S. N. (ed.) (1964), *Drug interactions*, Raven Press, New York.
Morselli, P. L., Rizzo, M. and Garattini, S. (1971), *Ann. NY Acad. Sci.*, **179**, 88.
Mountain, K. R., Hirsh, J. and Gallus, A. S. (1970), *Lancet*, **1**, 265.
Mowat, A. P. (1968), *J. Endocrinol.*, **42**, 585.
Mulder, G. J. (1970), *Biochem. J.*, **117**, 319.
Mumford, J. P. (1974), *Brit. Med. J.*, **2**, 333.
Nayak, R. K., Smith, R. D., Chamberlain, J. H., Polk, A., de Long, A. F., Herezeg, T., Chemburkar, P. B., Joslin, R. S. and Reavey-Cantwell, N. H. (1974), *J. Pharmacokinet. Biopharm.*, **2**, 107.
Nebert, D. W. Winkler, J. and Gelboin, H. V. (1969), *Cancer Res.* **29**, 1763.
Nelson, E. B., Raj, P. P., Belfi, K. J. and Masters, B. S. S. (1971), *J. Pharmacol. Exp. Ther.*, **178**, 580.
Nitti, V., Ninni, A., Meola, G., Iuliano, A. and Curci, G. (1973), *Chemotherapy*, **19**, 206.
Ohnhaus, E. E., Thorgeirsson, S. S., Davies, D. S. and Breckenridge, A. (1971), *Biochem. Pharmacol.*, **20**, 2561.
Okada, M., Matsui, M., Kaizu, T. and Abe, F. (1969), *Chem. Pharm. Bull. (Tokyo)*, **17**, 2625.
O'Malley, K., Browning, M., Stevenson, I. H. and Turnbull, M. J. (1973), *Eur. J. Clin. Pharmacol.*, **6**, 102.
O'Malley, K., Stevenson, I. H. and Crooks, J. (1972), *Clin. Pharmacol. Ther.*, **13**, 552.
O'Reilly, R. A. and Levy, G. (1970), *Clin. Pharmacol. Ther.*, **11**, 378.
Orme, M., Breckenridge, A. and Brooks, R. V. (1972), *Brit. Med. J.*, **3**, 611.
Palade, G. E. and Siekevitz, P. S. (1956), *J. Biophys. Biochem. Cytol.*, **2**, 171.
Pantuck, E. J., Hsiao, K. C., Maggio, A., Nakamura, K., Kuntzman, R. and Conney, A. H. (1974), *Clin. Pharmacol. Ther.*, **15**, 9.
Parke, D. V. (1968), *The biochemistry of foreign compounds*, Pergamon Press, Oxford.
Parke, D. V. (1972), in Rabin, B. R. and Freedman, R. B. (ed.), *Effects of drugs on cellular control mechanisms*, p. 69, University Park Press, Baltimore.

Parke, D. V. and Rahman, H. (1969), *Biochem. J.*, **113**, 12P.
Pelkonen, O., Kaltiala, E. H., Larmi, T. K. I. and Kärki, N. T. (1973), *Clin. Pharmacol. Ther.*, **14**, 840.
Pelkonen, O. and Kärki, N. T. (1973a), *Life Sci.*, **13**, 1163.
Pelkonen, O. and Kärki, N. T. (1973b), *Chem.-Biol. Inter.*, **7**, 93.
Peters, J. H. and Levy, L. (1971), *Ann. NY Acad. Sci.*, **179**, 660.
Peters, J. H., Miller, K. S. and Brown, P. (1965), *J. Pharmacol. Exp. Ther.*, **150**, 298.
Petruch, F., Schüppel, R. V. A. and Steinhilber, G. (1974), *Eur. J. Clin. Pharmacol.*, **7**, 281.
Poland, A., Smith, D., Kuntzman, R., Jacobson, M. and Conney, A. H. (1970), *Clin. Pharmacol. Ther.*, **11**, 724.
Potter, W. Z., Davis, D. C., Mitchell, J. R., Jollow, D. J., Gillette, J. R. and Brodie, B. B. (1973), *J. Pharmacol. Exp. Ther.*, **187**, 203.
Preis, C., Schaude, G. and Siess, M. (1966), *Arch. Pharmakol. Exp. Pathol.*, **254**, 489.
Prescott, L. F. (1969), *Lancet*, **2**, 1239.
Prescott, L. F., Newton, R. W., Swainson, C. P., Wright, N., Forrest, A. R. W. and Matthew, H. (1974), *Lancet*, **1**, 588.
Prescott, L. F. and Wright, N. (1973), *Brit. J. Pharmacol.*, **49**, 602.
Price-Evans, D. A. (1968), *Ann. NY Acad. Sci.*, **151**, 723.
Radzialowski, F. M. and Bousquet, W. F. (1968), *J. Pharmacol. Exp. Ther.*, **163**, 229.
Ramboer, C., Thompson, P. R. H. and Williams, R. (1969), *Lancet*, **1**, 966.
Rane, A. and Ackermann, E. (1972), *Clin. Pharmacol. Ther.*, **13**, 663.
Rane, A., von Bahr, C., Orrenius, S. and Sjöqvist F. (1973), in Boréus, L. O. (ed.), *Fetal pharmacology*, p. 287, Raven Press, New York.
Rawlins, M. D., Collste, P., Frisk-Holmberg, M., Lind, M., Östman, J. and Sjöqvist, F. (1974), *Eur. J. Clin. Pharmacol.*, **7**, 353.
Redinger, R. N. and Small, D. M. (1973), *J. Clin. Invest.*, **52**, 161.
Redman, D. R. and Prescott, L. F. (1973), *Diabetes*, **22**, 210.
Reimers, D. and Jezek, A. (1971), *Prax Pneumol.*, **25**, 255.
Remmer, H. (1958a) *Naturwissenschaften*, **45**, 189.
Remmer, H. (1958b), *Arch. Exp. Pathol. Pharmakol.*, **233**, 184.
Remmer, H. (1969), *J. Mond. Pharm.*, **12**, 169.
Remmer, H. (1970a), *Amer. J. Med.*, **49**, 617.
Remmer, H. (1970b), *Proc. Eur. Soc. Study Drug Toxicity*, **11**, 14.
Remmer, H. (1972), *Eur. J. Clin. Pharmacol.*, **5**, 116.
Remmer, H. and Merker, H. J. (1963), *Science*, **142**, 1657.
Remmer, H. and Merker, H. J. (1965), *Proc. Second Int. Pharmacol. Meet.*, **4**, 299, Pergamon Press, Oxford.
Remmer, H., Schoene, B. and Fleischmann, R. A. (1973), *Drug Metab. Disposition*, **1**, 224.
Reynolds, E. H. (1968), *Brain*, **91**, 197.
Reynolds, E. H. (1972), *Brit. Med. J.*, **2**, 656.
Reynolds, E. H., Preece, J., Chanarin, I. (1969), *Lancet*, **1**, 1264.
Reynolds, J. W. and Mirkin, B. L. (1973), *Clin. Pharmacol. Ther.*, **14**, 891.
Richens, A. and Rowe, D. J. F. (1970), *Brit. Med. J.*, **4**, 73.
Richens, A. and Waters, A. H. (1971), *Brit. J. Pharmacol.*, **41**, 414P.
Riegelman, S., Rowland, M. and Epstein, W. L. (1970), *J. Amer. Med. Ass.*, **213**, 426.
Roberts, R. J. and Plaa, G. L. (1967), *Biochem. Pharmacol.*, **16**, 827.
Robinson, D. S. and MacDonald, M. S. (1966), *J. Pharmacol. Exp. Ther.*, **153**, 250.
Robinson, J. and Roberts, M. (1969), *Food Cosmet. Toxicol.*, **7**, 501.
Rosalki, S. B., Tarlow, D. and Rau, D. (1971), *Lancet*, **2**, 376.
Rosenberg, I. H., Godwin, H. A., Streiff, R. R. and Castle, W. B. (1968), *Lancet*, **2**, 530.

Rowland, M. (1972), in Montagna, W., van Scott, E. J. and Stoughton, R. B. (ed.), *Pharmacology and the skin*, p. 235, Appleton–Century–Crofts, New York.
Rubin, E., Gang, H., Misra, P. S. and Lieber, C. S. (1970), *Amer. J. Med.*, **49**, 801.
Rubin, E. and Lieber, C. S. (1968), *Science*, **162**, 690.
Sandhoff, K., Andreae, U. and Jatzkewiz, H. (1968), *Life Sci.*, **5**, 283.
Schaefer, K., Flury, W. H., von Herrath, D., Kraft, D. and Schweingruber, R. (1972), *Schweiz. Med. Wschr.*, **102**, 785.
Schanker, L. S. (1964), *Adv. Drug. Res.*, **1**, 72.
Schlede, E., Kuntzman, R., Haber, S. and Conney, A. H. (1970), *Cancer Res.*, **30**, 2893.
Schmid, K., Cornu, F., Imhof, P. and Keberle, H. (1964), *Schweiz. Med. Wschr.*, **94**, 235.
Schneiderman, M. A. (1974), *Lancet*, **2**, 1085.
Schoene, B., Fleischmann, R. A., Remmer, H. and von Olderhausen, H. F. (1972), *Eur. J. Clin. Pharmacol.*, **4**, 65.
Sellers, E. M. and Koch-Weser, J. (1970), *New Engl. J. Med.*, **283**, 827.
Sellers, E. M., Lang, M., Koch-Weser, J., Le Blanc, E. and Kalant, H. (1972), *Clin. Pharmacol. Ther.*, **13**, 37.
Sereni, F., Perletti, L. and Marini, A. (1967), *Pediat.*, **40**, 446.
Sharp, H. L. and Mirkin, B. L. (1972), *J. Pediat.*, **81**, 116.
Sher, S. P. (1971), *Toxicol. Appl. Pharmacol.*, **18**, 780.
Sherlock S. (1972) in Orlandi, F. and Jezequel, A. M. (ed.), *Liver and drugs*, p. 193, Academic Press, London.
Sherwood, W. C., Martinez, J., Flegel, E. (1971), *Lancet*, **1**, 1075.
Shojania, A. M., Hornady, G. and Barnes, P. H. (1968), *Lancet*, **1**, 1376.
Sigell, L. T. and Flessa, H. C. (1970), *J. Amer. Med. Ass.*, **214**, 2035.
Silver, J., Neale, G. and Thompson, G. R. (1974), *Clin. Sci. Mol. Med.*, **46**, 433.
Sjöqvist, F. (1965), *Proc. Roy. Soc. Med.*, **58**, 967.
Sjöqvist, F. and von Bahr, C. (1973), *Drug Metab. Disposition*, **1**, 469.
Sjöqvist, F., Hammer, W., Ideström, C.-M., Lind, M., Tuck, D. and Asberg, M. (1968), *Proc. Eur. Soc. Study Drug Toxicity*, **9** 246.
Sladek, N. E. and Mannering, G. J. (1966), *Biochem. Biophys. Res. Commun.*, **24**, 668.
Sladek, N. E. and Mannering, G. J. (1969), *Mol. Pharmacol.*, **5**, 174.
Smith, S. E. and Rawlins, M. D. (1973), *Variability in human drug response*, Butterworth, London.
Smith, S. E. and Rawlins, M. D. (1974), *Eur. J. Clin. Pharmacol.*, **7**, 71.
Smith, S. E., Taylor, S. A., Brooks, R. V. and Rawlins, M. D. (1972), in *Abstracts 5th International Congress of Pharmacology*, p. 217.
Solomon, H. M. and Abrams, W. B. (1972), *Amer. Heart J.*, **83**, 277.
Sotaniemi, E. A., Isoaho, R., Huhti, E., Huikko, M. and Koivisto, O. (1972), *Ann. Allergy*, **30**, 254.
Sotaniemi, E. A., Kontturi, M. J. and Larmi, T. K. (1973), *Clin. Pharmacol. Ther.*, **14**, 413.
Sotaniemi, E. A., Medzihradsky, F. and Eliasson, G. (1974), *Clin. Pharmacol. Ther.*, **15**, 417.
Southren, A. L., Gordon, G. G., Tochimoto, S., Krikun, E., Krieger, D., Jacobson, M. and Kuntzman, R. (1969), *J. Clin. Endocrinol Metab.*, **29**, 251.
Southren, A. L., Tochimoto, S., Strom, L., Ratuschi, A., Ross, H. and Gordon, G. (1966), *J. Clin. Endocrinol. Metab.*, **26**, 268.
Spray, G. H. and Burns, D. G. (1972), *Brit. Med. J.*, **2**, 167.
Stamp, T. C. B., Round, J. M., Rowe, D. J. F. and Haddad, J. G. (1972), *Brit. Med. J.*, **4**, 9.

Steinfeld, J. L. (1971), *The health consequences of smoking. A report of the surgeon general: 1971*, p. 239, Department of Health, Education and Welfare, Publication no. (HSM) 71-7513.
Stenger, R. J. (1970), *Gastroenterology*, **58**, 554.
Stenger, R. J. and Johnson, E. A. (1972), *Gastroenterology*, **62**, 167.
Stocks, P. (1970), *Brit. J. Cancer*, **24**, 215.
Streiff, R. R. (1970), *J. Amer. Med. Ass.*, **214**, 105.
Swidler, G. (1971), *Handbook of drug interactions*, Wiley, London.
Syvälahti, E. K. G., Pihlajamäki, K. K., Iisalo, E. J. (1974), *Lancet*, **2**, 232.
Szczeklik, E., Orlowski, M. and Szewczuk, A. (1961), *Gastroenterology*, **41**, 353.
Tenhunen, R., Marver, H. S. and Schmid, R. (1969), *J. Biol. Chem.*, **244**, 6388.
Tephly, T. R. and Mannering, G. J. (1968), *Mol. Pharmacol.*, **4**, 10.
Thompson, R. P. H., Eddleston, A. L. W. F. and Williams, R. (1969a), *Lancet*, **1**, 21.
Thompson, R. P. H., Pilcher, C. W. T., Robinson, J., Stathers, G. M., MacLean, A. E. M. and Williams, R. (1969b), *Lancet*, **2**, 4.
Thorpe, E. and Walker, A. I. T. (1973), *Food Cosmet. Toxicol.*, **11**, 433.
Trolle, D. (1968), *Lancet*, **2**, 705.
Tschudy, D. P., Perlroth, M. G., Marver, H. S., Collins, A., Hunter, G. and Rechcigl, M. (1965), *Proc. Nat. Acad. Sci.*, **53**, 841.
Uehleke, H. (1969), *Proc. Eur. Soc. Study Drug Toxicity*, **10**, 94.
Valdes, O. S., Maurer, H. M., Shumway, C. N., Draper, D. A. and Hossaini, A. A. (1971), *J. Pediat.*, **79**, 1015.
Van Dam, F. E. and Gribnau-Overkamp, M. J. H. (1967), *Folia Med. Neerlandica*, **10**, 141.
Vas, C. J. and Parsonage, M. J. (1967), *Acta Neurol. Scand.*, **43**, 580.
Vesell, E. S. (ed.) (1971), *Ann. NY Acad. Sci.*, **179**.
Vesell, E. S. (1972a), *Fed. Proc.*, **31**, 1253.
Vesell, E. S. (1972b) in Orlandi, F. and Jezequel, A. M. (ed.), *Liver and drugs*, p. 1, Academic Press, London.
Vesell, E. S. and Page, J. G. (1969), *J. Clin. Invest.*, **48**, 2202.
Vesell, E. S., Page, J. G. and Passananti, G. T. (1971a), *Clin. Pharmacol. Ther.*, **12**, 192.
Vesell, E. S. and Passananti, G. T. (1973), *Drug Metab. Disposition*, **1**, 402.
Vesell, E. S., Passananti, G. T. and Greene, F. E. (1970), *New Engl. J. Med.*, **283**, 1484.
Vesell, E. S., Passananti, G. T., Greene, F. E. and Page, J. G. (1971b), *Ann. NY Acad. Sci.*, **179**, 752.
Vesell, E. S., Passananti, G. T. and Lee, C. H. (1971c), *Clin. Pharmacol. Ther.*, **12**, 785.
Vesell, E. S., Passananti, G. T., Viau, J. P., Epps, J. E. and DiCarlo, F. J. (1972), *Pharmacology*, **7**, 197.
Vessell, E. S. and Shively, C. A. (1974), *Science*, **184**, 466.
Virtanen, S. and Tala, E. (1974), *Clin. Pharmacol. Ther.*, **16**, 817.
von Wartburg, J. P. (1971), in Kissin, B. and Begleiter, H. (ed.), *The biology of alcoholism*, vol. 1, p. 63, Plenum Press, New York.
von Wartburg, J. P. and Rothlisberger, M. (1961), *Helv. Physiol. Acta*, **19**, 30.
Wagstaff, D. J. and Short, C. R. (1971), *Toxicol. Appl. Pharmacol.*, **19**, 54.
Walker, A. I. T., Stevenson, D. E., Robinson, J., Thorpe, E. and Roberts, M. (1969), *Toxicol. Appl. Pharmacol.*, **15**, 345.
Walker, A. I. T., Thorpe, E. and Stevenson, D. E. (1973), *Food Cosmet. Toxicol.*, **11**, 415.
Wattenberg, L. W. and Leong, J. L. (1971), in Brodie, B. B. and Gillette, J. R. (ed.), *Handbook of experimental pharmacology*, vol. 28, part 2, p. 422, Springer-Verlag, Berlin.

Waltman, R., Bonura, F., Nigrin, G. and Pipat, C. (1969), *Lancet*, **2**, 1265.
Watson, B. M. (1969), *Anaesthesia*, **24**, 230.
Watson, M., Gabica, J. and Benson, W. W. (1972), *Clin. Pharmacol. Ther.*, **13**, 186.
Weiner, I. M. (1971) in Brodie, B. B. and Gillette, J. R. (ed.), *Handbook of experimental pharmacology*, vol. 28, part 1, p. 328, Springer-Verlag, Berlin.
Welch, R. M., Harrison, Y. E. and Burns, J. J. (1967), *Toxicol. Appl. Pharmacol.*, **10**, 340.
Welch, R. M., Harrison, Y. E., Gommi, B. W., Poppers, P. J., Finster, M. and Conney, A. H. (1969), *Clin. Pharmacol. Ther.*, **10**, 100.
Welch, R. M., Levin, W., Kuntzman, R., Jacobson, M. and Conney, A. H. (1971), *Toxicol. Appl. Pharmacol.*, **19**, 234.
Weiss, C. F., Glazko, A. J. and Weston, J. K. (1960), *New Engl. J. Med.*, **262**, 787.
Welling, P. G., Craig, W. A., Amidon, G. L. and Kunin, C. M. (1974), *Clin. Pharmacol. Ther.*, **15**, 344.
Werk, jr. E. E., MacGee, J. and Sholiton, L. J. (1964), *J. Clin. Invest.*, **43**, 1824.
Werk, E. E., Sholiton, L. J. and Olinger, C. P. (1966), *Second International Congress on Hormonal Steroids, Milan*, in *Excerpta Medica Inter. Cong. Series*, No. 111, p. 301.
Werk, jr. E. E., Thrasher, K., Sholiton, L. J., Olinger, C. and Choi, Y. (1971), *Clin. Pharmacol. Ther.*, **12**, 698.
Whelton, M. J., Krustev, L. P. and Billing, B. H. (1968), *Amer. J. Med.*, **45**, 160.
White, T. A. and Price-Evans, D. A. (1968), *Clin. Pharmacol. Ther.*, **9**, 80.
Whitfield, J. B., Moss, D. W., Neale, G., Orme, M. and Breckenridge, A. (1973), *Brit. Med. J.*, **1**, 316.
Whittaker, J. A. and Price-Evans, D. A. (1970), *Brit. Med. J.*, **4**, 323.
With, T. K. (1968), *Bile pigments*, Academic Press, New York.
Wright, J. A. (1965), *Epilepsia*, **6**, 67.
Wright, N. and Prescott, L. F. (1973), *Scot. Med. J.*, **18**, 56.
Yaffee, S. J. and Juchau, M. R. (1974), *Ann. Rev. Pharmacol.*, **14**, 219.
Yaffee, S. J., Levy, G., Matsuzawa, T. and Baliah, T. (1966), *New Engl. J. Med.*, **275**, 1461.
Yeung, C. Y. and Field, C. E. (1969), *Lancet*, **2**, 135.

CHAPTER 5

Drug–serum protein interactions and their biological significance

J. W. Bridges and A. G. E. Wilson

INTRODUCTION

The interaction between a drug and protein molecules often profoundly influences its biological activity, for not only is such an association necessary for 'drug-receptor site' interactions and metabolism to take place, but it may also play a primary role in governing the drug's absorption, distribution and excretion, characteristics. A thorough understanding of the nature and magnitude of drug–protein binding is thus clearly fundamental to an accurate prediction of the therapeutic and toxic effect of drugs. In most instances the barrier to attaining success in this quest has been the inability to identify or isolate the proteins involved. However, such information has been, and will continue to be, gained from a detailed study of drug interactions with model or readily isolable protein.

Serum albumin and other plasma proteins have been particularly investigated not only as model proteins, but also because they often figure prominently in determining the onset, duration and intensity of drug action. The argument regarding the significance of the role of the protein here is based on the assumption that a drug cannot normally express its biological activity when bound to plasma proteins unless it acts by displacing pharmacologically active substances from their binding sites (see pages 232–234).

The purpose of this review is to examine our present state of knowledge of the nature and significance of drug–plasma proteins and especially drug–albumin binding. Other reviews on various aspects of this subject have been penned by Goldstein (1949), Scatchard (1949), Brodie and Hogben (1957), Thorp (1964), Brodie (1965), Desgrez and de Traverse (1966), Goldstein *et al* (1968), Meyer and Guttman (1968), Settle *et al* (1971), Cohen (1971), Davison (1971), Thorp (1972), Westphal and Knoefel (1972), and Anton and Solomon (1973).

Drugs, other xenobiotics and endogenous compounds, may be transported in the blood stream in simple solution, as a suspension or bound to plasma proteins or blood cells. Potentially, the interaction of a drug with plasma proteins may limit its availability to the receptor sites and to the drug metabolism and excretory systems (see figure 1). These interactions are

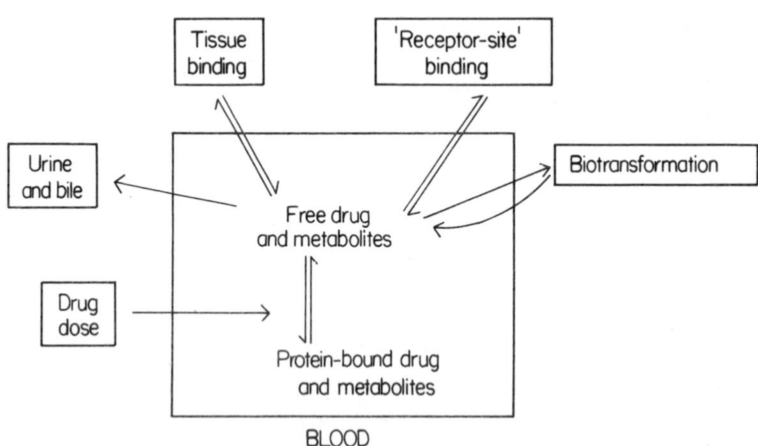

Figure 1 Influence of protein binding on drug distribution

probably completely reversible and relatively nonspecific in the majority of cases. It is likely therefore that for weakly bound drugs, plasma-protein binding is of little direct therapeutic significance, although for strongly bound drugs it may exert a strong influence over a drug's potential bioavailability and *in vivo* activity profile. It is tacitly assumed in the measurement and interpretation of drug–plasma protein binding that the process is invariably completely and rapidly reversible. Although this may be true, only rarely have studies been carried out to attempt to substantiate this basic concept. Experiments proving that, by dialysis or ultrafiltration, considerable quantities of drug can be dissociated from proteins, do not in themselves demonstrate that irreversible binding does not occur; they simply argue against it being the sole form of binding. Obviously this is an important area for further investigation because covalent binding of drugs to plasma proteins, in addition to modifying the binding characteristics of other drugs and endogenous compounds such as fatty acids (which normally associate with these proteins), could give rise to antigenic molecules which might produce hypersensitivity reactions.

THEORETICAL ASPECTS OF DRUG–PROTEIN BINDING

It is unfortunately common practice to express the results of drug-binding studies simply as the percentage of drug bound to the protein. The use of this value alone is, at best, misleading unless the concentrations of drug and protein involved are also given.

In discussing the relevance of drug–protein interactions, both the affinity or strength of binding (usually expressed as an apparent association constant k) and the capacity of the protein sites (n) should be considered. For completely reversible associations the interaction of a drug (D) with the unoccupied binding sites of a protein (P) may be considered to obey the law of mass action (equation 1).

$$\mathrm{D_f} + \mathrm{P} \underset{k_2}{\overset{k_1}{\rightleftharpoons}} \mathrm{DP}$$

where DP is the protein–drug complex and k_1 and k_2 are the rate constants of the forward and reverse reactions.

At equilibrium therefore

$$\frac{[\mathrm{D_f}][\mathrm{P}]}{[\mathrm{DP}]} = \frac{k_2}{k_1} = K \qquad (1)$$

where D_f is the molar concentration of unbound drug, P is the molar concentration of protein, DP the molar concentration of the drug–protein complex and K is the equilibrium or dissociation constant. The reciprocal of this latter term (k), the association constant, is a measure of the affinity of the drug for the protein.

This is obviously the simplest situation in which a homogenous binding protein with a single binding site for the drug is involved. In cases where several binding sites or proteins are concerned, a succession of such equilibria are required to describe the overall interaction (Thorp, 1964). Alternatively, if the general case is considered of the binding of a protein which contains n independent binding sites, each exhibiting a similar affinity k for the drug, then $n[\mathrm{P}]$ will be the total concentration of binding sites for the drug

$$\therefore \quad n[\mathrm{P}] = [\mathrm{DP}] + [\mathrm{P_f}]$$

$$\text{i.e.} \quad [\mathrm{P_f}] = n[\mathrm{P}] - [\mathrm{DP}] \tag{2}$$

Substitution of equation (2) into (1) yields:

$$\frac{(n[\mathrm{P}] - [\mathrm{DP}])[\mathrm{D_f}]}{[\mathrm{DP}]} = \frac{1}{k}$$

which by rearrangement gives:

$$n[\mathrm{P}][\mathrm{D_f}] = [\mathrm{DP}]\left(\frac{1}{k} + [\mathrm{D_f}]\right) \tag{3}$$

Now, if r = moles of drug bound per mole of protein

$$r = \frac{[\mathrm{DP}]}{[\mathrm{P}]}$$

Rearrangement of equation (3) gives:

$$r = \frac{nk[\mathrm{D_f}]}{1 + k[\mathrm{D_f}]} \tag{4}$$

It is presupposed here that all the binding sites are identical. If there are m classes of sites, all of which are independent but not equivalent, then for each class i having n_i sites with an apparent association constant k_i, equation (4) can be extended in the form:

$$r = \Sigma_{i=1}^{m} \frac{n_i k_i \mathrm{D_f}}{1 + k_i \mathrm{D_f}} \tag{5}$$

or

$$r = \frac{n_1 k_1 \mathrm{D_f}}{1 + k_1 \mathrm{D_f}} + \frac{n_2 k_2 \mathrm{D_f}}{1 + k_2 \mathrm{D_f}} \cdots\cdots + \frac{n_i k_i \mathrm{D_f}}{1 + k_i \mathrm{D_f}} \tag{6}$$

It is assumed in this equation that the binding of a drug molecule at one site does not influence the binding at another site. In practice this assumption is probably not entirely valid (see page 218). A modification of binding may potentially arise through either an induced conformational change in the protein or, in the case of ionized drugs, from a resultant overall change in the electrostatic environment of the protein; this may increase the difficulty of incorporating a similar ion, or competition for binding sites by constituents of the buffer solution. Ionic contributions can be corrected for (Scatchard *et al*, 1950) although this is seldom accomplished. Since it is also common practice to use concentration rather than activity coefficient terms to calculate the association constants for ionized molecules, most determinations of binding strength are best described as 'apparent association constants'.

Plotting of Data

Even in the age of the computer which largely pre-empts the need to plot results graphically, the visual presentation of data in this form has not lost its appeal. A number of different schemes are employed. The major difficulty with each is to give appropriate weighting to the individual points and to accurately determine multiple and interacting binding-site contributions.

The earliest approach to the plotting of protein-binding data was the adsorption-isotherm method of Freundlich (1907) and Langmuir (1917) where r is plotted against $[D_f]$. The approach is unsatisfactory since curved plots result and large changes in binding at high drug: protein ratios only result in a small alteration in curvature. A better approach is to use a reciprocal plot based on equation 3 in which either r^{-1} is plotted against $[D_f]^{-1}$, figure 2a (Klotz, 1946) or alternatively $r/[D_f]$ is plotted against r, figure 2b (Scatchard, 1949). In either the Klotz or Scatchard plots, deviations from linearity are taken to indicate the involvement of more than one type or class of binding site or the modification of one protein-binding site by drug interaction at the second site. The Klotz plot is generally less widely used than the Scatchard because it tends to excessively underemphasize the results obtained at low drug: protein ratios, frequently the most relevant *in vivo* (Kreiglstein, 1969; Meyer and Guttman, 1968). There is also an intrinsic danger in using a Klotz plot because it is analogous to the Lineweaver–Burk plot commonly used in enzyme kinetic studies and may be interpreted in a similar manner. In drug investigations, where a number of possible interacting binding sites may be

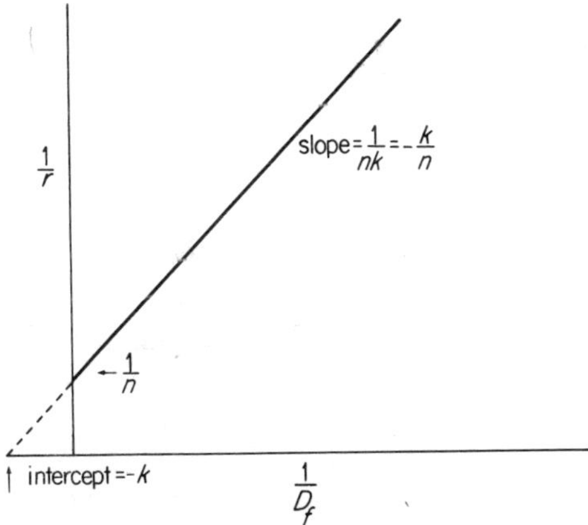

Figure 2a Klotz plot (for single class of binding site)

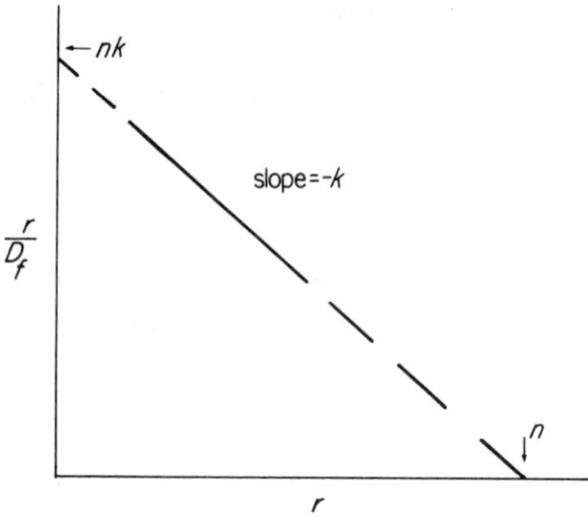

Figure 2b Scatchard plot (for single class of binding site)

involved (as opposed to substrate metabolism where a single site is normally considered), concepts such as competitive, noncompetitive and uncompetitive drug association must be used with great caution. Furthermore, whereas the affinity constant, k, or k^{-1} (determined from drug–albumin studies) is of direct physical significance, the interpretation of the Michaelis–Menten constant (K_m) for enzyme–substrate reactions depends on the prior establishment of the nature of the reaction mechanism.

A linear Scatchard plot will only be obtained if a single class of binding sites is involved, each site being totally independent of the others. Under these circumstances, extrapolation will permit the estimation of nk. Scatchard plots are frequently nonlinear. For binding involving either different classes of sites or interacting sites, no simple relationship exists between the slope and k value (Klotz and Hunston, 1971).

Other representations less frequently employed have included: plots of the degree of binding vs the unbound-drug concentration (Bjerrum, 1941), and logarithm of the saturation fraction vs the logarithm of the unbound-drug concentration (Thompson and Klotz, 1971). Klotz (1973) has stated that logarithmic or double logarithmic plots of binding data are far more reliable representations for determining whether one is approaching saturation of binding sites. A number of discussions of graphical methods have appeared (Goldstein, 1949; Edsall and Wyman, 1958; Rosenburg and Klotz, 1960; Sandberg *et al*, 1966; Goldstein *et al*, 1968; Meyer and Guttman, 1968; Baulieu and Raynaud, 1970; Karush, 1950a, b; Steinhardt and Reynolds, 1969; Deranleau, 1969; Davison, 1971; Gutfreund, 1972; Weder *et al*, 1974; Fletcher *et al*, 1970).

Several manual methods of curve fitting have been described (Hart, 1965; Rosenthal, 1967; Weder and Bickel, 1970; Feldman, 1972; Halfman and Nishida, 1972). However, the complexity and tediousness of such procedures has increasingly led to the development of computerized curve-fitting procedures based on linear regression analysis (Fletcher and Spector, 1968;

Crothers, 1968; Raz and Goodman, 1969; Rodbard *et al*, 1969; Feldman, 1972; Fletcher *et al*, 1973). Despite this sophistication, large differences in binding affinities are generally required in order to properly characterize individual binding sites. Computer analysis should be used in preference to manual methods wherever possible for use of a computer largely pre-empts arguments about which is the best plot, provided suitable weighting can be applied. However, it should be remembered that many computer methods assume a gaussian distribution of errors, which is not valid where an interdependent method of calculating r, n and k values is used.

To permit ready comparison of results it is desirable that standardization of data evaluation by the Scatchard plot is achieved. For this purpose, quoted n and k values should be qualified by the relevant r values over which the determinations are made and the experimental variance of these parameters, and the temperatures and pH values involved should be presented (Agren *et al*, 1970; Cohen, 1971). The calculation of the thermodynamic parameters—enthalpy and entropy—could perhaps eradicate some of these problems.

For investigations of binding to partially purified proteins where the amount, or molecular weight, of the protein involved in the binding may be unknown, neither the Scatchard nor the Klotz plots can be employed. In such instances a plot of $[D_b]/[D_f]$ against $[D_b]$, based on the equation:

$$\frac{[D_b]}{[D_f]} = nk[P_t] - k[D_b] \qquad (7)$$

where $[D_b]$ is the concentration of bound drug, and $[P_t]$ is the total molar concentration of protein, allows an estimation of $nk[P_t]$, $n[P_t]$ and k, from the intercepts and slope, without knowledge of the protein concentration (Sandberg *et al*, 1966; Rosenthal, 1967). In common with the Scatchard and Klotz graphical methods, curvature of the plot results when more than one species of binding protein is present or where there is more than one class of binding site on the protein.

Obviously, absolute n and k values can only be produced for pure homogenous proteins. Even low concentrations of contaminating ions may modify a drug's protein-binding characteristic. In blood there are many competing materials for binding to a single protein. Furthermore, since blood contains a complex protein mixture, n and k values can be considered to give only an overall measure of the affinity and capacity of binding.

For thorough estimation of the binding parameters it is essential that measurements are made over a wide drug-concentration range. Unfortunately, because of the insensitivity of many drug analyses at low concentrations, and drug-solubility problems at high concentrations, this is seldom accomplished. If studies at low concentrations are neglected, high-affinity site binding may be missed. Conversely, it is necessary to make measurements at high drug concentrations in order to ascertain the presence of low affinity (secondary) sites. Studies over a wide concentration range may also

Table 1a Principal methods of studying drug–protein binding

Technique	Advantages	Disadvantages	Selected references
Equilibrium dialysis	Thermodynamically sound, accurate reproducible quantitative data. Most used technique, therefore comparison easy.	Quantitative information only, which is subject to errors from binding to membrane and Donnan inequalities. Nonphysiological and prolonged equilibration time may cause bacterial contamination and protein denaturation. Equilibrium disturbed by dilution.	Klotz (1953) Rosenburg and Klotz (1960)
Dynamic dialysis	Rapid	Essentially same disadvantages as equilibrium dialysis. New method, therefore validity not fully established.	Stein (1965) Meyer and Guttman (1970a)
In vivo dialysis	Probably the most physiological method available.	Assumes unbound drug in serum ≡ peritoneal fluid ≡ concn in peritoneal dialysis sac. New method largely untested. Binding to membrane and quantitative data only.	McQueen (1968, 1969) Wilson, *et al* (1974)
Diafiltration	No protein dilution or concentration effects. More rapid than equilibrium dialysis.	New method, therefore validity not established. Membrane binding and Donnan inequalities. Calculations lengthy and involved.	Blatt *et al* (1968) Crawford *et al* (1972)
Ultrafiltration	Thermodynamically sound and rapid. Suggested to closely approximate *in vivo* situation. Specialized apparatus ideally suited for plasma samples. Up to 40% of fluid can be filtered without upset of equilibrium.	Quantitative data only. Binding to membrane and Donnan inequalities. Equilibrium disturbed by protein concentration.	Toribara *et al* (1957) Bennet and Kirby (1965)
Ultracentrifugation	No membrane binding or Donnan inequalities.	Theoretical basis not so well established as for dialysis or ultrafiltration. Prolonged experimental time. Quantitation more difficult. Cannot use protein mixtures.	Steinberg and Schachman (1966) Steinhardt and Reynolds (1969)
Gel chromatography	Separation of several binding proteins possible. Thermodynamically sound.	Adsorption to gel may disturb equilibrium; can largely be circumvented by frontal analysis and Hummel-Dreyer methods. Although these methods require large samples. Dilution occurs.	Scholtan (1964) Cooper and Wood, (1968) Wood and Cooper, (1970)

Electrophoresis	Qualitative data. Can separate multi-protein mixtures and only small samples required. Can be combined with autoradiography and immunoelectrophoresis.	Quantification difficult. Non-physiological. Interpretation can be difficult and may be complicated by binding to support medium.	Hummel and Dreyer (1962) Bickel and Bovet (1962) Clausen (1966) O'Reilly and Kowitz (1967)
Ultraviolet and visible spectrophotometry	Sensitive technique can monitor absorption changes in either drug or protein consequent upon binding. Can detect conformational changes and qualitative information on chromophore's binding site. Homogenous system, only microquantities of material required.	Cannot be used if interaction causes no spectral change. Non-physiological May need to compensate for compound's absorbance.	Klotz (1946) Herskovits (1967) Chignell (1971) Steinhardt and Reynolds (1969)
Fluorescence spectrophotometry	Sensitive technique. Can monitor fluoroescence changes in both drug and/or protein consequent upon binding. Can provide both qualitative and quantitative information, although quantification can involve lengthy calculation. Homogenous system and only microquantities of material required.	Cannot be used if interaction causes no spectral change. Non-physiological. 'Inner-filter' effects may occur and make interpretation difficult. Change not always directly related to alteration in the association or dissociation of protein drug complex.	Teale (1960) Attalah and Lata (1968) Radda (1971) Chignell (1972)
Optical rotatory dispersion and circular dichroism	Sensitive technique. Can serve as a probe for binding sites and provide both qualitative and quantitative data, although quantitation not simple.	Interaction must generate cotton effect. Non-physiological. Equipment expensive. Interpretation difficult. Change not always directly related to alteration in the association or dissociation of protein–drug complex	Chignell and Chignell (1972) Perrin and Hart (1970) Jirgensons (1962)
Nuclear magnetic resonance	Sensitive to changes in molecular geometry.	Interpretation may be difficult. Equipment expensive. Non-physiological.	Jardetzky and Wade-Jardetzky (1965) Steinhardt and Reynolds (1969) Burgen and Metcalfe (1970) Hollis (1972) Sykes and Hull (1973)

be of value in ascertaining whether irreversible binding is occurring. Investigations of the extent of binding against time are infrequently attempted. It is self-evident that two drugs could have identical high-affinity constants, but very different k_1 and k_2 values and hence very different equilibration times with plasma and tissue proteins. If this were the case the two drugs could well display dissimilar distribution and excretion profiles. Despite its potential practical importance in evaluating the significance of particular drug–protein interactions, only in a few instances has an attempt been made to directly measure the rate constants k_1 and k_2 (Thorp, 1964). The widely accepted assumption that these constants are in the millisecond to microsecond region may not always be justified. Furthermore, unless the case of thyroxine is unique (Robbins *et al*, 1965), it is likely that in some instances dissociation may be better described in terms of an initial fast phase followed by a slower secondary phase.

METHODS OF STUDYING PROTEIN BINDING

It is axiomatic that the results obtained and the validity of the interpretation that can be placed on them are only as good as the experimental method employed. Ideally, a technique for studying drug–protein binding should not only meet the obvious requirements of accuracy, precision, simplicity, inexpensiveness, ease of automation and application to a broad range of compounds, but also fulfil the following criteria:

(i) It must not upset the equilibrium between free and bound drug.
(ii) It should be valid over a wide range of drug and protein concentrations.
(iii) It should enable reliable control over pH, ionic concentration and temperature, while minimizing Donnan effects.
(iv) It must avoid denaturation or extraneous contamination of the protein, and also adsorption onto the apparatus walls, membranes and other components.
(v) It should be capable of detecting both reversible and irreversible binding, and fast and slow phase associations and dissociations of drug and protein.
(vi) It should not introduce interfering agents, such as organic solvents.
(vii) The method should allow extrapolation to the *in vivo* situation.
(viii) The protein should be homogeneous (see page 215).

None of the currently available techniques can be claimed to encompass all these demands. It is therefore important that the limitations of an individual method should be fully appraised before its selection for a particular purpose (see Table 1a and b). Thus, in studying the binding of a large concentration range of a highly lipophilic drug it is not possible to fulfil the criteria of accurate concentration control unless organic solvents or other extraneous agents (e.g. detergent) are used. In these instances it is obviously most important to carefully appraise the contribution of the drug solubilizing system to the observed protein binding.

A diverse range of methods have been used to investigate drug–protein interactions. It is not within the scope of this review to give a detailed evaluation of each one, but rather to consider the most widely employed methods. Chignell (1972) has reviewed a number of these techniques. Further information can be derived from the references given in Tables 1a and 1b. All the available methods utilize one of four basic principles (Goldstein, 1949):

(i) The concentration of free drug or its thermodynamic activity may be diminished in the presence of a binding protein.

(ii) The drug may show measurable changes in its properties other than

Table 1b Less commonly used methods for studying drug–protein interactions

Method	Reference
Biological action	Goldstein (1949)
Diffusion	Goldstein (1949)
Physical properties, e.g. osmotic pressure, vapour pressure, surface tension, viscosity, electrophoretic mobility, sedimentation of protein	Goldstein (1949)
Solubility of small molecules	Goldstein (1949) Westphal (1961)
Adsorption of small molecule	Goldstein (1949) Heyns *et al* (1967)
Precipitation	Goldstein (1949) Priestly and O'Reilly (1966)
Stabilization a) of small molecules b) of protein	 a) Goldstein (1949) b) Colombo *et al* (1968)
Equilibrium partition of small molecules	Goodman (1958) Spector *et al* (1969)
Autoradiography	Meyer and Guttman (1968)
Polarography	Steinhardt and Reynolds (1969)
Conductivity and e.m.f. methods	Goldstein (1949) Steinhardt and Reynolds (1969)
Pulse radiolysis	Phillips *et al* (1970)
ΔpH method	Scatchard and Black (1949) Steinhardt and Reynolds (1969)
Heatburst microcalorimetry	O'Reilly *et al* (1969) Reynolds *et al* (1973)
Refractive index	Steinhardt and Reynolds (1969)
Dielectric increment and dispersion	Steinhardt and Reynolds (1969)
X-ray diffraction	Steinhardt and Reynolds (1969)
Saturation analysis	Zettner (1973)
Isoelectric focussing	van Baelen and de Moor (1972)

those attributable to reduction in thermodynamic activity, e.g. biological activity.

(iii) Measurable alteration in the protein's properties may occur on drug binding.

(iv) The drug's interaction may be studied by its ability to displace a 'probe compound' from protein-binding site(s).

Equilibrium Dialysis, Ultrafiltration and Gel-Chromatography Methods

The most extensively used techniques at present are those of equilibrium dialysis, ultrafiltration and gel filtration, although spectroscopic methods are increasingly achieving popularity. The main value of the former methods lies in their direct quantitative application to drug–protein interaction measurements since their use in deriving structural information regarding the nature of the interaction is in general rather limited. Despite the theoretical pros and cons for individual methods (Goldstein, 1949; Edsall and Wyman, 1958; Rosenburg and Klotz, 1960; Scholtan, 1964; Steinhardt and Reynolds, 1969; Chignell, 1971), few practical comparisons of these methods have been attempted and where reports of such studies have been published they are frequently in apparent disagreement. For example, McArthur and Smith (1969) found a higher percentage binding of salicylate to bovine-serum albumin (BSA) using equilibrium dialysis compared with ultrafiltration or frontal-analysis gel chromatography, whereas in apparently similar experiments Kereszites-Nagy *et al* (1972) described good agreement between equilibrium dialysis and frontal-analysis gel-chromatography methods although they detected a greater variability in results obtained using equilibrium dialysis. Wilson and Bridges (unpublished data) have demonstrated close similarity between these three methods in the study of BSA binding of sodium salicylate (see figure 3). The n and k values derived by the three methods were also shown by these workers to be in good agreement for the binding of a number of other drugs displaying a range of physicochemical properties, including clofibrate (*Atromid-S*), sulphamethoxazole (*Gantanol*), sulphanilamide, sulphadimethoxine (*Madribon*), sulphaphenazole (*Orisulf*) and sulphormethoxine (*Fanasil*). In contrast, zonal and batch methods of gel chromatography were found to be unsuitable for ascertaining the protein-association characteristics of clofibrate, sulphadimethoxine and sulphormethoxine due to excessive adsorption of the drug onto the *Sephadex* gel. For highly lipophilic drugs no method was really satisfactory.

Although ultrafiltration, equilibrium dialysis and frontal gel chromatography frequently appear to produce comparable results, certain experimental considerations may predispose towards the selection of a particular method. For example, where studies involving plasma samples, using O_2–CO_2 gas mixture to control pH rather than a foreign buffer, are desired ultrafiltration using Toribara tubes (Toribara *et al*, 1957) is the preferred technique. Binding to the dialysis sac may for some compounds constitute a

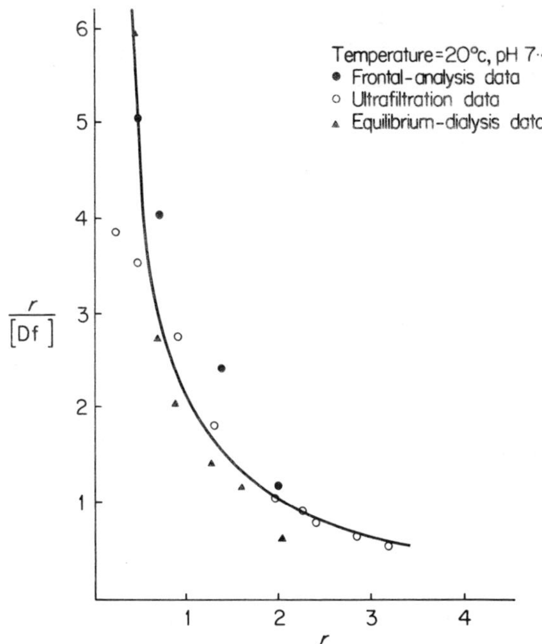

Figure 3 Comparison of Scatchard plots of data for the binding of sodium salicylate to bovine serum albumin by three techniques

major obstacle to the use of equilibrium dialysis or ultrafiltration although boiling the bag with deionized water followed by a thorough washing, with a solvent such as methanol or with acid, is often successful in overcoming this problem. If membrane binding is extensive either gel chromatography (provided adsorption onto the gel does not occur) or an organic-solvent partition method (Robertson and Madsen, 1974) may be more suitable. It is important to check that denaturation of the protein or chemical modification of the drug has not occurred in experiments involving a long time course.

For investigating binding of drugs to high molecular-weight proteins such as tissue proteins or to cells, membrane or solvent interfaces may be unnecessary. Often the drug can simply be added to a suspension of the protein followed by separation of the phases by differential centrifugation, although it should be realized that a firm 'pelleting' of protein may upset the equilibrium. Assessment of the degree of bag binding, adsorption onto the apparatus walls or gel adsorption, must always be made if confidence is to be placed on the results obtained. Furthermore, in equilibrium dialysis it is often necessary to correct for, or avoid contributions due to, Donnan effects. Unfortunately such elementary precautions are frequently neglected.

More recent developments of potential value include micro- and nonequilibrium-dialysis techniques which require much shorter experimental times than the conventional methods (Stein, 1965; Agren and Elofsson, 1967; Meyer and Guttman, 1970a, b; Colowick and Womack, 1969). Non-equilibrium methods usually incorporate an automatic flow-through system, controlled so that the rate at which unbound drug enters the buffer-containing compartment is proportional to the concentration of free drug in the protein-containing compartment. The use of continuous ultrafiltration methods involving *Diaflo* membranes (Amicon, Lexington, Mass., U.S.A.) also appears to be a promising approach (Blatt *et al*, 1968; Ryan and Hanna, 1971; Danon and Sapira, 1972; Crawford *et al*, 1972; Thompson, 1973). Particular advantages are the large range of concentration points which can be determined in one experiment and the fact that no concentration of protein occurs. However, denaturation may constitute a problem.

Spectroscopic Methods

Spectroscopic methods including circular dichroism, nuclear magnetic resonance, electron-spin resonance, ultra-violet and visible spectroscopy and fluorimetry are proving of increasing value in protein-binding studies, particularly for investigations on the nature of the binding sites. Since membranes and gels are not involved and measurements can frequently be made with rapidity, adsorption problems and worries concerning the disturbance of equilibrium conditions are often minimized (Jardetzky and Wade-Jardetzky, 1965; Steinhardt and Reynolds, 1969; Chignell, 1971, 1972; Fischer, 1971; Radda, 1971; Brand and Gohlke, 1972). On the other hand, spectroscopic methods are generally of rather limited application, frequently lacking in the required sensitivity (and hence unsuited to studies over a wide concentration range), commonly difficult to interpret and often not directly applicable to quantitative measurements. It is evident that such methods may be used to their best advantage in conjunction with conventional methods such as ultrafiltration, dialysis and gel chromatography. Spectroscopic methods can be employed either to examine changes in a drug's properties on binding or to examine modifications in the characteristics of the protein. Studies of drug-induced changes in the tryptophan environment of proteins have been fruitful in establishing the involvement of tryptophan in drug binding (see page 218).

An especially promising extension of the application of spectroscopic techniques has been their use in the estimation of a drug's protein binding through its ability to displace model 'probe' molecules from protein-binding sites. Displacement methods employing fluorescence spectroscopy have gained particular acceptance. Unlike dialysis and ultrafiltration approaches, probe analysis can give information on specific-site interactions. The major limitations to its extensive use has been the lack of a suitable range of probes. The most commonly used fluorescence probe is 1-anilino-8-naphthalene sulphonate (ANS). Recently the introduction of a number of new probes of biological relevance, including tetracycline (Popov *et al*, 1971 and 1972), kynurenine (Churchich, 1972), bilirubin (Krasner, 1973), dansyl amino acids (Wade, 1976) and warfarin (Chignell, 1970a, b; Wilson and Bridges, unpublished data) and iprindole (Wilson and Bridges, unpublished data) has markedly extended the scope of the displacement approach (see also page 234). Fluorescence probes can frequently be used over a wide concentration range and the method has particular virtue in that it allows the assessment of the protein-binding properties of even those drugs which are intrinsically difficult to assay (provided they will displace a suitable probe). Interpretation of the results must, however, be treated with caution in the absence of supporting data from more conventional methods, for a drug could cause a change in a spectroscopic probe's characteristics via a modification of the protein conformation rather than by its direct displacement from a specific-binding site. Alternatively a probe might be shifted from one binding site to another by addition of a drug without any obvious modification in the probe's spectroscopic properties becoming apparent.

In vivo Measurements of Binding

Although many studies have been made of drug binding on adding the drug *in vitro* to human-serum albumin, serum, plasma or blood, direct *in vivo* measurements of the amount of drug bound in blood samples from patients receiving a drug have seldom been carried out. The major reason for the lack of direct *in vivo* determinations has been the difficulty involved in specifically analysing very low concentrations of free drug, and the problem of competing metabolites. As a consequence, the validity of extrapolating from an *in vitro* to the *in vivo* situation has only recently been checked. *In vivo* measurements could prove of particular value in examining the reasons for the poor correlation frequently observed between drug-blood levels and therapeutic efficacy since a major potential contributor to this situation is a variation in protein bound drug but not total drug in the blood. The misconception appears in much published work on protein binding that measurements on human-serum albumin, plasma, serum and blood, are synonymous. Even when serum albumin is found to be the major binding component for a particular drug in blood, the higher solvation properties of blood compared with a simple buffer solution, and the presence in blood of many endogenous and exogenous compounds which may compete for protein-binding sites renders it unlikely that serum albumin and blood ever present identical binding conditions (see pages 211–213).

A possible means of making a limited evaluation of the validity of an extrapolation from the *in vitro* to the *in vivo* situation in animals has been described by McQueen (1968). The technique involves determining the drug concentration in a dialysis sac after it has been implanted for 24 h in the peritoneal cavity of a rat which has attained a steady-state plasma level of the drug. The assumption must be made that the drug partitions freely between tissue compartments and hence free-drug levels in the peritoneum are a direct reflection of those in the plasma. It is also obviously unsuited to compounds which may bind to the sac. Despite these potential limitations McQueen has observed that for sulphormethoxine (with a long half-life of ~40 h in which approximately steady-state conditions are readily attainable) good agreement with *in vitro* dialysis is obtained. Wilson *et al* (1974) have shown that for sodium salicylate which has a short half-life in the rat (~7 h) and hence probably does not reach a steady-state level, good agreement can also be achieved between equilibrium dialysis, ultrafiltration or frontal gel chromatography. This *in vivo* method has also been employed to demonstrate an increase in unbound tryptophan due to salicylate displacement *in vivo* (Wilson, 1974). In assessing the practical significance of an observed *in vitro* competitive binding situation, this kind of *in vivo* approach should have particular application. Further studies are required to establish whether the technique is generally suitable for drugs of relatively short half-life whose serum concentrations are rapidly changing. The successful extension of this type of *in vivo* approach also obviously necessitates more precise information regarding the relative rates of change of the drug concentration in the serum and peritoneal fluid compared with that of the dialysis-sac contents. The potential of the method could probably be enhanced, particularly for pharmacokinetic and pharmacodynamic studies, if either regular sampling or continual recirculation of the dialysis-sac contents employing flow-through monitoring devices, were perfected. The suggestion (Keen, 1971) that the concentration of drug in the dialysis sac does not represent that in the tissue fluid, because the effective diameter of the dialysis membrane pores is very much less than that of the capillary pores, must be considered. Experiments employing membranes with larger pore size are required to examine the correctness of this argument. The development of a technique recently described (Aziz and Dennhardt, 1973) of a continuous *in vivo* ultrafiltration of circulating blood could also prove to be a significant advance.

BLOOD PROTEINS

Before giving attention to the clinical nature of drug-plasma protein interactions it is necessary to first consider the qualitative and quantitative nature of the proteins involved. The plasma contains large quantities of protein which are able to bind to a considerable number and variety of ions and small molecules (figure 4). This is perhaps not surprising for Bennhold (1966) has calculated that five litres of blood contain plasma proteins having a minimum surface area of 336,700 km^2. Many detailed treatises on the composition, structure and function, of the plasma proteins have appeared (Schultze and Heremans, 1966; Putnam, 1960; Neurath, 1965; Turner and Hulme, 1971; Marks, 1972; Dettlebach and Ritzmann, 1968; Haaf, 1969; Scanu, 1972; Jonas, 1972; Mateau *et al*, 1972; Scanu and Wisdom, 1972) and only limited aspects of this topic therefore will be covered in this review.

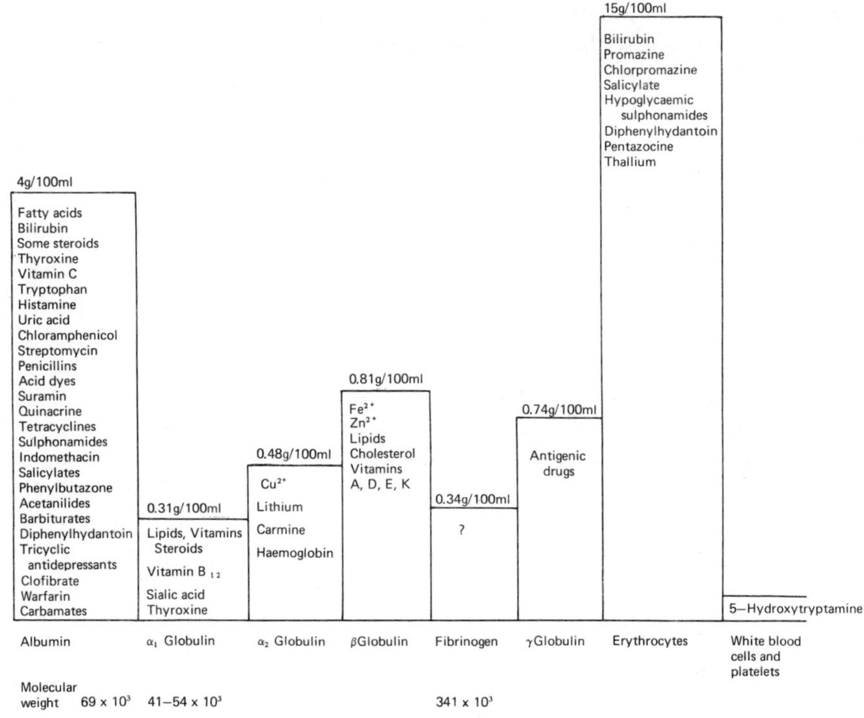

Figure 4 Concentrations and binding roles of major blood proteins

The red blood cells, despite their high protein concentration relative to that of the plasma proteins, appear in general not to be significantly involved in drug binding (see figure 4 and page 212). In part at least this may be due to the relatively very much smaller surface area of cellularly contained proteins compared with those in solution.

Albumin

Albumin, which is the principal plasma protein ($\simeq$ 50% of the total) makes the predominant contributions to the plasma-protein binding of most drugs, as well as interacting with many endogenous materials such as fatty acids and bilirubin (Goldstein *et al*, 1968). Indeed, with the possible exception of cytochrome P-450, albumin is probably unique in its capacity for binding with chemicals of diverse chemical and physical properties. It has been suggested that one of its major functions may be the transport of endogenous materials in the blood and for some compounds possibly across cell membranes (Bennhold, 1966). Since both drugs and endogenous materials when bound to proteins are normally considered to be biologically inactive, protein binding may also be regarded both as a means of suppressing the potential biological activity of a wide variety of compounds and as a reservoir of these materials. The albumin molecule consists of a single polypeptide chain with a molecular weight of about 69,000. In addition to its proposed transport function, its high concentration in plasma and relatively low molecular weight make it the major determinant of intravascular-colloid osmotic pressure (oncotic pressure). Albumin has an isoelectric point at about pH 5 when it carries about 100 each of positive and negative charges. It therefore has many potential sites for interaction with ionic species such as charged drug molecules. At plasma pH 7·4 (Table 2), it has a net negative charge of 18 (White *et al*, 1968), but it can nevertheless interact strongly at this pH with anions as well as cations; indeed acidic drugs are generally more avidly bound.

The albumin of the blood (which constitutes 30–40% of the total body albumin) is involved in very active exchange with that of the other body fluids. Thus of the circulating mass of intravascular albumin (approximately 140 g for a 75 kg man), ten per cent or more per hour passes into the interstitial fluid, from whence it is returned to the blood via the lymphatic system. Furthermore, the half-life of albumin in the body is about 10–25 days, and approximately 13 g of albumin is normally synthesized and catabolized per day. The liver appears to be the only site of synthesis (Miller and Bale, 1954; Rothschild *et al*, 1972), but catabolism takes place at several sites, notably the liver, kidneys and gastrointestinal tract (Schultze and Heremans, 1966; Turner and Hulme, 1971).

It is now generally accepted that in most normal healthy adults, albumin concentration in plasma is between 3·5 and 4·5 g/100 ml (Marks, 1972). In common with other plasma proteins, albumin shows a 10–20% change in concentration with posture and during exercise, the higher level being found within 10–30 minutes of assuming the standing position (Poortmans, 1971). Serum-albumin levels are lower during infancy, pregnancy and senility, and in disease such as nephrosis, hepatitis, cirrhosis, cancers, gastrointesti-

Table 2 Ionized groups present on the albumin molecules at pH 7.4 (after Tanford *et al*, 1955)

Residue	Group	Number of groups per molecule	pKa	Number ionized at pH 7.4
		acidic groups		
C-terminal	α carboxyl	1	3·75	1
Aspartic	β carboxyl	99	3·97	99
Glutamic	γ carboxyl			
Tyrosine	Phenolic	19	10·35	0
		Basic groups		
Histidine	Imidazole	16	6·9	6
N-terminal	α amino	1	7·75	0·8
Lysine	ϵ amino	57	9·8	57
Arginine	Guanidine	22	12	22

nal diseases, hypergammaglobulinaemia, malnutrition (e.g. Kwashiorkor), heart disease and hypothyroidism. In addition, stress, injury, alcohol, carbon tetrachloride and acclimatization to heat, are known to decrease albumin production (Rothschild *et al*, 1972). With highly bound drugs such albumin changes could lead to a significant enhancement of free-drug blood levels and hence an enhancement of the therapeutic and/or toxicological effects if similar drug doses as those given to normal healthy adults are administered (Goldstein, 1949; Reynolds and Cluff, 1960; Wishinsky *et al*, 1962; Rolinson and Sutherland, 1965; Anton, 1968). Apart from lower levels of serum albumin, additional factors such as an increase in circulating endogenous metabolites, e.g. bilirubin, fatty acids, the presence of other drugs or altered protein structure (Pruit and Dayton, 1971) may also give rise to a decrease in drug–protein binding. Thus subjects with prehepatic or hepatic jaundice or those on a high-lipid diet are likely to show a reduced serum-albumin binding capacity for anionic drugs such as sulphonamides and salicylates. Anton and Corey (1971) have indicated that lower concentrations of serum albumin are responsible for observed decreases in sulphonamide binding in anephric patients. Andreasen (1973), recently reported decreased binding of acetylsalicylic acid, salicylic acid, phenylbutazone, diphenylhydantoin, sulphadiazine and thiopental, in patients with acute renal failure. Such decreases in protein binding could, however, not be completely explained by lower albumin concentrations, although it has been demonstrated that these drugs do not bind significantly to other plasma proteins. Similarly Congo red (Ehrstrom, 1937), thyroxine (Arango *et al*, 1968), tryptophan (Gulassay *et al*, 1971), clofibrate (Bridgman *et al*, 1972) and fluorescein (Reidenberg and Affrime, 1973) have been shown to have reduced binding in various disease states. Serum-albumin variants can occur in some subjects. These proteins may have different binding properties from normal albumin, for example Kawasaki *et al* (1973) have demonstrated considerable modifications in indocyanine-green binding in one patient compared with normal subjects. Interestingly, most of the basic drugs studied appear to bind normally to plasma from uremic patients (Reidenberg and Affrime, 1973). Reidenberg *et al* (1971) demonstrated decreased plasma-protein binding for diphenylhydantoin in uremic patients, but found no effect on the binding of desmethylimipramine. Similarly, quinidine binding has been found to be normal in various subjects with renal failure (Skuterud *et al*, 1972).

Globulins and Lipoproteins

The α, β and γ globulins also constitute an important group of binding proteins (Westphal, 1961; Sandberg *et al*, 1966; Seal and Doe, 1966). Several α and β globulins have a high affinity, but relatively low capacity, for a number of endogenous substances and chemically related synthetic compounds. The physiological importance of these high-affinity binding globulins is not clear, but they may act as transporters and regulators of biological activity (Salvatore, 1966; Keller *et al*, 1969). The metal-binding globulins, transferrin and ceruloplasmin, interact strongly and specifically with iron and copper respectively, and are essential to the transport of these ions. Binding globulins have also been identified for other endogenous compounds including corticosteroids (Westphal, 1971), testosterone (Rosner and Deakins, 1968; Clark *et al*, 1971; Lea and Støa, 1972), oestradiol (Raynaud *et al*, 1971), progesterone (Ryan and Westphal, 1972), vitamin B_{12} (Retief *et al*, 1967; Hippe and Olesen, 1971), vitamin A (Kanai *et al*, 1968), vitamin D (Morgan *et al*, 1958) and thyroxine (Rall *et al*, 1964; Salvatore *et al*, 1966; Tritsch, 1972). It has been observed that thyroxine also displays a higher affinity interaction with prealbumin than to thyroxine-binding globulin (Tritsch, 1972; Davis and Gregerman, 1971).

The plasma γ globulins have not so far been found to interact significantly with drugs (Goldstein *et al*, 1968), except where they occur as specific antibodies to them. The production of antibodies to protein hormones such as insulin and gonadotrophins is well known as a cause of lessening therapeutic efficacy in cases where these drugs have been used for a long time. With growing recognition that many chemically simpler drugs are capable of behaving as haptens or antigens, the possibility that some patients might develop circulating antibodies capable of binding a drug avidly and extensively must be considered.

Most plasma lipids are transported bound to certain proteins known collectively as lipoproteins. At low concentrations free fatty acids are transported preferentially by serum albumin, but at higher levels binding to α and β lipoproteins also occurs (Mora *et al*, 1965; Polonovski, 1966). The formation of a bilirubin–lipoprotein complex has also been reported to occur at high plasma-bilirubin levels (Cooke and Roberts, 1969), although the preferential association of bilirubin is with albumin as is the binding of endogenous prostaglandins (Raz, 1972a). The drug tetrahydrocannabinol and its metabolites are also reported to bind to lipoproteins (Wahlqvist *et al*, 1970; Widman *et al*, 1973). It is apparent that other proteins may often take up free drug if the albumin sites become saturated, e.g. methadone (Olsen, 1973), sulphonylureas (Judis, 1972)).

Blood Cells

The interaction with erythrocytes of both endogenous and exogenous compounds has been reported and includes promazine and chlorpromazine (Jähnchen *et al*, 1971), steroids (Brinkmann and van der Molen, 1972), bilirubin (Bratlid, 1972), salicylate and phenobarbital (McArthur *et al*, 1971), sulphonamides (Maren, 1967) and pentazocine (Ehrnebo *et al*, 1974). Although usually the amount bound is small, the significance of erythrocyte binding should not be overlooked. Borondy *et al* (1973) have shown that diphenylhydantoin binds to red cells, but they concluded that the passage of the drug from plasma into the red cells appears to be influenced much more by the binding properties of the plasma than by the erythrocytes. The binding of chlorpromazine to rat erythrocytes and also rat-brain synaptosomes has led Manian *et al* (1974) to postulate that binding to erythrocytes may represent a transport system for phenothiazines to the brain, where they exert their pharmacological response. Little is known about drug binding to platelets or white blood cells although it has been shown that blood platelets can accumulate monoamines (e.g. 5-hydroxytryptamine) and that this uptake can be inhibited by phenothiazines and tricyclic antidepressants (Ahtee *et al*, 1974). Marked species differences have been observed for the binding of triethyltinchloride. This compound binds very tightly (probably via histidines) to rat red-blood cells but only weakly to those from rabbit, hamster and man (Rose and Aldridge, 1968). Krieglstein's group has presented evidence that erythrocyte binding of chlorpromazine may cause a modification in its expected albumin binding.

Species and Individual Differences in Protein Binding

In general, no obvious consistent pattern of drug-binding characteristics between species has yet emerged. Goldstein (1949) has surveyed a number of reported interspecies differences in the serum-binding capacity of a variety of drugs. Despite the fact that no constant trend was apparent, rabbit sera often appeared to exhibit superior binding capabilities to that of other species. Rieder (1963) has detected a similar trend for the albumin binding of a series of sulphonamide drugs. For particular series of compounds a reproducible pattern may be observed. For example, Keen (1965) examined the binding of three penicillins and showed that for each penicillin the amount bound decreased in the order horse > goat > ox > sheep > pig, while Peets *et al* (1969) demonstrated that betamethasone and dexamethasone were more highly bound to rat plasma than to plasma for dog or cow. However, they noted that whereas betamethasone was bound more strongly to dog than cow plasma, for dexamethasone the reverse situation occurred. The binding of salicylate to monkey, rabbit and guinea-pig plasma has been shown to be similar to human plasma, and significantly higher than plasma from rat and dog (Kurtz and Friemel, 1967; Sturman and Smith, 1967; Kucera and Bullock, 1969). Witiak and Whitehouse (1969) on the basis of their observation of species differences in binding of several acidic drugs have suggested that the rat may be an unrepresentative species as far as drug binding to albumin is concerned. These authors also observed differences between drug binding to rat serum and isolated rat albumin.

Other drugs, e.g. warfarin and salicylate, also vary in their binding to different preparations of albumin (crystalline and fraction V) (Kostenbauder *et al*, 1970; Meyer and Guttman, 1970b; O'Reilly and Motley, 1971; Wilson, 1974). An added complication from a prediction viewpoint is the finding that species differences occur not only in the affinities of binding but also in binding sites, such as with phenylbutazone, between the albumin of rat, dog and rabbit (Chignell and Starkweather, 1971).

Species differences in the binding of the basic drugs desipramine (Borgå *et al*, 1968) and amphetamine (Baggot *et al*, 1972) have also been found. Borgå *et al* (1968) showed the amount of bound desipramine to decrease in the order cat > dog > man > rat > rabbit. Such differences could contribute to the reported differences in the pharmacological effect of this and other similar tricyclic antidepressants.

In contrast, the binding of a series of phenothiazines to defatted serum albumins has been shown by spectroscopic methods to be qualitatively similar in man, cow, dog, rat, rabbit, pig, horse, sheep, goat and chicken, but no consistent quantitative pattern emerged (Gabay and Huang, 1974). But it was apparent that for most of the phenothiazines, human-serum albumin (HSA) bound less strongly than the albumin of most other species except for trifluoromazine and trifluperazine where a stronger binding was observed to HSA than to other albumins except those of the pig and horse. The binding of chlorpromazine was found to be highest in the rat, followed by the cow, rabbit, horse, dog, goat, man, sheep, pig and chicken. The binding of chlorpromazine to rat albumin was found to be nearly 80% higher than to human albumin. It is worthy of note that different preparations of different albumins were used in this study; this may have contributed to some of the observed differences.

These species differences must arise through variations both in the concentration of albumin in plasma and in amino-acid sequence between species. For example, two tryptophans are found in bovine-serum albumin whereas only one occurs in human-serum albumin (see figure 5). The exact relationship between structure and binding still remains obscure. However, Thorp (1972) concluded that the amino-acid composition of rat albumin corresponds most closely to the average or 'normal' species situation. Since the rat shows anomalous behaviour in binding of a number of drugs (e.g. Witiak and Whitehouse, 1969) it is apparent that the relationship between primary protein structure and binding ability is a highly complex one.

Knowledge of strain and interindividual differences in protein binding (see also pages 212–213) is even more limited (Thorp, 1972). Interindividual differences in the plasma protein binding in man of the tricyclic antidepressant drug, nortriptyline, have been observed (Alexanderson and Borgå, 1972). It has also been reported that protein-bound iodine in Negro preadolescent children is significantly greater than that of white children (Starr *et al*, 1967). Difference in the thyroxine-binding globulin, total gamma globulin and albumin concentration, but not thyroxine-binding prealbumin were noted. Apparent individual differences, determined by the levels of circulating fatty acids, must also be expected (Spector and Imig, 1971).

STRUCTURE OF SERUM ALBUMIN

Despite the fact that bovine- and human-serum albumins have been two of the most widely investigated proteins, knowledge of their structures is still

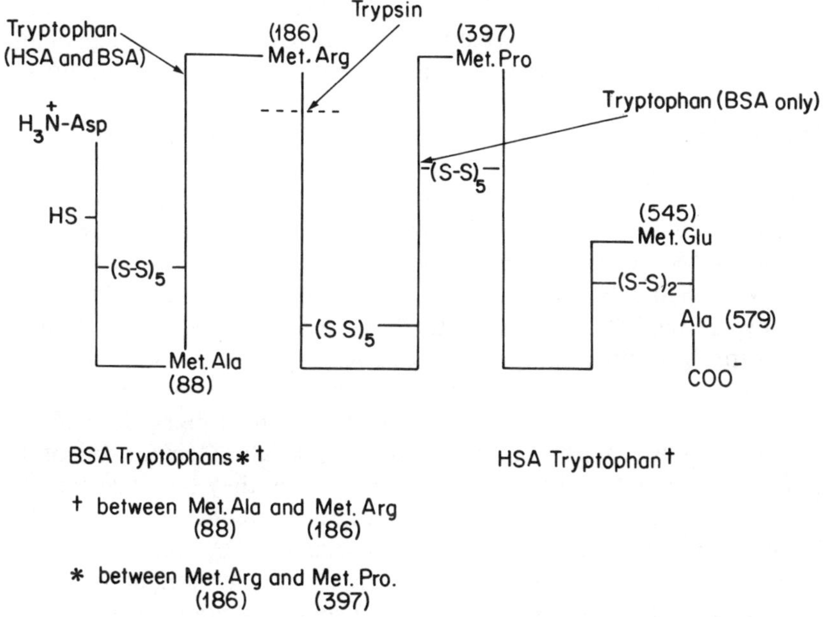

Figure 5 Diagrammatic representation of human- and bovine-albumin structures

relatively limited. In part this stems from the heterogeneity of serum albumins which frequently becomes exacerbated during isolation and purification. Changes in SH group bonding appear to make a major contribution to this heterogeneity. Commercially obtainable albumins tend to vary between one manufacturer and another and even between different batches from the same manufacturer. Traces of other proteins, e.g. α and β globulins and endonucleases, together with small amounts of fatty acids, metal salts and other chemicals, are frequently found (Janatová, 1974).

The primary structure of albumin has only been partly resolved. Albumin to exist partly as an α-helix (for human-serum albumin, about 45–50%) and partly as a random coil. Relatively little is known about the tertiary and quaternary structure of the albumin molecule although it may exist to some extent in solution as a dimer. It has been established that at pH 4, albumin undergoes a conformational transition which results in an increased viscosity and greater electrophoretic mobility (normal to fast, hence N–F transition). Optical rotatory (Sogami and Foster, 1968) and viscosity studies (Tanford *et al*, 1955) have revealed that at low pH, three albumin transition forms are distinguishable. Using the model of Harrington *et al* (1956) as modified by Foster (1960), of four compact fragments held together in pairs by hydrophobic bonds and linked by short randomly coiled polypeptide chains, the three forms can be considered to arise from an increase of the distance between these fragments from pH 4·5 to 3·9, a more or less stable situation between 3·9 and 3·6 and a further partial unfolding at lower pHs (acid-expanded form). Obviously, other more subtle changes in conformation and surface changes are occurring at other pH values and great caution must be used in interpreting binding data based on comparisons at different pHs.

The first 24 amino acid residues of the N-terminal end of human, rat and bovine albumin have been sequenced and a high degree of similarity shown (Shearer *et al*, 1967; Bradshaw and Peters, 1969). Recently King and Spencer (1970), using cyanogen-bromide cleavage of plasma albumin in 75% formic acid, obtained two fragments which could be further reduced to fragments of 88, 98, 211, 148 and 34, amino-acid residues. The single sulphydryl group of albumin was found to be located in the 88 amino-acid residue peptide which occupies the N-terminal position of the molecule. These workers also found that defatted bovine albumin subjected to limited tryptic hydrolysis gave a fragment of molecular weight *ca* 40,000, the fragment being derived from the C-terminal two thirds of the albumin molecule. Comparison of this tryptic fragment and defatted albumin showed that they both had the same primary binding site for both octanoate and L-tryptophan.

Using similar methods, Sjoholm and Ljungstedt (1973) split human-serum albumin into three parts, A, B and C, with molecular weights of 32,000, 13,900 and 18,100, respectively. Only the A and C positions were found to bind tryptophan. It was suggested that the binding to fragment A, the secondary site, involves mainly a strong electrostatic interaction, whereas the binding to fragment C (which contains the sole tryptophan residue), is markedly hydrophobic in nature. The affinity constants obtained were comparable to those found in intact human-serum albumin indicating that the primary peptide structure in the fragment was sufficient to enable the adoption of secondary and tertiary structures which closely resemble those of the native albumin. The role of the tryptophan residue in fragment C in binding free tryptophan remains to be determined.

Recently, Meloun and Küsnir (1972) sequenced the 37 residues at the C-terminal end of human-plasma albumin and the residues between the first and second methionine residues (Küsnir and Meloun, 1973). Studies with such 'fragmented' albumins (Means and Feeney, 1971; Wilson, 1974) are likely to play a very important role in characterizing binding sites for drugs and other small molecules. The considerable body of knowledge gained in producing albumin-drug antigens for radioimmunoassay purposes could also be used to good effect for the synthesis of covalently bound probes to albumin in order to examine conformational forms of albumin.

Nature of Binding Sites

Potentially a drug may bond to serum albumin through the establishment of covalent, ionic, charge transfer, hydrophobic, van der Waals or hydrogen-bond linkages. For the binding of many if not all drugs, several of these bond types are probably involved. The stability of a particular binding interaction is obviously not only dependent on the nature of the drug and amino acid(s) concerned but is likely to be considerably modified by the environment created by the peptide chain in the vicinity of the bonding amino acid(s). The energy value for bond strengths given in Table 3 should therefore be taken only as guidelines. All the amino acids in albumin are potential binding sites for drugs and many are capable of interacting via several types of bonds. Thus there are 86 possible binding sites for anions and 100 theoretically available binding sites for cationic drugs. It is perhaps surprising that although there are numerous interaction sites on the albumin surface for small ions (Klotz, 1949), for most drugs the highest affinity (primary) binding sites number less than ten (Jones and Weber, 1971), and for many no more than two (Thorp, 1964). Many compounds also bind to lower affinity (secondary) binding sites, but again the number of such interactions is often less than ten. It should be noted that in instances in which more than one binding site of a particular class is detected, unless these sites are truly identical, which is unlikely, the n value will be an average term without true physical meaning.

It is self-evident that the peptide residues which provide the surrounding environment for a particular bonding amino acid must be a major governing influence on the feasibility of a drug bonding to it. Furthermore, it is likely that the interaction of a drug with a particular binding site may result in a modification of the conformation of the albumin molecule as a consequence of which the protein's potential to associate with drug molecules at other sites may be changed. This concept is analogous to that of the induced fit and allosteric transition theories of enzyme-activity modification (Koshland,

Table 3 Bonds involved in drug–protein interactions

Bond type	Bond energy (kJ/mol^{-1})	Major amino acids concerned
Covalent	210–460	Serine, tyrosine, cysteine, lysine, arginine.
Ionic	up to 210	For cations aspartate, glutamate For anions lysine, arginine, histidine
Hydrogen bonds	8–21	Electron donors, aspartate, glutamate, serine, tyrosine and tryptophan Electron acceptors nitrogen heterocycles, also lysine, arginine, tyrosine and serine.
Charge transfer	8–21	Phenylalanine, tyrosine, tryptophan
Hydrophobic per —CH—CH—	2·9–3·6	All aliphatic amino acids
van der Waals	2·1–4·2	All amino acids

1958; Monod *et al*, 1963) and the mode of antigen–antibody interactions (Roitt, 1974). Assuming that such conformational changes are commonly involved in drug–albumin binding it may be rather misleading to consider a specific number and structure of binding sites for a particular group of drugs.

In order to account for its binding to a wide range of chemicals a high, if not unique, conformational adaptivity would appear to be necessary. Thus, although only a limited number of sites appear to be involved in drug–albumin interactions, many drugs and endogenous materials which bind to the same sites would be expected to produce different conformational changes in the albumin.

Thorp (1972) has suggested that there are potentially only three separate primary binding sites for organic acids on human albumin. One or more of these sites may become uncovered through local changes in the conformation of the albumin molecule which are induced specifically by certain structural features of the compound. However such a site might be essentially 'inaccessible' to related compounds incorporating even minor structural changes. Thorp (1964) considered that the N-terminal amino-acid group (aspartic acid for bovine and human albumin) acts as a binding site for fatty acids, co-enzymes (e.g. pyridoxal phosphate) and hormones (e.g. thyroxine and steroid sulphates or glucuronides), while Whitehouse *et al* (1967) have suggested that the ϵ-amino group of lysine is a binding site for a number of triterpenoid acids (see figure 4). Swaney and Klotz (1970) have investigated the properties of the peptides surrounding the tryptophan of human-serum albumin (HSA), which earlier workers (Reynolds *et al*, 1967; Herskovits, 1967) had suggested might be associated with a potential binding site. Following chymotrypsin hydrolysis and tryptic digestion they were able to determine the primary structure adjoining the lone tryptophan in HSA as:

Lys.Ala.Trp.Ala.Val.Ala.Arg.

They suggested that the highly apolar character of the region and the presence of the two basic residues, arginine and lysine, made it especially suitable for the binding of organic ions, particularly those which contain both apolar and electronegative regions. The same reasoning would apply to the neighbourhood of the 'reactive' tyrosine (Sanger, 1960):

Arg.Tyr.Thr.Arg in BSA and Arg.Tyr.Thr.Lys in HSA

The finding that the interaction of anions, such as dodecyl sulphate with HSA, quenches the fluorescence of tryptophan (Steinhardt *et al*, 1971) may support the hypothesis that tryptophan is in close proximity to the binding site although neutral molecules such as the long-chain aliphatic carbamates produce a blue shift in the tryptophan fluorescence indicating that they too modify its environment (A. G. E. Wilson and J. W. Bridges, unpublished data). It is suggested that in the case of BSA, which has two tryptophans, only one is embedded in the protein structure (Ivkova *et al*, 1971). Initial studies (Sugae and Jirgensons, 1964) would imply that the portion of the protein containing both tryptophans lacks appropriate positive charges, at least on the C-terminal side, although they may be found on the N-terminal side. Whether or not the environs of both tryptophan molecules enable the binding of anions with equal avidity is difficult to ascertain, but it appears unlikely since the determined numbers of primary binding sites on BSA for anions is often less than two.

Little information is available on potential binding sites for basic compounds in either BSA or HSA. It is generally thought that albumin has different binding sites for acidic and basic drugs (Brodie, 1966). However, Franz *et al* (1969) have shown that promazine can apparently be displaced by acidic drugs, although interestingly it is neither displaced by, nor displaces, chlorpromazine (Borgå *et al*, 1969). While this does not necessarily imply a common binding site for acidic and basic drugs, it does suggest that the view that basic drugs never replace acidic drugs at the same site (Brodie, 1965) may require modification.

Gabay and Huang (1974) have suggested that whereas the phenothiazines are in a hydrophobic environment, imipramine and chlorprothixene are bound at hydrophilic sites on the albumin surface. Preliminary fluorescent probe studies with the tricyclic antidepressant iprindole (A. G. E. Wilson and J. W. Bridges, unpublished data) suggest a binding site with a hydrophilic environment, although the nature of this binding site still remains to be fully characterised. Few reports on the number of binding sites on the albumin molecule for basic drugs appear to have been published. Krieglstein *et al* (1972a) have, however, reported a single primary binding for phenothiazines. In contrast, values quoted by other workers range from 1 to 23 (Brodie, 1965; Noval and Mao, 1970; Gabay and Huang, 1974). Clearly these conflicting findings need to be resolved.

Recently the technique of photoaffinity labelling has greatly improved the prospects of identifying the binding sites of many compounds (Knowles, 1972). The basis of this approach is that a molecule containing a photoreactive group, such as an azide or ketone function (Galardy *et al*, 1974; Kiefer *et al*, 1970), is allowed to bind to the protein. On exposure to ultra-violet light the molecule becomes activated and combines covalently with amino acid(s) of the binding site through an interaction with a C—H bond. The protein can then be fragmented and the labelled site fully characterized.

It is conceivable that, in solution, serum albumin may exist in a variety of different but approximately energetically equivalent conformational forms (Karush, 1950; Janatová, 1974). If this is indeed the case, then a number of different sites could potentially be in a suitable configuration to permit interaction with a particular drug structure. The existence of this heterogeneity of conformational forms might help to explain the great binding versatility of serum albumin (if it could be demonstrated that albumin was outstanding in the range of conformational forms it adopted) it would, of course, also seriously hamper attempts to identify a specific binding site or sites.

INFLUENCE OF DRUG PROPERTIES ON ALBUMIN BINDING

Although the binding of acidic compounds to albumin has been extensively studied (Goldstein, 1949; Meyer and Guttman, 1968), the binding of neutral (Steinhardt and Reynolds, 1969), and basic compounds (Borgå *et al*, 1969; Franksson and Anggard, 1970), has not. At one time, binding to plasma protein was attributed to simple electrostatic attraction between the ionic form of the drug and a charged group on albumin. However, additional forces must be involved to explain the observed relationship between degree of binding and chemical structure. In a series of barbiturates, for example, all of which have the same pK_a(7·6), barbitone is hardly bound, but as the chain length is extended the binding increases to 55% with pentobarbitone (Brodie, 1966). It seems likely that even for highly ionized drugs, hydrogen bonds, charge-transfer bonds, van der Waal forces and hydrophobic bonds are considerably involved in their association with albumin (Goldstein *et al*, 1968; Korolkovas, 1970; Nemethy and Laiken, 1970).

Few albumin-binding studies have been made on series of drugs in which the individual contributions of these bonds to the drug–protein interaction can be properly evaluated. Thus the predictability of binding from knowledge of drug structure and conformation is still poorly developed. Based on a diverse range of drugs certain rough guidelines for the effects of substitution on drug–protein associations can, however, be discerned.

(i) Substituents which cause an enhancement in hydrophobicity (e.g. aromatic ring, methylene group or halogen substitution) tend to elevate binding (Scholtan, 1968) although the tendency for micelle formation with highly lipid-soluble compounds may detract from this trend.

(ii) Substituents which produce an increase in the degree of electrolytic dissociation of an ionizable drug, at the pH of the plasma, increase binding whereas addition of an amino group or N-heterocycle frequently causes a diminution in binding (Dearden and Tomlinson, 1970).

(iii) Substitution by polar groups may also increase binding. Affinities have also been shown to be in the order of $(SO_4)^{2-} > (SO_3)^{2-} > COO^- = OH$ (Reynolds *et al*, 1968).

(iv) *Ortho* substitution tends to produce considerably greater changes in binding than *meta* or *para* substituents (Davison and Smith, 1961; Moriguchi *et al*, 1968), probably because *ortho* substitution confers more propensity for intermolecular hydrogen bonding, whereas *meta* and *para* substituents can interact more with surrounding water molecules, thereby decreasing binding to the protein (Klotz *et al*, 1948).

Useful as these rules are, they must be applied with caution; thus hydroxylation of warfarin in the 6, 7 or 8 positions leads to diminution rather than enhancement of binding to albumin. Conversely, hydroxylation in position 5 increases binding, possibly due to intramolecular hydrogen-bond formation (O'Reilly and Motley, 1971). Similarly hydroxylation also decreases binding for the *p*-substituted acetanilides (Dearden and Tomlinson, 1970).

Relationship between Drug Lipophilicity and Protein-binding Ability

Hydrophobic bonding probably makes the major contribution to the interaction of protein with most neutral drugs, and is usually significantly involved in the binding of ionized drugs. The concept of hydrophobic bonding has largely arisen from the early work of Frank and Wen (1957). However, despite a number of other fundamental studies on the thermodynamic properties of hydrocarbons in aqueous solution (Nemethy and Scheraga, 1962a, b, c and 1963; Crothers and Ratner, 1968; Hermann, 1971; Tanford, 1972), differences of opinion exist as to the nature of these interactions (Klotz, 1958; Pauling, 1961; Hildebrand, 1968; Nemethy *et al*, 1968; Holtzer and Emerson, 1969; Tanford, 1974). Hydrophobic bonding has been broadly defined as the tendency of nonpolar groupings, particularly hydrocarbons, to aggregate together in aqueous solution. The structure of water in close proximity to hydrophobic groups is believed to play a significant role in this bonding (Nagwekar and Kostenbauder, 1970). The disruption of the quasi-crystalline water structure ('ice-berg') around the nonpolar groups in aqueous solution with a concomitant entropy gain has been suggested to be the driving force for the formation of hydrophobic bonding (Kauzmann, 1959; Schachman, 1963; Molyneux and Frank, 1969). However, it should be emphasized (Frank and Evans, 1945) that the structure of these 'ice-bergs' may be variable and need not be typical of ordinary ice.

While a drug–protein interaction accompanying a positive entropy change is consistent with a mechanism involving hydrophobic bonding, thermodynamic parameters do not by themselves necessarily provide diagnostic criteria, for example Klotz (1973) has suggested that electrostatic interactions such as the binding of Cu^{2+} to albumin are also entropically driven. Furthermore, conformational changes in either drug or protein could also give rise to entropy changes (Dearden and Tomlinson, 1970). Similarly, although drug–protein interactions frequently accompany large negative enthalpies (ΔH) (Steinhardt and Reynolds, 1969), this observation alone does not unequivocally establish a role for London (van der Waal) forces.

Hydrophobic bonding could explain the increasing positive entropies with longer chain length observed for the binding of the anions octyl, decyl and dodecyl sulphates (Karush and Sonenberg, 1949). More recently a number of studies have substantiated the significance of the role of hydrophobic bonding in drug–protein interactions. Hansch and his co-workers have studied the binding of a wide variety of compounds to bovine-serum albumin (Hansch *et al*, 1965; Hansch, 1969, 1971). A good correlation was found between log *p* (a term related to the partition coefficient between octanol and water) and the molar concentration of a compound necessary for it to form a one-to-one complex with protein. Scholtan (1968), using a variety of drugs including sulphonamides, antibiotics, cardenolides and steroid hormones, showed that the affinity of binding increased for each series when the hydrophobic character of the drug was increased by the introduction of nonpolar substituents such as alkyl groups, halogen atoms or aromatic rings. Correlations between binding and lipophilic character have also been obtained for a number of other compounds, e.g. penicillins (Bird and Marshall, 1967), *p*-hydroxybenzoic acid esters (Patel *et al*, 1968), a homologous series of fatty acids (Teresi and Luck, 1952; Goodman, 1958); sulphates, sulphonates and alcohols (Ray *et al*, 1966; Reynolds *et al*, 1967), hydrocarbons (Wildnauer and Canady, 1966; Mohammadzadeh-K., 1969a, b) aromatic compounds and alkanes (Wetlaufer and Lovrien, 1964; Sahyun, 1966). Wishnia and Pinder (1964), in a detailed account of hydrophobic interactions of a homologous series of alkanes with BSA have suggested that the binding of these compounds to protein could arise through either penetration of the alkane into the interior of the protein or into surface clusters, or binding to the protein surface with the formation of a more favourable ice-cage or clathrate cage. Correlations have also been found between partition coefficients and the interaction of basic compounds such as phenothiazines with BSA (Krieglstein *et al*, 1972a, b; Nambu and Nagai, 1972), but not for the binding of eight tricyclic antidepressants (Jorgensen *et al*, 1973).

Hansch (1971) has concluded from calculations of the free energy of binding for a wide variety of drugs, e.g. sulphonamides, tetracyclines, penicillins, cardenolides, steroid bisguanylhydrazones, acridines and steroid hormones, that steric effects and specific hydrogen bonding (not accounted for in the partitioning reference model) are not generally important in the binding of drugs to albumin.

In order to try and resolve the importance of the contribution of hydrophobic bonding to protein binding, Wilson *et al* (1974) examined the albumin binding of a homologous series of simple aliphatic carbamates in which interactions from H bonding are relatively constant and ionic binding cannot occur. They demonstrated that for these carbamates there was a good linear correlation between binding and the lipophilic character of the carbamate (see figure 6). The slope of the graph may represent a fundamental relationship between hydrophobic binding and lipid solubility. If this interpretation is correct then departure from this linear relationship can be considered to be due to the superimposition of other variables. On this assumption the slopes of nk vs $\log p$ plots should be similar for other series of compounds whose binding is largely hydrophobic in nature, providing that similar experimental conditions prevail. Interestingly the correlation between the association constant (k) and lipid solubility for the carbamates is much poorer than that using nk, indicating that the number of binding sites for the carbamates on albumin varies with chain length. This illustrates the need to determine both the n and k values when investigating suspected correlations between binding and physicochemical parameters; where con-

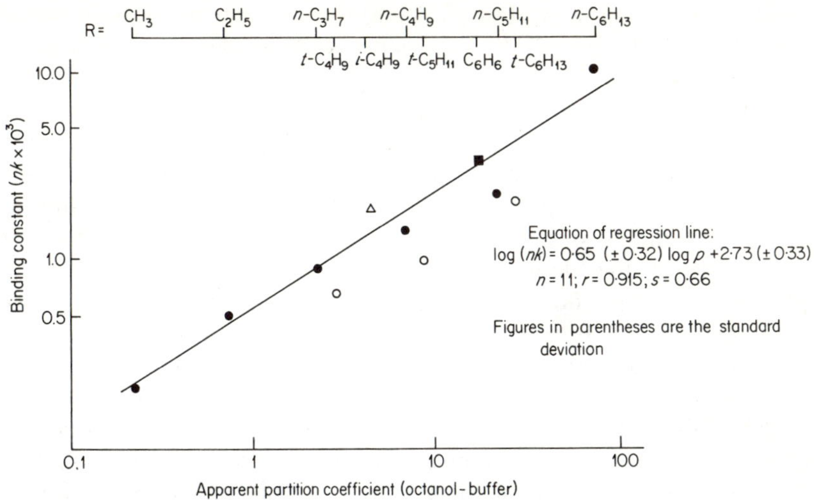

Figure 6 The relationship between carbamate binding constants (nk) for bovine-serum albumin and apparent partition coefficient for the series R—O—CO—NH_2

siderable variation in n is apparent for a homologous series the parameter nk is to be preferred. Calculation of the free-energy change for a single $\geq CH_2 \ldots\ldots CH_2 \leq$ interaction in the carbamates ($\Delta G = 86{\cdot}2$ kJ/mol where ΔG is the free energy of binding) indicates reasonable agreement with that reported in the literature from studies on the aqueous solubility of hydrocarbons, thus implying that the hydrophobic bonding is analogous to a partitioning effect. A possible complicating factor is that the estimation of the thermodynamic contribution of hydrophobic groups to form a drug–protein complex may sometimes be obscured by the simultaneous contribution of protein molecules due to their 'conformational adaptability' (Nagwekar and Kostenbauder, 1970). This phenomenon may perhaps partially explain the marked increase in k values for the high-affinity binding of fatty acids on extending the carbon-chain length from C_6 (hexanoic acid) to C_8 (octanoic acid) (N. Brown and J. W. Bridges, unpublished observations).

Calculation of the free-energy change may often be used as an approximate indication of hydrophobic bonding in, for example, the interaction of long-chain compounds. Furthermore in some instances it may be possible to calculate the approximate free energy of interaction for substituent groups such as aromatic rings and hence derive theoretical protein-binding affinities. The feasibility of such an extrapolation awaits further systematic data collection.

Attempts to use water solubility (Vandenbelt *et al*, 1954; Sahyun, 1966) of the small molecule as an extrathermodynamic reference generally appear to give less reliable correlation with protein-binding ability than partition coefficients. This is perhaps surprising in view of the finding of Saracco and

Marchetti (1958) and later Hansch (1968) that a linear correlation between p^{-1} (partition coefficient) and s^{-1} (aqueous solubility) existed for a number of compounds.

Deviations from a linear relationship between serum-albumin binding and log p has recently been reported for a series of carboxylic-acid and p-aminobenzenesulphonamide antiinflammatory and uricosuric agents (Dunn, 1973, based on the data of Whitehouse *et al*, 1971). Using as a parameter of binding strength the concentration of drug required for a 50% displacement of the fluorescence probe 5-dimethylaminonaphthalene-1-sulphonamide, it was shown that there was a parabolic relationship between binding and the partition coefficient of the drug with optimum log p values of 5·48 for the carboxylic acids and 1·10 for the sulphonamides. This parabolic relationship is of particular interest because a similar type of situation has been shown to pertain for a wide variety of biological systems including drug absorption (Houston *et al*, 1974) and anaesthetic activity (Glave and Hansch, 1972). However, the general significance of this phenomenon for drug protein interactions remains uncertain. One partial explanation of the results of Whitehouse *et al* is that at log p values above the optimum point the drug may commence binding to a second, lower affinity site.

Tanford (1972) has shown that the hydrophobic parts of the binding site(s) are limited in the length of hydrocarbon chain that can be accommodated. It is important that the possibility of the hydrophobic part of the binding site not being a single contiguous area is considered when evaluating the binding characteristics of long-chain hydrocarbon groups. For example it may involve separated areas, and binding to such areas by an 'inch-worm' type of attachment may occur (Laiken and Nemethy, 1970a, b; Tanford, 1972). Tanford (1974) has also pointed out that the competition between the binding of molecules to albumin and their incorporation into micelles will shift in favour of micelle formation as the size of the hydrophobic portion of the molecule increases. This is particularly relevant for compounds such as anionic phospholipids, since it may prevent association with albumin, especially at lower-affinity sites. It is possible that some highly lipophilic drugs may bind through the endogenous lipids associated with serum proteins rather than via a direct interaction with protein itself. However, this concept must await experimental verification.

Sulphonamide Binding

The sulphonamide drugs have frequently been used as models to elucidate the importance of the various binding forces in drug–protein interactions. While the view that most of the energy of sulphonamide–albumin interactions is due to hydrophobic forces is receiving increasing support (Clausen, 1966; Fujita and Hansch, 1967; Scholtan, 1968), other experimental evidence has suggested an important role for electrostatic interactions between the sulphonamide anion and the positive charge on the protein surface (Klotz and Walker, 1948; Nakagaki *et al*, 1964). Moriguchi *et al* (1968) determined the binding of 19 sulphonamides to BSA and showed binding to be correlated with the pK_a of the N^1 nitrogen of the sulphonamides.

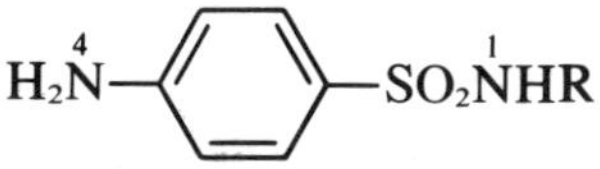

$$H_2\overset{4}{N}-C_6H_4-SO_2\overset{1}{N}HR$$

They suggested that this may indicate that electrostatic forces are dominant in the binding of such anions. Nakagaki *et al*, (1964), who determined the binding of six sulphonamides to BSA at various pHs, similarly concluded that electrostatic forces are the most important factor in sulphonamide binding. However they did not consider the hydrophobic character of the sulphonamides. Subsequently Fujita (1972) has re-examined their data and concluded that the hydrophobicity of the drug largely determines binding to BSA through interaction of the neutral drug molecule with the hydrophobic fraction of the protein surface, the hydration shell over which is uncovered by dissociation of cationic bases on the BSA. Agren *et al* (1971) demonstrated a direct relationship between lipophilicity and binding of 26 sulphonamides to HSA, but a much better correlation was found between binding and electron distribution using the extended Hückel method. They concluded that the major determinant in sulphonamide binding is electrostatic attraction between the anionic-drug species and the primary binding site of HSA (consisting of a sequence of amino acids containing positively charged lysine and arginine). A secondary role was ascribed to attraction between the tryptophan residues of HSA and the *para* atom of the heterocyclic ring in the sulpha ring, with hydrophobic bonding being of lesser importance. Jardetzky and Wade-Jardetzky (1965), using n.m.r. methods, concluded that a hydrophobic part of the sulphonamide structure, probably the *p*-aminobenzene moiety, participates in binding.

The above studies clearly illustrate the problem of data interpretation when more than one potential binding force is involved. They further indicate that unless the various physicochemical effects can be separated, true correlations of physicochemical significance may be obscured.

Phenothiazine Binding

Studies of particular groups of basic drugs such as phenothiazines, although less numerous than for acidic compounds, have provided valuable indications of the interactions between basic drugs and albumins. Several workers have demonstrated the importance of hydrophobic bonding in albumin–phenothiazine interactions (Krieglstein *et al*, 1972a, b; Nambu and Nagai, 1972; Gabay and Huang, 1974). Huang and Gabay (1974) have suggested that neither hydrogen bonding nor dipolar interactions play major roles in the binding process although they may make some contribution (Krieglstein *et al*, 1972b).

The albumin binding of 2-substituted phenothiazines; promazine, chlorpromazine, triflupromazine and bromopromazine, has been shown to be directly related to the hydrophobic character of the 2 substituent on the phenothiazine nucleus. (Krieglstein *et al*, 1972b; Nambu and Nagai, 1972; Gabay and Huang, 1974).

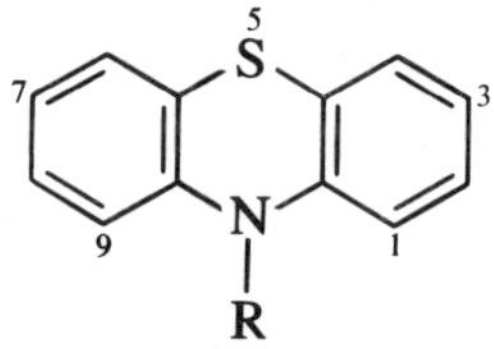

Nambu and Nagai (1972) have demonstrated that the binding of chlorpromazine to BSA accompanied a positive entropy change, which is suggested to be consistent with such a hydrophobic-bonding mechanism (Kauzmann, 1959).

From studies of the effect of simple aromatic substances and series of acidic and basic drugs on the binding of promazine and chlorpromazine, Jähnchen *et al* (1969) have claimed that only one of the phenothiazine benzene rings is inserted into a hydrophobic crevice in the albumin. However, Gabay and Huang (1974) have recently proposed that all three rings of the phenothiazine nucleus are essential to the binding. They suggest that this site is quite specific for the phenothiazine molecule, such that an alteration in the spatial relationship of a molecule, as in the case of chlorpromazine sulfoxide, imipramine or chlorprothixene, excludes them from this particular albumin-binding site. The incorporation of any hydrophilic groups into the chlorpromazine structure either into the ring nucleus or side-chain tends to cause a reduction of binding (Huang and Gabay, 1974). For example chlorpromazine-N-oxide exhibits less than half the binding of chlorpromazine while 7-hydroxychlorpromazine is also less well bound than chlorpromazine. However, the degree of substituent effect appears to differ according to the ring position, the 6 position being least sensitive, while a 7 grouping has most influence. The insertion of a 7-methoxyl substituent is quite similar in effect to that of a 7-hydroxyl group.

Hydrophobic forces also appear to influence, to a certain extent, the interaction of N-10 substituted phenothiazines. For instance, promethazine is bound to a greater extent than promazine (Krieglstein *et al*, 1972b) which is inexplicable in terms of simple lipophilicity since it differs from promazine only in the position of the dimethylamino group in the N-10 propyl side-chain. It is apparent that steric considerations must also be invoked to explain this type of observation. In addition Krieglstein *et al* (1972a) have suggested that the similarity between the binding of desmethylchlorpromazine and that of promazine and chlorpromazine, indicates the involvement of ionic bonding through the side-chain position 10 of the phenothiazine nucleus. Further support for some ionic contribution is provided by the pH sensitivity of the chlorpromazine–albumin interaction (Huang and Gabay, 1974). This is readily understandable in that the pK_a of chlorpromazine is about 9·3, and therefore at pH 7·4 it exists largely in ionized form. Evidence of the involvement of the side-chain in binding has also been provided by Krieglstein *et al* (1972a) who showed that hydroxine, which like perazine possesses a piperazine ring, displaces perazine but not chlorpromazine from its albumin-binding site.

Binding of Other Compounds

Dearden and Tomlinson (1970) have studied the binding of a series of *p*-substituted acetanilides to BSA. The free energy of binding (ΔG) was found to be negative in all cases, although little variation of ΔG amongst the different derivatives was apparent. Binding accompanied a negative enthalpy and, with the exception of *p*-aminoacetanilide, all entropy changes in binding were found to be positive. They demonstrated a good correlation between the thermodynamics of binding (ΔH, ΔS) and Hammett's substituent constant (σ), a reasonable agreement with the Hansch partition coefficient (π) was also found. On this basis they suggested that the interaction between acetanilides and BSA is nonspecific, involving only London (van der Waals) forces, rather than hydrogen bonding, binding occurring to a hydrophobic region of the BSA molecule.

Sellers and Koch-Weser (1974) recently studied the binding of a series of benzothiadiazines to human albumin. They were found to bind extensively to human albumin and the effects of deuterium substitution and of pH, temperature, ionic strength and cations, on the binding were consistent with a mechanism involving mainly hydrophobic bonding and to a lesser extent hydrogen bonding. Chu (1974) in a study of the binding of ochratoxins to BSA concluded that both ionic and hydrophobic forces played a major role in the interaction.

The above examples demonstrate that for widely differing molecular structures hydrophobic bonding usually plays a major role in the protein binding but other forces are also normally involved.

IMPLICATIONS OF PLASMA PROTEIN BINDING

Although studying a drug's fate by organ perfusion experiments using variable concentrations of protein would appear to be the most direct approach to ascertain the role of binding on drug distribution, metabolism and excretion, few definitive studies of this nature have been reported.

Absorption

A high degree of plasma protein binding could enhance the intestinal absorption of a drug by rendering its concentration gradient favourable for absorption. This may be of particular importance with drugs having a poor water solubility, e.g. dicoumarol (bishydroxycoumarin), since it will enable larger concentrations of drug to be carried in the plasma (Brodie, 1966). There are unfortunately few clear-cut illustrations to substantiate the role of plasma protein binding in influencing intestinal absorption. Kakemi *et al* (1969) using *in vitro* methods have demonstrated a correlation between intestinal absorption rate and protein binding for a series of barbituric-acid derivatives in the rat. They concluded, however, that for these compounds binding to the mucosal surface is of more significance in affecting absorption rate than plasma protein binding. More recently Dearden and Tomlinson (1971) have suggested that protein binding may be important in determining the rate of buccal absorption for a series of *p*-substituted acetanilides. Tregear (1966) has shown that perfusing of skin with serum enhances absorption of dieldrin and parathion through the skin surface compared with that observed with saline. He ascribed this difference to the protein-binding capacity of the serum for these compounds.

Distribution and Pharmacological Activity

Most drugs probably distribute through the body water and tissue by passive distribution down a concentration gradient. It is generally considered that only the unbound plasma concentration of the drug is available for transport to extravascular sites (Goldstein, 1949; Brodie, 1966). Among the experimental observations supporting this view are the reduced potency of drugs such as sulphonamides (Davis, 1943; Anton, 1960; Krüger-Thiemer *et al*, 1965), penicillins (Rolinson and Sutherland, 1965) and prostaglandin E_2 (Raz, 1972b), when bound to serum albumin. Mikkelson *et al* (1973) have demonstrated that high concentration of protein in the lacrimal fluid from the eye in both *in vivo* and *in vitro* normal and diseased states leads to a considerable loss of local activity of drugs such as sulphisoxazole and pilocarpine.

However, it is by no means certain that a protein-bound drug is invariably therapeutically and toxicologically inactive. Indeed, the fact that drugs which are deliberately covalently bound to serum albumin often cause specific antibodies to be produced when the drug–protein complex is injected into experimental animals implies that drugs bound to protein may still be able to at least partially interact with some receptor sites. Bennhold (1938) suggested that in order to pass into cells, drugs should be bound to plasma proteins. Although this view is largely discounted nowadays, it is not beyond the bounds of possibility that large polar-drug molecules which are normally unable to pass across cell membranes may be taken into cells bound to proteins by pinocytosis. Indeed Barbanti-Brodano *et al* (1974) have shown that the hepatotoxic action of the toxic cyclopeptide phalloidin is due to its uptake bound to serum albumin. For cells active in protein uptake the possibility of drug absorption in the albumin-bound form should be given serious consideration.

Providing they do not bind preferentially or irreversibly to tissue sites, highly protein-bound drugs are likely to be located initially in the plasma compartment, particularly at doses where the high-affinity binding sites are not saturated (Brodie and Hogben, 1957; Martin, 1965a, b). Under these circumstances protein-bound drugs can serve potentially as a reservoir replenishing (by dissociation) some of the drug that is lost by metabolism and excretion, thus tending to maintain the concentration of unbound drug at a therapeutically useful concentration, over a considerable range of total-plasma concentrations. Furthermore, plasma protein binding could reduce the free concentration of some drugs below that required to elicit a toxic response, thus rendering the drug safe for therapeutic use. The plasma proteins may thus have an important buffering role for many drugs, enabling them to be given only a few times a day instead of by continual infusion. In the steady state the concentration of unbound drug in the tissues, and tissue compartments of the extracellular fluid, such as synovial fluid, can equal that in the plasma (Howell *et al*, 1972).

Martin (1965a) has discussed a theoretical model describing the binding of four hypothetical drugs ranging from weakly bound to strongly bound from which it can be calculated that only for drugs with association constants (k) greater than $10^4\ M^{-1}$ will binding have an appreciable effect on distribution. At low-plasma levels a drug with a high association constant ($k = 10^5\ M^{-1}$) will be almost completely bound to plasma proteins. When the concentration of the drug increases, however, the available plasma protein binding sites become fewer as saturation approaches with the result that more of the drug diffuses into the tissues and the fraction of drug remaining within the vasculature is reduced. For such drugs there will be a concentration range over which small changes in the plasma level may exert a profound influence on the distribution of the drug within the body. Martin's model is highly simplified, but illustrates that the controllable therapeutic-dose range may be narrow for highly bound drugs which undergo large dose-dependent changes in distribution. It also assumes, as do other models, that drug–protein complexes are invariably completely and rapidly reversible, which may not always be valid (see page 195). A number of theoretical models concerning the effect of protein binding on the pharmacokinetics of drug action have been made (Coffey, 1972; Coffey *et al*, 1971 and Schoenemann *et al*, 1973). Levy and Nagashima (1969) and Levy (1973) have demonstrated that the distribution and elimination of the highly bound drug dicoumarol is affected by its plasma-protein binding, but they emphasize that such effects are likely to be less pronounced for drugs not so extensively bound. Curry (1970a,b) has reported that the plasma concentration of chlorpromazine fluctuates after intravenous doses in dogs and man, possibly due to drug exchange between the plasma and tissue-bound compartments. Although tissue binding has not yet been intensively investigated, it seems likely that some highly bound drugs have even higher affinities for certain tissue proteins. The cardiac glycosides, for example, have been found *in vitro* to have a higher affinity for cardiac actin and myosin than for bovine-serum albumin (Genazzani and Santamaria, 1969), such that *in vivo* their concentration in the heart is about twenty to thirty times that in plasma. From the foregoing considerations it is apparent that it is usually only the free drug and drug metabolite concentration in the plasma which could be expected to directly correlate with the therapeutic or toxicological effects of the drug. Almost invariably, however, it is the total drug blood level which is measured in clinical pharmacology studies. Interpretation of data based on total blood levels generally rests on the assumption that free-drug levels and total drug blood levels are directly correlatable. For moderately or poorly bound drugs this may be valid but it is frequently not justified for highly bound drugs in which large changes in total-drug level with only minor changes in free level may occur (e.g. when changes in endogenous or exogenous displacing agents arise), if the free drug is readily tissue bound. Conversely when protein-binding sites of a highly bound drug are nearly saturated, small changes in total blood level may mask very significant increases in free-drug level. The presence of metabolites may also considerably modify the levels of free drug in the plasma.

It is therefore scarcely surprising that for many strongly bound drugs poor correlations have been reported between biological effects and total drug blood levels particularly when it is borne in mind that many of the analytical and clinical appraisal methods used lack accuracy and precision. It is to be hoped that the use of displacement techniques (cf radioimmunoassay) in which a very small quantity of the labelled drug is added to the blood and the binding of this radiolabel is then studied *in vitro*, as a monitor of the degree of *in vivo* binding, will overcome some of these difficulties (e.g. ^{14}C-warfarin, G. Levy, unpublished data). Alternatively, suitable fluorescence probes could be employed for this purpose. Problems in anticipating the likely involvement of protein binding in modifying a drug's pharmacokinetic profile from *in vitro* data are frequently compounded by the fact that many workers measure binding parameters at drug concentrations well removed from those found *in vivo*.

Metabolism

It is generally thought that only unbound drug is available for metabolism and filtration at the glomerulus. However, assuming that the rates of association and dissociation are very rapid, it would seem unlikely that protein binding is normally the limiting factor in determining the rate of metabolism of most drugs (Meyer and Guttman, 1968).

A theoretical consideration of the effect of protein binding on metabolism has recently been made by Gillette (1971). He suggests that if the activity of the drug-metabolizing enzymes in liver is so high that virtually all the drug is cleared from the blood as it passes through the liver (i.e. extraction ratio nearly one), then an elevation in binding of the drug by plasma proteins could accelerate its metabolism, by increasing the rate at which it is carried to the liver. Alternatively, if very little of the drug is metabolized as it passes through the liver (i.e. extraction ratio nearly zero), an increase in the binding of the drug in the blood may either decrease its metabolism or have little effect. Thus for drugs with a short half-life, protein binding may have a transport function whereas for those with a long half-life it may serve as a storage form. The effect of protein binding on half-lives of drugs which are entirely metabolized has not been elucidated, largely because variations in drug clearance (extraction ratio) tend to obscure the effects of drug binding. Investigation of the effect of protein binding on the metabolism of drugs is further complicated because changes in chemical structure, which can effect the extent of protein binding, may also modify the nature and rate of metabolism. Dayton *et al* (1973) recently discussed the influence of protein binding on drug metabolism and distribution.

Newbould and Kilpatrick (1960) found that addition of plasma to the fluid perfusing a rabbit-liver preparation, reduced the rate of acetylation of two 'long-acting' sulphonamides, and that the rate of metabolism was dependent on the concentration of unbound drug. Later Anton and Boyle (1964) and Wiseman and Nelson (1964) reported a correlation between the rate of metabolism of a sulphonamide and the extent of protein binding. Raz (1972c) has shown that both the rate of metabolism of prostaglandins (F_2 and A_2) and the nature of the metabolites formed, can be affected by plasma-protein binding. The higher affinity of digitoxin ($k = 10^5\ M^{-1}$) for serum albumin compared to digoxin ($k = 10^3\ M^{-1}$) has been held responsible for the higher plasma concentration, lower urinary excretion rate and longer plasma half-life for the former drug in man (Lukas and de Martino, 1969). The presence of warfarin in the plasma and the absence of unchanged drug in urine has also been suggested to result from both its binding to albumin and its nonpolar character (O'Reilly, 1969). On the other hand, hydroxylated metabolites of warfarin, which are more weakly protein bound, are virtually absent from plasma but present in urine. Strong binding, however, does not necessarily result in slower metabolism, for highly protein-bound drugs such as sulphobromophthalein ($k = 10^7\ M^{-1}$) are rapidly metabolized (Brodie and Hogben, 1957).

As large quantities of serum albumin are synthesized on the hepatic endoplasmic reticulum and secreted out of the cell, it is possible that this newly synthesized albumin might bind drug metabolites which are being formed on the endoplasmic reticulum thus enabling their clearance from liver cells. This could constitute an explanation for the lack of hepatic damage caused by some active metabolites formed by the liver cells. However, serum albumin binding does not necessarily enhance chemical stability for in some instances it may act as a 'pseudo enzyme' encouraging metabolic degradation (Brown *et al*, 1974; Tildon and Ogilvie, 1972).

Excretion

Considering the importance of this subject surprisingly few experimental studies have been made. Kakemi *et al* (1962) found an approximate inverse correlation between the binding of a series of salicylates and their rates of excretion. However, such a correlation is likely to hold only for drugs, for which the renal excretion is predominantly determined by the rate of glomerular filtration. For drugs which are actively secreted, e.g. penicillins, protein binding may only have a minimal influence on the excretion rate. Several authors have considered from a theoretical viewpoint the elimination of drugs possessing high binding affinities for plasma proteins, but without complete agreement (Martin, 1965b; Krüger-Thiemer, 1968; Keen 1971).

Rieder (1963), in a study of a number of sulphonamides, was unable to observe a correlation between their protein-binding characteristics and their rate of disappearance from plasma through renal excretion, although Arita *et al* (1971) in an investigation involving two sulphonamides reported that protein binding did affect their glomerular filtration rate. Penicillins have a very high clearance value reflecting tubular secretion which would explain the finding that their $t_{1/2}$ values are relatively insensitive to protein binding (Notari, 1973). In contrast it has been stated that the renal clearance of a series of tetracyclines decreases with increasing protein binding (Fabre *et al*, 1971). Bluestone *et al* (1969) have reported the increased excretion of urate following its displacement from plasma-binding sites by aspirin and phenylbutazone.

The effect of plasma protein binding on biliary excretion is still largely a matter of conjecture (Keen, 1971; Smith, 1971). Several highly bound anions (e.g. bromosulphthalein, bilirubin) have been shown to be rapidly excreted in the bile (Bradley *et al*, 1952). Furthermore, a number of highly protein bound radio-opaque compounds were excreted in the bile, whereas related poorly bound compounds were excreted in the urine (Lasser *et al*, 1962). This would tend to suggest that protein binding may assist biliary excretion, however, the situation is complex for the structural requirements for biliary excretion (Smith, 1973) are largely features which also tend to encourage protein binding independent of a relationship between these two phenomena. In addition, Czok *et al* (1970) have shown that a number of poorly bound compounds (phenolphthalein glucuronide, succinylsulphathiazole) are readily excreted in the bile in the unchanged form. It has also been suggested that binding to plasma proteins may affect the uptake of the drug by the liver cells (Priestly and O'Reilly, 1966; Osorio and Myant, 1965).

Competition for Binding Sites

Binding of an exogenous compound to plasma proteins may potentially increase or decrease the protein binding capacity for other endogenous and exogenous compounds. Alternatively an increase in levels of endogenous materials may lead to changes in drug binding. Displacement phenomena are most frequently noted. Thus competition between endogenous and exogenous compounds such as steroid hormones has been shown to occur (Keller *et al*, 1966), although its significance remains to be ascertained. A number of examples of displacement of endogenous compounds by drugs are known. Odell (1959) has demonstrated that bilirubin can be displaced from serum albumin by sulphonamides with resultant toxicity. This displacement can be of particular significance in premature infants with low plasma-albumin concentrations or in individuals with an impaired capacity to metabolize bilirubin. The view that the antirheumatic activity of certain drugs, e.g. salicylate, phenylbutazone, indomethacin, prednisolone, chloroquine, may be mediated through their ability to displace endogenously plasma protein bound tryptophan and other small peptides has been proposed (McArthur *et al*, 1971; Smith *et al*, 1971). It has also been suggested (Brodie, 1965) that some antiinflammatory drugs may act by displacing steroids from plasma binding sites.

Numerous drugs have been shown *in vitro* and in animal experiments to compete for plasma protein binding sites (Meyer and Guttman, 1968) and many potential drug–drug interactions have been reviewed (Hussar, 1969; Hartshorn, 1970; Sellers and Koch-Weser, 1970a, b; Sher, 1971; Swidler, 1971; Baker and Neuhaus, 1972). Competition between compounds for protein-binding sites is likely to be of particular importance when the drug's distribution volume is small. If the drug on displacement is readily taken up by other tissue-binding sites then this biological efficacy may not be significantly modified. The data relating to human subjects, is unfortunately very limited and largely anecdotal. This type of interaction has been suggested to be the cause of clinically undesirable side effects in a number of instances. The most frequently cited cases are the displacement of the anticoagulant drug warfarin by highly bound drugs such as phenylbutazone, chlorophenoxyisobutyric acid, indomethacin, salicylate, fatty acids and various sulphonamides (Solomon and Schrogie, 1967; Solomon *et al*, 1967), from both plasma and tissue-binding sites, such as the liver, leading to increased anticoagulant effect which may give rise to spontaneous haemorrhage, and the displacement of the oral hypoglycaemic drug, tolbutamide by bishydroxycoumarin causing a sudden hypoglycaemic crisis. Displacement phenomena may be of particular potential importance in the case of those drugs which are frequently self-prescribed and not regarded as drugs by patients. Drug displacement might, in certain circumstances, also be of potential clinical value (Mroszczak *et al*, 1969). Thus highly albumin-bound pharmacologically relatively inert excipients such as sodium trichloroacetate, which lower the dose of a drug necessary to produce a given pharmacological response, might be included in a pharmaceutical preparation of a drug such as warfarin in order to give stable blood levels even when other highly bound drugs known to displace warfarin are concurrently administered. Because of the complexity of protein binding and our lack of a thorough understanding of it, this approach could only be used in special controlled circumstances.

For a clinical standpoint it is important to distinguish between potential and actual drug interactions since competitive phenomena, which are readily demonstrable *in vitro*, may not be of sufficient magnitude to have a clinical effect or may be obscured by other factors *in vivo*. It is unfortunately difficult to predict the displacement of one drug by another merely from a knowledge of binding data and plasma concentrations. Yesair *et al* (1972) have recently discussed the mechanisms by which drug interactions can occur.

Wardell (1974) has suggested that the following criteria should be met before it can be accepted that an observed drug interaction in man is primarily operating via the displacement of a drug from plasma-protein binding site(s).

(i) Demonstrate displacement of the drug from human plasma *in vitro*.

(ii) Establish that an *in vivo* fall in total plasma concentration of the displaced drug occurs and that it is partially offset by a rise in free drug.

(iii) Show that the whole body gain in free drug is equal to or less than the loss of bound drug.

(iv) Prove quantitatively whether redistribution alone can wholly account for the observed pharmacokinetic changes. Useful indicators being:

(a) the mimicking of the effect by another chemically dissimilar displacer with comparable displacing activity.
(b) a rapid and short-lived onset of enhanced pharmacological activity.
(c) elimination of other interaction possibilities such as modified absorption, metabolism, excretion, receptor-site response and competition at tissue-binding sites.

It must be emphasized that a drug with a higher association constant (k) does not necessarily displace a drug of lower affinity unless both share common binding sites. It is axiomatic, however, that until such mechanisms are better understood, great caution must be exercised when administering novel combinations of drugs known to be highly protein bound. Reports that hospitalized patients in America (Seidl *et al*, 1965) received an average of 13 different drugs during a patient's stay, emphasizes this need for caution. Appropriate *in vitro* screening tests must be sought since it is unrealistic to test all combinations in the far more complex *in vivo* experiments.

A potentially suitable rapid *in vitro* interaction-assessment method for warfarin has been devised by Wilson and Bridges (unpublished data) based on the red shift the reduction in warfarin fluorescence when a drug displaces it from its albumin-binding site. Using this approach it was found that phenylbutazone, sulphormethoxine and clofibrate appeared to interact competitively, biphenyl noncompetitively, while diazepam, chlordiazepoxide, iprindole, pentobarbital and hexyl carbamate did not significantly displace warfarin.

Binding of Drugs to Tissues

The major contributor to competitive protein binding with blood constituents is undoubtedly tissue protein binding, unfortunately knowledge of this binding is still in a primitive state compared with that of albumin binding. Since the ratio of tissue mass to albumin mass is of the order of 100 : 1, it is apparent that for many compounds tissue binding may be of more importance than albumin binding. It is usually assumed that the fraction of unbound drug in the tissues is the same as the unbound fraction in the plasma. However, the situation *in vivo* may be complicated by binding to tissue proteins, which will entail a series of equilibria being established between the tissues of various organs and the tissue fluids. Furthermore, whereas tissue uptake after a single dose of a drug may be rapid, disappearance is often slow (Wagner, 1973). Evidence to support the similarity of tissue fluid concentration with the unbound plasma level in the case of protein-bound drugs comes from a number of sources. Verwey and Williams (1962a, b) used dogs to show that the concentration of protein-bound penicillins in lymph was directly related to that of the plasma concentrations. Furthermore, Scholtan and Schmid (1962) provided experimental evidence in mice which indicated that the levels of unbound penicillin and propicillin in serum were very similar to those in tissue fluid, even though levels of total drug were quite different. Kunin (1965) demonstrated that the distributions of penicillins in the tissues of rabbit was inversely related to their known binding to rabbit serum. Further support has come from the work of McQueen (1968) who, using an *in vitro* dialysis technique, has reported that the concentration of sulphormethoxine in the peritoneal fluid of the rat corresponded well with the unbound fraction in serum. However, in the case of drugs which are highly bound to tissues, drug levels per unit weight of tissue may well be in excess of the concentration of free drug in the plasma. Brodie (1952) demonstrated that three hours after an intravenous injection of the ultra short-acting barbiturate, thiopentone, levels in the fat were ten times higher than in plasma, while Burns *et al* (1953) reported higher unbound phenylbutazone levels in lung, heart and muscle than in plasma. Lullman and van Zweiten (1969) have shown that the cardiac glycosides were both highly bound to plasma proteins and to isolated atria, and demonstrated that tissue binding was not directly proportional to biological activity, thus indicating that plasma binding and tissue binding may be similar processes, each sequestering drug and thereby lowering free-drug concentration.

Drug displacement from the tissue binding sites can also occur, and has been demonstrated by the interaction between the antimalarial drugs, mepacrine and pamaquine, in patients (Brodie, 1966). This interaction appeared to be the cause of the potentiation of the toxic effects of pamaquine, which exhibits only a small safety margin between the concentrations causing its therapeutic and toxic effects. It is apparent that consideration of redistributional drug interactions must take into account both displacement from plasma protein, and tissue-binding sites. The possibility of displacement from both intravascular and extravascular albumin, which is approximately three times that of the intravascular pool (Sellers *et al*, 1966), should be considered.

The driving force for the exchange of compounds between plasma proteins and tissue proteins is poorly understood. If the affinity of the tissue binding sites for a compound is much greater than that of the blood proteins, or if the time of exposure of the blood protein-bound drug to unsaturated tissue binding sites is relatively long, then fo further explanation need be sought. However, for many compounds neither situation pertains. A possible explanation of the means by which albumin fulfils its transport role to specific tissues is that the conformation of albumin is altered by its combination with 'receptor sites' on the surface of the cells of such tissues thus weakening the binding of the compound to the albumin and enabling its release into the cell. The validity or otherwise of this concept awaits experimental verification.

Binding may occur to the cell-membrane nucleus, other cytoplasmic organelles or cytosol. This binding may be with proteins, polypeptides, lipids or polysaccharides (Woolley and Gommi, 1966). A number of binding proteins to which both endogenous and exogenous molecules are known to associate have been isolated from cells of various organs. Rat kidneys have been found to contain aldosterone-binding proteins (Guidollet and Louisot, 1969). Two hepatic cytoplasmic proteins Y (ligandin, which may constitute up to 5·10% of the cytosol protein) and Z, have been isolated, purified and characterized (Levi *et al*, 1969; Reyes *et al*, 1971) and shown to bind sulphobromophthalein, bilirubin, haem, corticosteroids, carcinogens and various dyes. The amount of ligandin (Litwack *et al*, 1971) increases significantly in rat liver following phenobarbitone pretreatment (Reyes *et al*, 1969). The cytoplasmic proteins Y and Z are found largely in the liver in a great variety of animals although they may also be present in other tissues (Reyes *et al*, 1971; Ockner *et al*, 1972). Their function is unclear but they could be involved in the uptake of small molecules by exchange with plasma proteins, in intracellular transport or as an essential mediator via the compound bound complex, of the biological action of endogenous (and perhaps some exogenous) compounds. It is likely that a number of specific and nonspecific cellular binding proteins will be isolated and characterized in the future which will enable a more sophisticated interpretation of tissue-binding phenomena.

In embryonic serum and in many subjects with carcinoma, α-foetoprotein, a protein which has been claimed to serve as the foetal equivalent of serum albumin occurs. Although its drug-binding capability remains to be established, it has been demonstrated to display a high affinity for oestradiol (Uriel *et al*, 1972).

Many drugs bind to microsomal components, particularly to cytochrome

P-450. For neutral molecules the extent of binding correlates very well with the log p value indicating predominantly hydrophobic bonding (Al-Gailany *et al*, 1976). Comparison of the structure-binding relationships suggests that the so called 'type I' association of drug with cytochrome P-450 is mainly through an interaction largely similar to that involved in drug binding to serum albumin, although the binding protein may represent only a small proportion of the total-protein content of microsomes. Bickel and Steele (1974) showed that chlorpromazine and imipramine irreversibly bind *in vitro* to both the microsomes and mitochondria of a wide variety of tissues including liver, lung, brain, kidney, erythrocytes and skeletal muscle, through both high affinity ($k = 10^5\ M^{-1}$) and low affinity ($k = 10^3\ M^{-1}$) interactions. The dissociation constant for the high-affinity site(s) were considerably larger than those reported for serum albumin. Conversely they showed that acidic drugs such as warfarin, sulphadimethoxine, salicylic acid and phenylbutazone, which show strong binding to serum albumin showed only weak binding to either microsomes or mitochondria.

It is apparent from these and other studies that although the binding of a drug to serum albumin may often mirror the tissue binding, for a number of drugs at least, the nature of the interactions between drug and albumin are quite different from those involved in drug-tissue binding. Further investigations on selective tissue binding of particular drugs could well take us further towards Ehrlich's goal of the 'magic-bullet' drug.

CONCLUSIONS

With the possible exception of cytochrome P-450, the ability of serum albumin to bind a diverse range of compounds with apparently unrelated chemical and physical properties appears to be unique.

The quest for a thorough comprehension of the nature and mechanism of drug binding to serum albumin and other serum proteins is worthwhile from two major standpoints:

(i) It should serve as an important model in anticipating and understanding other drug–protein interactions such as enzyme (including cytochrome P-450), receptor site and tissue binding.

(ii) It would enable more accurate prediction of the pharmacokinetic behaviour of protein-bound drugs to be made.

If a protein binding mechanisms are to be elucidated it is apparent that a systematic approach, using homologous series of compounds, will be necessary. It appears from the few systematic investigations which have been carried out that hydrophobic interactions are usually the predominant binding force although contributions from other bonds may assume a major role for particular classes of compounds. The characterization of these binding sites requires more detailed information on the primary, secondary and tertiary, protein structures. Some considerable caution in interpretation of such data may be necessary, because serum albumin may exist in a number of energetically equivalent conformational forms in solution, in which case information on its tertiary structure and potential binding sites derived from studies on the crystalline protein, may be misleading. However, studies on chemically modified albumins and albumin fractions and employment of techniques such as photoaffinity labelling, which can be used in a number of instances to covalently binding compounds to amino acids, thus enabling the amino acids concerned to be identified, would also appear to be particularly relevant approaches. Valuable information could also be derived from tailor-made fluorescent, phosphorescent electron-spin resonant or light-polarizing probe molecules.

The likely significance of protein binding in a particular clinical context is dependent on a number of factors including the level of drug in the blood, the ability of the excretory and biotransformation mechanisms to clear it, the spectrum of blood and tissue proteins to which it binds and their relative affinity constants and the concentration of endogenous and exogenous compounds which are competing for binding sites.

On theoretical grounds, plasma-protein binding affinity constants greater than $10^{-4}\,M^{-1}$ would appear to be necessary for protein binding to be of prime importance in influencing drug fate. It is unfortunate that even for such highly bound drugs total blood levels rather than free blood levels are normally recorded. It is scarcely surprising that measurement of total blood levels in these cases frequently gives poor correlation with therapeutic or toxicological effects. In part the disinclination to measure free blood levels stems from the technical difficulties involved. In many cases these problems could be overcome by displacement methods (cf radioimmunoassay) in which a very small amount of the high activity radiolabelled drug or a strongly fluorescent compound which competes for the drug-binding sites is added to blood from a patient receiving the drug followed by a microscale dialysis or ultrafiltration and estimation of the free radioactivity or fluorescence recovered. Hopefully the adoption of these approaches will become more widespread in the future thus permitting a more realistic appraisal of the relationship between drug-blood levels and biological efficacy.

REFERENCES

Agren, A. and Elofsson, R. (1967), *Acta Pharm. Suec.*, **4**, 281.
Agren, A., Elofsson, R., Meresaar, U. and Nilsson, S.-O. (1970), *Acta Pharm. Suec.*, **7**, 105.
Agren, A., Elofsson, R. and Nilsson, S.-O. (1971), *Acta Pharmacol. Toxicol.*, **29**, 48.
Ahtee, L., Boullin, D. J., Saarnivaara, L. and Paasonen, M. K. (1974), in Forrest, I. S., Carr, C. J. and Usdin, E. (ed.), *The phenothiazines and structurally related drugs*, pp. 379–388, Raven Press, New York.
Alexanderson, B. and Borgå, O. (1972), *Eur. J. Clin. Pharmacol.*, **4**, 196.
Al-Gailany, K., Houston, J. B., Bridges, J. W. and Netter, K. J. (1976), in press.
Andreasen, F. (1973), *Acta Pharmacol. Toxicol.*, **32**, 417.

Anton, A. H. (1960), *J. Pharmacol. Exp. Ther.*, **129**, 282.
Anton, A. H. (1968), *Clin. Pharmacol. Ther.*, **9**, 561.
Anton, A. H. and Boyle, J. J. (1964), *Can. J. Physiol. Pharmacol.*, **42**, 809.
Anton, A. H. and Corey, W. T. (1971), *Acta Pharmacol. Toxicol.*, **29**, 134.
Anton, A. H. and Solomon, H. M. (ed.) (1973), *Ann. NY Acad. Sci.*, **226**, 1–362.
Arango, G., Mayberry, W. E., Hockert, T. J. and Elveback, L. R. (1968), *Mayo Clin. Proc.*, **43**, 503.
Arita, T., Hori, R., Takada, M. and Misawa, A. (1971), *Chem. Pharm. Bull.*, **19**, 937.
Attalah, N. A. and Lata, G. F. (1968), *Biochim. Biophys. Acta*, **168**, 321.
Aziz, O. and Dennhardt, R. (1973), *Pflugers Arch.*, **341**, 347.
Baggot, J. D., Davis, L. E. and Neff, C. A. (1972), *Biochem. Pharmacol.*, **21**, 1813.
Baker, S. B. de C. and Neuhaus, G. A. (ed.) (1972), *Proc. Eur. Soc. Drug. Tox.*, **13**.
Barbanti-Brodano, G., Derenzini, M. and Fiume, L. (1974), *Nature*, **248**, 63.
Baulieu, E. E. and Raynaud, J. P. (1970), *Eur. J. Biochem.*, **13**, 293.
Bennett, J. V. and Kirby, W. M. M. (1965), *J. Lab. Clin. Med.*, **66**, 721.
Bennhold, H. (1938), in Bennhold, H., Kylin, E. and Rusznyak, S. (ed.), *Die Eiweisskörper des Butplasmas*, Steinkopf, Leipzig.
Bennhold, H. (1966), in Desgrez, P. and De Traverse, P. M. (ed.), *Transport function of plasma proteins*, pp. 1–12, Elsevier, Amsterdam.
Bickel, M. H. and Bovet, D. (1962), *J. Chromatogr.*, **8**, 466.
Bickel, M. H. and Steele, J. W. (1974), *Chem.-Biol. Inter.* **8**, 151.
Bird, A. E. and Marshall, A. G. (1967), *Biochem. Pharmacol.*, **16**, 2275.
Bjerrum, J. (1941), in *Metal amine formation in aqueous solution*, P. Hassa & Son, Copenhagen.
Blatt, W. F., Robinson, S. M. and Bixler, H. J. (1968), *Anal. Biochem.*, **26**, 151.
Bluestone, R., Kippen, I. and Klinenberg, J. R. (1969), *Brit. Med. J.*, **4**, 590.
Borgå, O., Azarnoff, D. L. and Sjöqvist, F. (1968), *J. Pharm. Pharmacol.*, **20**, 571.
Borgå, O., Azarnoff, D. L., Forshell, G. P. and Sjöqvist, F. (1969), *Biochem. Pharmacol.*, **18**, 2135.
Borondy, P., Dill, W. A., Chang, T., Buchanan, R. A. and Glazko, A. J. (1973), *Ann. NY Acad. Sci.*, **226**, 82.
Bradley, S. E., Ingelfinger, F. J. and Bradley, G. P. (1952), *Circulation*, **5**, 419.
Bradshaw, R. A. and Peters, T. J. (1969), *J. Biol. Chem.*, **244**, 5582.
Brand, L. and Gohlke, J. R. (1972), *Ann. Rev. Biochem.*, **41**, 843.
Bratlid, D. (1972), *Scand. J. Clin. Lab. Invest.*, **29**, 91.
Bridgman, J. F., Rosen, S. M. and Thorp, J. M. (1972), *Lancet*, **11**, 505.
Brinkmann, A. O. and van der Molen, H. J. (1972), *Biochim. Biophys. Acta*, **274**, 370.
Brodie, B. B. (1952), *Fed. Proc.*, **11**, 632.
Brodie, B. B. (1965), *Proc. Roy. Soc. Med.*, **58**, 946.
Brodie, B. B. (1966), in Desgrez, P. and De Traverse, P. M. (ed.), *Transport function of plasma proteins*, pp. 137–145, Elsevier, Amsterdam.
Brodie, B. B. and Hogben, C. A. M. (1957), *J. Pharm. Pharmacol.*, **9**, 345.
Brown, N. A., King, R. F. G. J., Shillcock, M. E. and Brown, S. B. (1974), *Biochem. J.*, **137**, 135.
Burgen, A. S. V. and Metcalfe, J. C. (1970), *J. Pharm. Pharmacol.*, **22**, 153.
Burns, J. J., Rose, R. K., Chenkin, T., Goldman, A., Schulert, A. and Brodie, B. B. (1953), *J. Pharmacol. Exp. Ther.*, **109**, 346.
Chignell, C. F. (1970a), *Mol. Pharmacol.*, **6**, 1.
Chignell, C. F. (1970b), *Fluorescence News*, **5**, 1.
Chignell, C. F. (1971), in Brodie, B. B. and Gillette, J. R. (ed.), *Handbook of experimental pharmacology*, vol. 27 (part 1), pp. 187–211, Springer-Verlag, Berlin.
Chignell, C. F. (1972), in Chignell, C. F. (ed.), *Methods in pharmacology*, vol. 2, pp. 33–61, Appleton–Century–Crofts, New York.

Chignell, C. F. and Chignell, D. A. (1972), in Chignell, C. F. (ed.), *Methods in pharmacology*, vol. 2, pp. 111–156, Appleton–Century–Crofts, New York.
Chignell, C. F. and Starkweather, D. K. (1971), *Pharmacology*, **5**, 235.
Chu, F. S. (1974), *Biochem. Pharmacol.*, **23**, 1105.
Churchich, J. E. (1972), *Biochim. Biophys. Acta*, **285**, 91.
Clark, A. F., Calandra, R. S. and Bird, C. E. (1971), *Clin. Biochem.*, **4**, 89.
Clausen, J. (1966), *J. Pharmacol. Exp. Ther.*, **153**, 167.
Coffey, J. J. (1972), *J. Pharm. Sci.*, **61**, 138.
Coffey, J. J., Bullock, F. J. and Schoenemann, P. T. (1971), *J. Pharm. Sci.*, **60**, 1623.
Cohen, Y. (1971), "Radionuclides in Pharmacology", *Int. Encycl. Pharmacol. Ther.*, section 78, p. 241.
Colombo, C., Piliero, S. J. and Grosso, L. (1968), *J. Pharm. Sci.*, **57**, 1526.
Colowick, S. P. and Womack, F. C. (1969), *J. Biol. Chem.*, **244**, 774.
Cooke, J. R. and Roberts, L. B. (1969), *Clin. Chim. Acta*, **26**, 425.
Cooper, P. F. and Wood, G. C. (1968), *J. Pharm. Pharmacol.*, **20**, Suppl. 150S.
Crawford, J. S., Jones, R. L., Thompson, J. M. and Wells, W. D. E. (1972), *Brit. J. Pharmacol.*, **44**, 80.
Crothers, D. M. (1968), *Biopolymers*, **6**, 575.
Crothers, D. M. and Ratner, D. I. (1968), *Biochemistry*, **7**, 1823.
Curry, S. H. (1970a), *J. Pharm. Pharmacol.*, **22**, 193.
Curry, S. H. (1970b), *J. Pharm. Pharmacol.*, **22**, 753.
Czok, G., Hirom, P., Millburn, P., Smith, R. L. and Williams, R. T. (1970), unpublished observations cited by Smith, R. L. (1971), in Brodie, B. B. and Gillette, J. R. (ed.), *Handbook of experimental pharmacology*, vol. 28 (part 1), Springer-Verlag, Berlin.
Danon, A. and Sapira, J. D. (1972), *J. Pharm. Exp. Ther.*, **182**, 295.
Davis, B. D. (1943), *J. Clin. Invest.*, **22**, 753.
Davis, P. J. and Gregerman, R. I. (1971), *J. Clin. Endocrinol. Metab.*, **33**, 699.
Davison, C. (1971), in La Du, B. N., Mandel, H. G. and Way, E. L. (ed.), *Fundamentals of Drug Metabolism and Drug Disposition*, pp. 63–75, Williams and Wilkins, Baltimore.
Davison, C. and Smith, P. K. (1961), *J. Pharmacol. Exp. Ther.*, **133**, 161.
Dayton, P. G., Israili, Z. M. and Perel, J. M. (1973), *Ann NY Acad. Sci.*, **226**, 172.
Dearden, J. C. and Tomlinson, E. (1970), *J. Pharm. Pharmacol.*, **22**, Suppl. 53S.
Dearden, J. C. and Tomlinson, E. (1971), *J. Pharm. Pharmacol.*, **23**, Suppl. 68S.
Deranleau, D. A. (1969), *J. Amer. Chem. Soc.*, **91**, 4044.
Desgrez, P. and De Traverse, P. M. (ed.) (1966), *Transport function of plasma proteins*, Elsevier, Amsterdam.
Dettlebach, H. R. and Ritzmann, S. E. (ed.) (1968) *Laboratory notes for medical diagnostics*, Hoechst Pharmaceuticals, Brentford (Middlesex).
Dunn, W. J. (1973), *J. Pharm. Sci.*, **62**, 1575.
Edsall, J. T. and Wyman, J. (1958), *Biophysical chemistry*, **1**, p. 591, Academic Press, New York.
Ehrnebo, M., Agurell, S. Boreus, L. O., Gordon, E., and Lonroth, U. (1974), *Clin. Pharmacol. Ther.*, **16**, 424.
Ehrstrom, M. C. H. (1937), *Acta Med. Scand.*, **91**, 191.
Fabre, J., Milek, E., Kalfopoulos, P. and Merier, G. (1971), *Schweiz. Med. Wochenschr.*, **101**, 625.
Feldman, H. A. (1972), *Anal. Biochem.*, **48**, 317.
Fischer, J. J. (1971), in A. Schwartz (ed.), *Methods in pharmacology*, vol. 1, (pp. 431–453), Appleton-Century-Crofts, New York.
Fletcher, J. E. and Spector, A. A. (1968), *Comput. Biomed. Res.*, **2**, 164.
Fletcher, J. E., Ashbrook, J. D. and Spector, A. A. (1973), *Ann. NY Acad. Sci.*, **226**, 69.
Fletcher, J. E., Spector, A. A. and Ashbrook, J. D. (1970), *Biochemistry*, **9**, 4580.

Foster, J. F. (1960) in Putnam, F. W. (ed.), *The Plasma Proteins*, Academic Press, New York.
Franksson, G. and Anggård, E. (1970), *Acta Pharmacol. Toxicol.*, **28**, 209.
Frank, H. S. and Wen, W. Y. (1957), *Discuss. Faraday Soc.*, **24**, 133.
Frank, H. S. and Evans, M. W. (1945), *J. Chem. Phys.*, **13**, 507.
Franz, J. W., Jähnchen, E. and Kreiglstein, J. (1969), *Arch. Pharmakol.*, **264**, 462.
Freunlich, H. (1907), *Z. Physik. Chem.*, **57**, 385.
Fujita, T. (1972), *J. Med. Chem.*, **15**, 1049.
Fujita, T. and Hansch, C. (1967), *J. Med. Chem.*, **10**, 991.
Gabay, S. and Huang, P. C. (1974), in I. S. Forrest, Carr, C. J. and Usdin, E. (ed.), *The phenothiazines and structurally related drugs*, Raven Press, New York.
Galardy, R. E., Craig, L. C., Jamieson, J. D. and Printz, M. P. (1974), *J. Biol. Chem.*, **249**, 3510.
Genazzani, E. and Santamaria, R. (1969), *Pharmacol. Res. Commun.*, **1**, 249.
Glave, W. R. and Hansch, C. (1972), *J. Pharm. Sci.*, **61**, 589.
Gillette, J. R. (1971), *Ann. NY Acad. Sci.*, **179**, 43.
Goodman, D. S. (1958), *J. Amer. Chem. Soc.*, **80**, 3892.
Goldstein, A. (1949), *Pharmacol. Rev.*, **1**, 102.
Goldstein, A., Aronow, L. and Kalman, S. M. (1968), in *Principles of drug action*, Hoeber, New York.
Guidollet, J. and Louisot, P. (1969), *Clin. Chim. Acta*, **23**, 121.
Gulassay, P. F., Peters, J. H. and Schoenfeld, P. (1971), *Fifth Ann. Meet. Amer. Chem. Soc., Nephrol. Abstr. 29.*
Gutfreund, H. (1972), in *Enzymes: Physical Principles*, John Wiley, London.
Haaf, E. (ed.) (1969), *Laboratory notes for medical diagnostics*, Hoechst Pharmaceuticals, Brentford (Middlesex).
Halfman, C. J. and Nishida, T. (1972), *Biochemistry*, **11**, 3493.
Hansch, C. (1968), *J. Med. Chem.*, **11**, 920.
Hansch, C. (1969), *Acta Chem. Res.*, **2**, 232.
Hansch, C. (1971), in Ariens, E. J. (ed.), *Drug design*, vol. 1, pp. 271–337, Academic Press, New York.
Hansch, C., Kiehs, K. and Lawrence, G. L. (1965), *J. Amer. Chem. Soc.*, **87**, 5770.
Harrington, W. F., Johnson, P. and Ottewill, R. H. (1956), *Biochem. J.*, **62**, 569.
Hart, H. E. (1965), *Bull. Math. Biophys.*, **27**, 87.
Hartshorn, E. A. (1970), *Handbook of Drug Interactions*, Wiley–Interscience, New York.
Hermann, R. B. (1971), *J. Phys. Chem.*, **75**, 363.
Herskovits, T. T. (1967), in Colowick, S. P. and Kaplan, N. O. (ed.), *Methods in Enzymology*, vol. 2, pp. 748–775, Academic Press, New York.
Heyns, W., van Baelen, H. and de Moor, P. (1969), *J. Endocrinol.*, **43**, 67.
Hildebrand, J. H. (1968), *J. Phys. Chem.*, **72**, 1841.
Hippe, E. and Olesen, H. (1971), *Biochim. Biophys. Acta*, **243**, 83.
Hollis, D. P. (1972), in Chignell, C. F. (ed.), *Methods in Pharmacology*, vol. 2, pp. 191–221, Appleton Century Crofts, New York.
Holtzer, A., and Emerson, M. F. (1969), *J. Phys. Chem.*, **73**, 26.
Houston, J. B., Upshall, D. G. and Bridges, J. W. (1974), *J. Pharmacol. Exp. Ther.*, **189**, 244.
Howell, A., Sutherland, R. and Rolinson, G. N. (1972), *Clin. Pharmacol. Ther.*, **13**, 724.
Huang, P. C. and Gabay, S. (1974), *Biochem. Pharmacol.*, **23**, 957.
Hummel, J. P. and Dreyer, W. J. (1962), *Biochim. Biophys. Acta*, **63**, 530.
Hussar, D. A. (1969), *Amer. J. Pharm.*, **141**, 109.
Ivkova, M. N., Vedenkina, N. S. and Burstein, E. A. (1971), *Molekul. Biologiya*, **5**, 214.
Jähnchen, E., Krieglstein, J. and Kuschinsky, G. (1969), *Arch. Pharmacol.*, **263**, 375.

Jähnchen, E., Krieglstein, J., Kunkel, F., Samuelis, W. J. and Wollert, U. (1971), *Arch. Pharmacol.* **269**, 67.
Janatovā, J. (1974), *J. Med.* **5**, 149.
Jardetzky, O. and Wade-Jardetzky, N. G. (1965), *Mol. Pharmacol.*, **1**, 214.
Jirgensons, B. (1962), *Arch. Biochem. Biophys.*, **96**, 321.
Jonas, A. (1972), *J. Biol. Chem.*, **247**, 7767.
Jonas, A. and Weber, G. (1971), *Biochemistry*, **10**, 1335.
Jorgensen, A., Hansen, V. and Overø, K. F. (1973), *Acta Pharmacol. Toxicol.*, **33**, 81.
Judis, J. (1972), *J. Pharm. Sci.*, **61**, 89.
Kakemi, K., Arita, T., Hori, R., Konishi, R. and Nishimura, K. (1969), *Chem. Pharm. Bull.*, **17**, 248.
Kakemi, K., Arita, T., Yamashina, H. and Konishi, R. (1962), *J. Pharm. Soc.* (*Japan*), **82**, 536.
Kanai, M., Raz, A. and Goodman, D. S. (1968), *J. Clin. Invest.*, **47**, 2025.
Karush, F. (1950a), *J. Amer. Chem. Soc.*, **72**, 2705.
Karush, F. (1950b), *J. Amer. Chem. Soc.*, **72**, 2714.
Karush, F. and Sonenburg, M. (1949), *J. Amer. Chem. Soc.*, **71**, 1369.
Kauzmann, W. (1959), *Adv. Protein Chem.*, **14**, 1.
Kawasaki, H., Oma, H., Sakaguchi, S., Tominaga, K. and Hirayama, C. (1973) **47**, 39.
Keen, P. M. (1965), *Brit. J. Pharmacol.*, **25**, 507.
Keen, P. M. (1971), in Brodie, B. B. and Gillette, J. R. (ed.), *Handbook of experimental pharmacology*, vol. 28 (part 1), pp. 213–239. Springer-Verlag, Berlin.
Keller, N., Richardson, U. I. and Yates, F. E. (1969), *Endocrinol.*, **84**, 49.
Keller, N., Sendelbeck, L. R., Richardson, U. I., Moore, C. and Yates, F. E. (1966), *Endocrinol.*, **79**, 884.
Keresztes-Nagy, S., Mais, R. F., Oester, Y. T. and Zaroslinski, J. F. (1972), *Anal. Biochem.*, **48**, 80.
Kiefer, H. J., Lindstrom, J., Lennox, E. S. and Singer, S. J. (1970), *Proc. Nat. Acad. Sci. USA*, **67**, 1688.
King, T. P. and Spencer, M. (1970), *J. Biol. Chem.*, **245**, 6134.
Klotz, I. M. (1946), *J. Amer. Chem. Soc.*, **68**, 2299.
Klotz, I. M. (1949), *Cold Spring Harbor Symp. Quant. Biol.*, **14**, 97.
Klotz, I. M. (1953), in Neurath, H. and Bailey, K. (ed.), *The proteins*, 1st ed, vol. 1, p. 727, Academic Press, New York.
Klotz, I. M. (1958), *Science*, **128**, 815.
Klotz, I. M. (1973), *Ann. NY Acad. Sci.*, **226**, 18.
Klotz, I. M., Triwush, H. and Walker, F. M. (1948), *J. Amer. Chem. Soc.*, **70**, 2935.
Klotz, I. M. and Walker, F. M. (1948), *J. Amer. Chem. Soc.*, **70**, 943.
Klotz, I. M. and Hunston, D. L. (1971), *Biochemistry*, **10**, 3065.
Knowles, J. R. (1972), *Accts. Chem. Res.*, **5**, 155.
Koshland, D. E. (1958), *Proc. Nat Acad. Sci.*, U.S.A., **44**, 98.
Korolkovas, A. (1970), *Essentials of molecular pharmacology*, Wiley–Interscience, New York.
Kostenbauder, H. B., Bahal, S. M. and Jadwad, M. J. (1970), *J. Pharm. Sci.*, **59**, 1047.
Krasner, J. (1973), *Biochem. Med.*, **7**, 135.
Krieglstein, J. (1969), *Klin. Wochenschr.*, **40**, 153.
Krieglstein, J., Lier, F. and Michaelis, J. (1972a), *Arch. Pharmacol.*, **272**, 121.
Krieglstein, J., Meiler, W. and Staab, J. (1972b), *Biochem. Pharmacol.*, **21**, 985.
Krüger-Thiemer, E. (1968), in *Physico-chemical aspects of drug actions*, p. 63, Pergamon, Oxford.
Krüger-Thiemer, E., Bunger, P., Dettli, L., Spring, P. and Wempe, E. (1965), *Chemotherapia*, **10**, 325.
Kucera, J. L. and Bullock, F. L. (1969), *J. Pharm. Pharmacol.*, **21**, 293.
Kunin, C. M. (1965), *J. Lab. Clin. Med.*, **65**, 406.

Kurtz, H. and Friemel, G. (1967), *Arch. Exp. Path. Pharmak.*, **257**, 35.
Küsnir, J. and Meloun, B. (1973), *Biochim. Biophys. Acta*, **310**, 124.
Laiken, N. and Nemethy, G. (1970a), *J. Physical Chem.*, **74**, 4421.
Laiken, N. and Nemethy, G. (1970b), *J. Physical Chem.*, **74**, 4431.
Langmuir, I. (1917) *J. Amer. Chem. Soc.*, **39**, 1848.
Lasser, E. C., Farr, R. S., Fujimagari, T. and Tripp, W. N. (1962), *Amer. J. Roentgenol.*, **87**, 338.
Lea, O. A. and Støa, K. F. (1972), *J. Steroid Biochem.*, **3**, 409.
Levi, A. J., Gatmaitan, Z. and Arias, I. M. (1969), *J. Clin. Invest.*, **48**, 2156.
Levy, G. (1973), *Ann. NY Acad. Sci.*, **226**, 195.
Levy, G. and Nagashima, R. (1969), *J. Pharm. Sci.*, **58**, 1001.
Litwack, G., Ketterer, B. and Arias, I. M. (1971), *Nature*, **234**, 466.
Lukas, D. S. and DeMartino, A. G. (1969), *J. Clin. Invest.*, **48**, 1041.
Lullman, H. and van Zweiten, P. A. (1969), *J. Pharm. Pharmacol.*, **21**, 1.
Manian, A. A., Piette, L. H., Holland, D., Grover, T. and Leterrier, F. (1974), in Forrest, I. S., Carr, C. J. and Usdin, E. (ed.), *The phenothiazines and structurally related drugs*, pp. 149–161, Raven Press, New York.
Maren, T. H. (1967), *Physiol. Rev.*, **47**, 595.
Marks, V. (1972), *Teach-in*, (Aug., p. 641; Sept., p. 711; Nov., p. 861; Dec., p. 909).
Martin, B. K. (1965a), *Nature*, **207**, 274.
Martin, B. K. (1965b), *Nature*, **207**, 959.
Mateau, L., Tardieu, A., Luzzati, V., Aggerback, L. and Scanu, A. M. (1972), *J. Mol. Biol.*, **70**, 105.
McArthur, J. N. and Smith, M. J. H. (1969), *J. Pharm. Pharmacol.*, **21**, 589.
McArthur, J. N., Dawkins, P. D., Smith, M. J. H. and Hamilton, E. B. D. (1971), *Brit. Med. J.*, **2**, 677.
McQueen, E. G. (1968), *Brit. J. Pharmacol.*, **33**, 312.
McQueen, E. G. (1969), *Brit. J. Pharmacol.*, **36**, 29.
Means, G. E. and Feeney, R. E. (1971), *Chemical modification of proteins*, Holden–Day Inc., San Francisco.
Meloun, B. and Küsnir, J. (1972), *FEBS Lett.*, **27**, 121.
Meyer, M. C. and Guttman, D. E. (1968), *J. Pharm. Sci.*, **57**, 895.
Meyer, M. C. and Guttman, D. E. (1970a), *J. Pharm. Sci.*, **59**, 33.
Meyer, M. C. and Guttman, D. E. (1970b), *J. Pharm. Sci.*, **59**, 39.
Mikkelson, T. J., Chrai, S. S. and Robinson, J. R. (1973), *J. Pharm. Sci.*, **62**, 1648.
Miller, L. L. and Bale, M. F. (1954), *Medicine*, **99**, 125.
Mohammadzadeh-K, A., Feeney, P. E. and Smith, L. M. (1969a), *Biochim. Biophys. Acta*, **194**, 246.
Mohammadzadeh-K, A., Smith, L. M. and Feeney, P. E. (1969b), *Biochim. Biophys. Acta*, **194**, 256.
Molyneux, P. and Frank, H. P. (1969), *J. Amer. Chem. Soc.*, **83**, 3169.
Monod, J., Changeux, J. P. and Jacob, F. (1963), *J. Mol. Biol.*, **6**, 306.
Mora, R., Rebeyrotte, P. and Polonovski, J. (1955), *Bull. Soc. Chim. Biol.*, **37**, 957.
Morgan, H. G., Thomas, W. C. jr., Haddock, L. and Howard, J. E. (1958), *Trans. Assoc. Amer. Physicians*, **71**, 93.
Moriguchi, I., Wada, S. and Nishizawa, T. (1968), *Chem. Pharm. Bull.*, **16**, 601.
Mroszczak, E. J., Vallner, J. and Perrin, J. H. (1969), *J. Pharm. Sci.*, **58**, 1567.
Nakagaki, M., Koga, N. and Terada, H. (1964), *Yakugaku Zasshi*, **84**, 516.
Nambu, N. and Nagai, T. (1972), *Chem. Pharm. Bull.*, **20**, 2463.
Nagwekar, J. B. and Kostenbauder, H. B. (1970), *J. Pharm. Sci.*, **59**, 751.
Nemethy, G. and Laiken, N. (1970), *Il Farmaco*, **25**, 999.
Nemethy, G., Scheraga, H. A. and Kauzmann, W. (1968), *J. Phys. Chem.*, **72**, 1842.
Nemethy, G. and Scheraga, H. A. (1962a), *J. Chem. Phys.*, **36**, 3382.
Nemethy, G. and Scheraga, H. A. (1962b), *J. Chem. Phys.*, **36**, 3401.

Nemethy, G. and Scheraga, H. A. (1962c), *J. Phys. Chem.*, **66**, 1773.
Nemethy, G. and Scheraga, H. A. (1963), *J. Phys. Chem.*, **67**, 2888.
Neurath, H. (ed.) (1965), *The proteins; composition, structure and function*, vol. 3, 2nd ed., Academic Press, New York and London.
Newbould, B. B. and Kilpatrick, R. (1960), *Lancet*, **1**, 887.
Noval, J. J. and Mao, T. S. S. (1970), *Bull. Inst. Chem. Acad.*, **18**, 82.
Notari, R. E. (1973), *J. Pharm. Sci.*, **62**, 865.
Ockner, R. K., Manning, J. A., Poppenhausenm, R. B. and Ho, W. K. L. (1972), *Science*, **177**, 56.
Odell, G. B. (1959), *J. Clin. Invest.*, **38**, 823.
Olsen, G. D. (1973), *Clin. Pharmacol. Ther.*, **14**, 338.
O'Reilly, R. A. (1969), *J. Clin. Invest.*, **48**, 193.
O'Reilly, R. A. and Kowitz, P. E. (1967), *J. Clin. Invest.*, **46**, 829.
O'Reilly, R. A., Ohms, J. I. and Motley, C. H. (1969), *J. Biol. Chem.*, **244**, 1303.
O'Reilly, R. A. and Motley, C. H. (1971), *Mol. Pharmacol.*, **7**, 209.
Osorio, C. and Myant, N. B. (1965), *Endocrinol.*, **76**, 938.
Patel, N. K., Sheen, P-C. and Taylor, K. E. (1968), *J. Pharm. Sci.*, **57**, 1370.
Pauling, L. (1961), *Science*, **134**, 15.
Peets, E. A., Staub, M. and Symchowicz, S. (1969), *Biochem. Pharmacol.*, **18**, 1655.
Perrin, J. H. and Hart, P. A. (1970), *J. Pharm. Sci.*, **59**, 431.
Phillips, G. O., Power, D. M., Robinson, C. and Davies, J. V. (1970), *Biochim. Biophys. Acta*, **215**, 491.
Polonovski, J. (1966), in Desgrez, P. and de Traverse, P. M. (ed.), *Transport function of plasma proteins*, pp. 45–55, Elsevier, Amsterdam.
Poortmans, J. H. (1971), *J. Appl. Physiol.*, **30**, 190.
Popov, P. G., Vaptzarova, K. I., Kossekova, G. P. and Nikolov, T. K. (1971), *Compt. Rend. Acad. Bulg. Sci.*, **24**, 1357.
Popov, P. G., Vaptzarova, K. I. Kossekova, G. P. and Nikolov, T. K. (1972), *Biochem. Pharmacol.*, **21**, 2363.
Priestly, B. G. and O'Reilly, W. J. (1966), *J. Pharm. Pharmacol.*, **18**, 41.
Pruitt, A. W. and Dayton, P. G. (1971), *Eur. J. Clin. Pharmacol.*, **4**, 59.
Putnam, F. W. (ed.) (1960), *The plasma proteins*, vol. 2, Academic Press, New York and London.
Radda, G. K. (1971), *Curr. Topics Bioenerg.*, **4**, 81.
Rall, J. E., Robbins, J. and Lewallen, C. G. (1964), in Pincus, G., Thimann, K. V. and Ashwood, E. B. (ed.), *The homones*, vol. 5, p. 159, Academic Press, New York.
Raynaud, J. P., Mercier-Bodard, C. and Baulieu, E. E. (1971), *Steroids*, **18**, 767.
Ray, A., Reynolds, J. A., Polet, H. and Steinhardt, J. (1966), *Biochemistry*, **5**, 2606.
Raz, A. (1972a), *Biochem. J.*, **130**, 631.
Raz, A. (1972b), *Biochim. Biophys. Acta*, **280**, 602.
Raz, A. (1972c), *Life Sci.*, **11**, 965.
Raz, A. and Goodman, D. (1969), *J. Biol. Chem.*, **244**, 3230.
Reidenberg, M. M. and Affrime, M. (1973), *Ann. NY Acad. Sci.*, **226**, 115.
Reidenberg, M. M., Odar Cederlöf, I., Bahr, C. von, Borgå, O. and Sjöqvist, F. (1971), *New Eng. J. Med.*, **285**, 264.
Retief, F. P., Gottlieb, C. W., Kochwa, S., Pratt, P. W. and Herbert, V. (1967), *Blood*, **29**, 501.
Reyes, H., Levi, A. J., Gatmaitan, Z. and Arias, I. M. (1969), *Proc. Nat. Acad. Sci.*, U.S.A., **64**, 168.
Reyes, H., Levi, A. J., Levine, R., Gatmaitan, Z. and Arias, I. M. (1971), *Ann NY Acad. Sci.*, **179**, 520.
Reynolds, R. C., and Cluff, L. E. (1960), *Bull. J. Hopkins Hosp.*, **107**, 278.
Reynolds, J. A., Herbert, S., Polet, H. and Steinhardt, J. (1967), *Biochemistry*, **6**, 637.
Reynolds, J. A., Herbert, S. and Steinhardt, J. (1968), *Biochemistry*, **7**, 1357.

Reynolds, F. H. jr., Burkhard, R. K. and Mueller, D. D. (1973), *Biochemistry*, **12**, 359.

Rieder, J. (1963), *Arzneim.-Forsch.*, **13**, 81.

Robertson, J. S. and Madsen, B. W. (1974), *J. Pharm. Sci.*, **63**, 234.

Rodbard, D., Bridson, W. and Rayford, P. L. (1969), *J. Lab. Clin. Med.*, **74**, 770.

Roitt, I. (1974), *Essential Immunology*, 2nd ed., Blackwell, Oxford.

Rolinson, G. N. and Sutherland, R. (1965), *Brit. J. Pharmacol.*, **25**, 638.

Rose, M. S. and Aldridge, W. N. (1968), *Biochem. J.*, **106**, 821.

Rosenburg, R. M. and Klotz, I. M. (1960), in Alexander, P. and Block, R. J. (ed.), *A laboratory manual of analytical methods of protein chemistry*, vol. 2, pp. 131–168.

Rosenthal, H. (1967), *Anal. Biochem.*, **20**, 525.

Rosner, W. and Deakins, S. M. (1968), *J. Clin. Invest.*, **47**, 2109.

Rothschild, M. A., Oratz, M. and Schreiber, S. S. (1972), *New Eng. J. Med.*, **286**, 816.

Ryan, M. F. and Westphal, U. (1972), *J. Biol. Chem.*, **247**, 4050.

Ryan, M. T. and Hanna, N. S. (1971), *Anal. Biochem.*, **40**, 364.

Saracco, G. and Marchetti, E. S. (1958), *Ann. Chimica*, **48**, 1357.

Sahyun, M. R. V. (1966), *Nature*, **209**, 613.

Salvatore, G., Andreoli, N. and Roche, J. (1966), in Desgrez, P. and de Traverse, P. M. (ed.), *Transport function of plasma proteins*, pp. 57–73, Elsevier, Amsterdam.

Sandberg, A. A., Rosenthal, H., Schneider, S. L. and Slaunwhite, W. H. (1966), in Pincus, G., Nakao, T. and Tait, J. F. (ed.), *Steroid Dynamics*, pp. 1–61, Academic Press, New York.

Sanger, F. (1960), *Proc. Chem. Soc.*, **76**.

Scanu, A. M. (1972), *Ann. NY Acad. Sci.*, **195**, 390.

Scanu, A. M. and Wisdom, C. (1972), *Ann. Rev. Biochem.*, **41**, 703.

Scatchard, G. (1949), *Ann. NY Acad. Sci.*, **51**, 660.

Scatchard, G. and Black, E. S. (1949), *J. Phys. Colloid. Chem.*, **53**, 88.

Scatchard, G., Scheinberg, I. H. and Armstrong, S. H. (1950), *J. Amer. Chem. Soc.*, **72**, 535.

Schachman, H. K. (1963), *Cold Spring Harbor Symp. Quant. Biol.*, **28**, 409.

Schoenemann, P. T., Yesair, D. W., Coffey, J. J. and Bullock, F. J. (1973), *Ann. NY Acad. Sci.*, **226**, 162.

Scholtan, W. (1964), *Arzneim.-Forsch.*, **14**, 146.

Scholtan, W. (1968), *Arzneim.-Forsch.*, **18**, 505.

Scholtan, W. and Schmid, J. (1962), *Arzneim.-Forsch.*, **12**, 741.

Schultze, H. W. and Heremans, J. F. (1966), *Molecular biology of human proteins with special reference to plasma proteins*, vol. 1, Elsevier, Amsterdam.

Seal, U. S. and Doe, R. P. (1966), in Pincus, G., Nakao, T. and Tait, J. F. (ed.), *Steroid dynamics*, pp. 62–90 Academic Press, New York.

Seidl, L. G., Thorton, G. F. and Cluff, L. E. (1965), *Amer. J. Public Health*, **55**, 1170.

Sellers, A. L., Katz, J. K., Bonorris, G. and Okuyama, S. (1966), *J. Lab. Clin. Med.*, **68**, 177.

Sellers, E. M. and Koch-Weser, J. (1970a), *Clin. Pharmacol. Ther.*, **11**, 524.

Sellers, E. M. and Koch-Weser, J. (1970b), *Clin. Res.*, **18**, 344.

Sellers, E. M. and Koch-Weser, J. (1974), *Biochem. Pharmacol.*, **23**, 553.

Settle, W., Hegeman, S. and Featherstone, R. M. (1971), in Brodie, B. B. and Gillette, J. R. (ed.), *Handbook of experimental pharmacology*, vol. 28 (part 1), pp. 175–186, Springer-Verlag, Berlin.

Shearer, W. T., Bradshaw, R. A., Gurd, F. R. N. and Peters, T. (1967), *J. Biol. Chem.*, **242**, 5451.

Sher, S. P. (1971), *Toxicol. Appl. Pharmacol.*, **18**, 780.

Sjöholm, I. and Ljungstedt. I. (1973), *J. Biol. Chem.*, **248**, 8434.

Skuterud, B., Enger, E., Halvorsen, J., Jacobsen, S. and Lunde, P. K. M. (1972), *Fifth Int. Cong. Pharmacol. Abstr.*, **79**, 80.

Smith, M. J. H., Dawkins, P. D. and McArthur, J. N. (1971), *J. Pharm. Pharmacol.*, **23**, 451.
Smith, R. L. (1971), in Brodie, B. B. and Gillette, J. R. (ed.), *Handbook of experimental pharmacology*, vol. 28 (part 1), pp. 354–385, Springer-Verlag, Berlin.
Smith, R. L. (1973), *The excretory function of bile—the elimination of drugs and toxic substances in bile*, Chapman and Hall, London.
Sogami, M. and Foster, J. F. (1968), *Biochemistry*, **7**, 2172.
Solomon, H. M. and Schrogie, J. J. (1967), *Biochem. Pharmacol.*, **16**, 1219.
Solomon, H. M., Schrogie, J. J. and Williams, D. (1967), *Biochem. Pharmacol.*, **17**, 143.
Spector, A. A., John, K. M. and Fletcher, J. E. (1969), *J. Lipid Res.*, **10**, 56.
Spector, A. A. and Imig, B. (1971), *Mol. Pharmacol.*, **7**, 511.
Starr, P., Nicholoff, J. T. and Pilleggi, V. J. (1967), *Clin. Res.*, **15**, 127.
Stein, H. H. (1965), *Anal Biochem.*, **13**, 305.
Steinberg, I. Z. and Schachman, H. K. (1966), *Biochemistry*, **5**, 3728.
Steinhardt, J. and Reynolds, J. A. (1969), in *Multiple equilibria in proteins*, Academic Press, London and New York.
Steinhardt, J., Krijn, J. and Leidy, J. G. (1971), *Biochemistry*, **10**, 4005.
Sturman, J. A. and Smith, M. G. H. (1967), *J. Pharm. Pharmacol.*, **19**, 621.
Sugae, K. and Jirgensons, B. (1964), *J. Biochem. (Tokyo)*, **56**, 457.
Swaney, J. B. and Klotz, I. M. (1970), *Biochemistry*, **9**, 2570.
Swidler, G. (1971), *Handbook of drug interactions*, Wiley–Interscience, New York and London.
Sykes, B. D. and Hull, W. E. (1973), *Ann. NY Acad. Sci.*, **226**, 60.
Tanford, C., Swanson, S. A. and Shore, W. S. (1955), *J. Amer. Chem. Soc.*, **77**, 6414.
Tanford, C. (1972), *J. Mol. Biol.*, **67**, 59.
Tanford, C. (ed.) (1974), *The hydrophobic effect*, Wiley–Interscience, New York.
Teale, F. W. J. (1960), *Biochem. J.*, **76**, 381.
Teresi, J. D. and Luck, J. M. (1952), *J. Biol. Chem.*, **194**, 823.
Thompson, C. J. and Klotz, I. M. (1971), *Arch. Biochem. Biophys.*, **147**, 178.
Thompson, J. M. (1973), *Brit. J. Pharmacol.*, **47**, 133.
Thorp, J. M. (1964), in Binns, T. B. (ed.), *Absorption and distribution of drugs*, pp. 64–76, E. S. Livingstone, London.
Thorp, J. M. (1972), *Proc. Eur. Soc. Drug Tox.*, **12**, pp. 98–109, Excerpta Medica, The Hague.
Tildon, J. T. and Ogilvie, J. W. (1972), *J. Biol. Chem.*, **247**, 1265.
Toribara, T. Y., Terepka, A. R. and Dewey, P. A. (1957), *J. Clin. Invest.*, **36**, 738.
Tregear, R. T. (1966), *Physical functions of skin*, Academic Press, New York.
Tritsch, G. L. (1972), *J. Med.*, **3**, 129.
Turner, M. W. and Hulme, B. (1971), *The plasma proteins*, Pitman Medical and Scientific Publishing Co., London.
Uriel, J., Nechaud, B. and Dupiers, M. (1972), *Biochem. Biophys. Res. Commun.*, **46**, 1175.
Van Baelen, H. and De Moor, P. (1972), *J. Steroid Biochem.*, **3**, 321.
Vandenbelt, J. M., Childs, C. E., Lundquest, D. and Saladonis, H. (1954), *Science*, **119**, 514.
Verwey, W. F. and Williams, H. R. jr. (1962a), *Antimicrobial agents and chemotherapy*, 476.
Verwey, W. F. and Williams, H. R. jr. (1962b), *Antimicrobial agents and chemotherapy*, 484.
Wade, D. (1976), in press.
Wagner, J. G. (1973), *J. Pharmacokinet. Biopharm.*, **1**, 363.
Wahlqvist, M., Nilsson, I. M., Sandberg, F. and Agurell, S. (1970), *Biochem. Pharmacol.*, **19**, 2579.

Wardell, W. (1974), unpublished.
Weder, H. G. and Bickel, M. H. (1970), *J. Pharm. Sci.*, **59**, 1563.
Weder, H. G., Schildknecht, J., Lutz, R. A. and Kesselring, P. (1974), *Europ. J. Biochem.*, **42**, 475.
Westphal, U. (1961), in Engel, L. and Villee, C. H. (eds.) *Mechanisms of Action of Steroid Hormones*, p. 33, Pergamon, Oxford.
Westphal, U. and Knoefel, P. K. (1972), in Knoefel, P. K. (ed.) *Absorption, Distribution, Transformation and Excretion of Drugs* pp. 56–76, Thomas, U.S.A.
Westlaufer, D. B. and Lovrien, R. (1964), *J. Biol. Chem.*, **239**, 596.
Whitehouse, M. W., Dean, P. O. G. and Halsall, T. G. (1967), *J. Pharm. Pharmac.*, **19**, 533.
White, A., Handler, P. and Smith, E. G. (1968), *Principles of Biochemistry*, McGraw-Hill, New York.
Widman, M., Nilsson, I. M., Nilsson, J. L. G., Agurell, S., Borg, H. and Grandstrand, B. (1973), *J. Pharm. Pharmac.*, **25**, 453.
Wildnauer, R. and Canady, W. J. (1966), *Biochemistry* **5**, 2885.
Wilson, A. G. E., Brown, N. and Bridges, J. W. (1976), (in press).
Wilson, A. G. E. (1974), Ph.D. Thesis, University of Surrey.
Wiseman, E. H. and Nelson, E. (1964), *J. Pharm. Sci.*, **53**, 992.
Wishinsky, H., Glasser, E. J. and Perkal, S. (1962), *Diabetes*, **11**, 18.
Wishina, A. and Pinder, T. (1965), *Biochemistry*, **5**, 2885.
Witiak, D. T. and Whitehouse, M. W. (1969), *Biochem. Pharmacol.*, **18**, 971.
Wood, G. C. and Cooper, P. F. (1970), *Chromatog. Rev.*, **12**, 88.
Wooley, D. W. and Gommi, B. W. (1966), *Arch. Int. Pharmacodyn.*, **159**, 8.
Yesair, D. W., Bullock, F. J. and Coffey, J. J. (1972), *Drug Metabolism Review*, vol. 1, pp. 35–70.
Zettner, A. (1973), *Clin. Chem.*, **19**, 699.

Author index

Subject index